This book focuses on the basic techniques of cookery. It is intended to introduce the learner to a range of recipes that can be used and adapted to all sectors of the hospitality industry. It also introduces the learner to the industry, and includes the principles of health and safety. It is also aimed at those currently working in the industry, especially those who work in schools and colleges. It acknowledges the School Food Trust's training initiative, FEAST (Food Excellence and Skills Training).

This initiative is a major leap forward in recognising the importance of food in schools and that you have to educate young people from a very early age in food appreciation, diet, nutrition and health, so that they can fight against disease, and promote a healthy lifestyle. School cooks play an important part in the future food choices of young people. The book also recognises the importance of Licence to Cook food partnerships and other initiatives that aim to change eating habits and promote good food and cooking for all.

This book also covers healthy eating and does not encourage excessive use of salt, which is detrimental to health. It is anticipated that a high percentage of the population will suffer as a result of too much salt in their diet. For this reason, the recipes included here encourage the use of a range of fresh herbs such as parsley, fennel, coriander, chervil, tarragon, mint, chives, sage, marjoram and oregano. The book also provides the opportunity to learn more about the use of spices such as cumin, chillies, ginger and sesame seeds to make food tastier and more interesting. The use of herbs and spices can give flavour to many dishes that would otherwise taste bland, and can lessen the need for salt.

Two other ingredients need to be used in moderation to help prevent health problems such as obesity, heart problems and diabetes. These are sugar and fat. This book takes care to limit these ingredients and to suggest menus and food combinations that contribute to a balanced diet without loss of flavour.

To make some of the recipes more interesting for a wider range of learners, we asked Zamzani Abdul Wahab, a celebrity chef and teacher in Malaysia, to include some recipes. Zamzani is famous in South East Asia and appears regularly on television in Malaysia and Singapore. He is an expert on the use of spices.

The book clearly identifies the basic cookery processes for each recipe. It is intended to introduce young people in schools and colleges to cookery and to the importance of maintaining a healthy diet, encouraging the use of fresh fruit and vegetables.

The contents of the book can be cross-referenced to the **VRQ** and **NVQ** at **Level 1**. All subject areas are covered by the book in a user-friendly style. The VRQ theory chapters are clearly justifiable, with the VRQ processes incorporated throughout the book, and a separate section on methods of cookery. The book is also intended for the new Diplomas in Hospitality, to be offered in schools and colleges from September 2009.

This book has been written to cover everything you need for the Level 1 NVQ and VRQ courses. It is also a great resource for catering students on other courses, and for anyone training in a hospitality and catering workplace.

The book is divided into two parts: Theory and Practice.

Part 1, Theory, covers all the things you need to know when you work with food, including hygiene and safety, kitchen equipment and nutrition.

Part 2, Practice, explains the different methods of cookery, from boiling to baking, and provides more than 150 recipes, plus lots of information about choosing and handling ingredients. Whether you want to try out a particular method of cookery or a new ingredient, produce evidence for assessment or plan a meal, there will be a recipe here that's right for you.

To help make sure that you cover all the practical skills you need for your course, each recipe has icons showing which method(s) of cookery it uses. So if you want to practise shallow frying, look for that icon in Part 2. The icons look like this:

Boiling		Baking		Grilling	
Roasting		Steaming		Shallow frying	
Stewing or casserole		Deep frying		Poaching	

The NVQ and the VRQ

If you are studying for an NVQ or VRQ at Level 1, this book contains the facts you need, and recipes to develop your practical skills.

On this page you can see the units that make up each qualification, and where in the book they are covered. On the next page is a grid to help you find recipes that use different cookery skills.

NVQ Level 1 Food Preparation and Cooking is assessed through short knowledge tests and practical observation assessments. For VRQ Level 1 Diploma in Professional Cookery, theory units are assessed by short tasks and assignments. Practical units are assessed by short answer questions and practical tests.

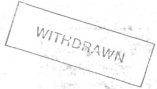

FOUNDATION PRACTICAL COOKERY

David Foskett, Victor Ceserani, John Campbell

With contributions from:
Zamzani Abdul Wahab, Patricia Paskins, Jacqueline Parks

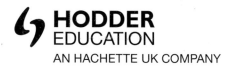
HODDER
EDUCATION
AN HACHETTE UK COMPANY

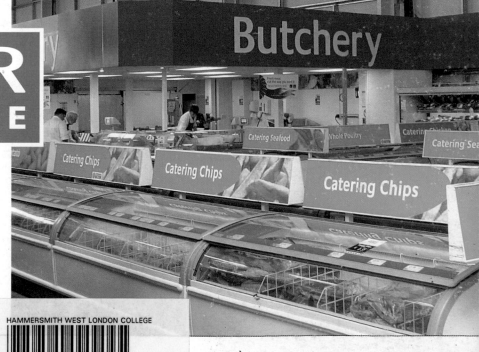

Every effort has been made to trace the copyright holders of material reproduced here. The authors and publishers would like to thank the following for permission to reproduce copyright illustrations:

p.2 © erwinova – Fotolia.com; p.3 © Photodisc/Getty Images; p.6 © Rob Bouwman – Fotolia.com; p.8 Sally & Richard Greenhill/Alamy; p.9 Crown copyright; p.15 Phil Cole/Getty Images; p.16 © Wollwerth Imagery – Fotolia.com; p.20 © erwinova – Fotolia.com; p.28 George Diebold/Photographer's Choice/Getty Images; p.29 © Karen Struthers – Fotolia.com; p.31 t © a4stockphotos – Fotolia.com; p.34 © Nikolay Okhitin – Fotolia.com; p.37 © BVDC – Fotolia.com; p.40 Charvet Premier Ranges; p.41 t Enodis, (others) Sam Bailey/Hodder Education; p.42 Enodis; p.43 m © Tatar – Fotolia.com, (others) Enodis; p.44 t Sam Bailey/Hodder Education, b Russums; p.45 b Enodis; p.46 t Sam Bailey/Hodder Education, b Ted Morrison/Photolibrary.com; p.47 Enodis; p.48 Maximilian Stock Ltd/Photolibrary.com; pp.49–51 Russums; p.52 m © orsoo – Fotolia.com, t, b Russums; p. 56 t l © Cimbal, Walter/StockFood UK, (others) Russums; p.57 Russums; p.70 t l Booker, t r © Fiolika – Fotolia.com, b Lester Lefkowitz/Stone/Getty Images; p.71 l Booker, r © Scott T. Smith/CORBIS; p.72 Booker; p.73 t l © Sumnersgraphicsinc – Fotolia.com, t r © MJPHOTO – Fotolia.com, b l © Maria Brzostowska – Fotolia.com, b r © Janusz Z. Kobylanski – Fotolia.com; p.74 © Monkey Business – Fotolia.com; p.79 © Visuals Unlimited/Corbis; p.82 Russums; p.85 t Booker, b Oxford Designers & Illustrators; p.87 Russums; pp.91 r, 94 Sam Bailey/Hodder Education; p.95 t © Fotoliall – Fotolia.com, b © Mewes, K./StockFood UK; pp.96–7 Sam Bailey/Hodder Education; pp.98–9 Donald Russell; p.101 © Patricia Hofmeester – Fotolia.com; p.104 Bon Appetit/Alamy; p.105 Sam Bailey/Hodder Education; p.106 © ImageShop/Corbis; p.109 Foodcollection/Getty Images; p.111 Donald Russell; p.112 Zamzani Abdul Wahab; p.113 Fancy/Photolibrary.com; pp.116 Donald Russell; p.118 t © Lucky Dragon – Fotolia.com, b Sam Bailey/Hodder Education; p.122 Frances M. Roberts/Alamy; p.154 Sarah Bailey/Hodder Education; p.156 t Sam Bailey/Hodder Education; pp.171, 179 Sarah Bailey/Hodder Education; p.181 Zamzani Abdul Wahab; p.187 Sarah Bailey/Hodder Education; p.206 Zamzani Abdul Wahab; p.207 Donald Russell; p.208 r Meat and Livestock Commission, (others) Donald Russell; p.209 Donald Russell; p.210 (except top) Sam Bailey/Hodder Education; p.211 Sam Bailey/Hodder Education; pp.226–32, 234 b, 235–6 Donald Russell; p.237 Meat and Livestock Commission; pp.238–41, 242 (except bottom) Donald Russell; p.247 m Meat and Livestock Commission, (others) Donald Russell; p.248 Donald Russell; p.256 Meat and Livestock Commission; p.271–3 Sam Bailey/Hodder Education; pp.281, 283 b Zamzani Adbul Wahab; p.297 Sarah Bailey/Hodder Education; p.314 b, 316 b Sam Bailey/Hodder Education; p.321 Zamzani Abdul Wahab; p.325 Sam Bailey/Hodder Education; p.326 t © Monkey Business – Fotolia.com, b Graham Kirk/Photolibrary.com; p.327 © photlook – Fotolia.com; p.328 m © Obak – Fotolia.com; p.329 © Paul Cowan – Fotolia.com; p.330 t © Jorge Chaves – Fotolia.com, b Martin Brigdale/Photolibrary.com.

Except where stated above, photos of plated dishes are by Andrew Callaghan and photos of recipe techniques are by Sarah Bailey. Illustrations by Barking Dog Art. Icons designed by Art Construction. Crown copyright material is reproduced with the permission of the Controller of HMSO and the Queen's Printer for Scotland.

t = top, m = middle, b = bottom, l = left, r = right of page

Orders: please contact Bookpoint Ltd, 130 Milton Park, Abingdon, Oxon OX14 4SB. Telephone: (44) 01235 827720. Fax: (44) 01235 400454. Lines are open from 9.00 – 5.00, Monday to Saturday, with a 24-hour message answering service. You can also order through our website www.hoddereducation.co.uk

If you have any comments to make about this, or any of our other titles, please send them to educationenquiries@hodder.co.uk

British Library Cataloguing in Publication Data
A catalogue record for this title is available from the British Library

ISBN: 978 0 340 98399 7

First Edition Published 2009
Impression number   10 9 8 7 6 5 4 3 2 1
Year   2012 2011 2010 2009

Copyright © 2009 David Foskett, Victor Ceserani and John Campbell

Hachette UK's policy is to use papers that are natural, renewable and recyclable products and made from wood grown in sustainable forests. The logging and manufacturing processes are expected to conform to the environmental regulations of the country of origin.

Cover photo © Banana Stock/Photolibrary.
Typeset by Fakenham Photosetting, Fakenham, Norfolk.
Printed in Italy for Hodder Education, an Hachette UK Company, 338 Euston Road, London NW1 3BH

Contents

336992

Jeremy Macveigh
International Cuisine.
USA
Yale
Delmar
Cengage learning

Foreword by Prue Leith OBE

When we think of chefs, cooking schools or colleges, and of 'gastronomy', we tend to think of trendy male TV chefs showing off their skills, or rather intimidating chaps in tall toques making fancy restaurant food, or amateurs learning how to produce the perfect dinner party. But few of us eat expensive, elaborate or 'fancy' food very often, and many more cooks are engaged in producing ordinary fare for ordinary people, out of ordinary ingredients, to a very ordinary budget.

And most of those cooks are working in commercial kitchens, feeding many people: in hospitals, schools, in works canteens, in prisons, in conference centres or in central production units preparing food for airlines, trains or ships.

This book is for them, and high time too! My special interest in this area is that I have been a cook and caterer all my life and, believe me, it takes more skill to make a good sandwich than it does to dish up a pot of caviar or a plate of smoked salmon. Simple food requires knowledge, skill and, above all, the desire to do it right – to make it look, smell and taste delicious while providing food that is nourishing and will not harm the health of the customer.

Now I chair the School Food Trust, which is charged with getting children at school to eat the new healthy school dinners. And of course children who have been brought up on a diet of chips and chocolate will need some persuading. Our best allies in this are the school cooks.

But school cooks, just like restaurant chefs, doctors, lawyers or IT buffs, need updating. They need to know what's new, what's fashionable, what's healthy, how to manage on a tight budget, how to 'sell' food to new customers, how to use modern equipment. And some of them, who were hired at a time when many schools only required them to reheat bought-in products, need to learn, or re-learn, the basic techniques of cooking.

This book concentrates on simple dishes (some familiar, some excitingly different) made with affordable ingredients, that can be produced in large quantities, that are healthy and, above all, that taste great. It's a good book and will, I hope, become the bible of many a cook.

501 (1GEN1) Maintain a safe, hygienic and secure working environment (Ch. 3, 6, 7, 8, Part 2)

504 (1GEN4) Contribute to effective teamwork (Ch. 6)

515 (1FP1) Prepare vegetables (Part 2)

516 (1FP2) Prepare and finish simple salad and fruit dishes (Part 2)

517 (1FP3) Prepare hot and cold sandwiches (Part 2)

520 (1FPC2) Prepare and cook meat and poultry (Ch. 5, Part 2)

518 (1FC1) Cook vegetables (Part 2)

521 (1FPC3) Prepare and cook pasta (Ch. 5, Part 2)

NVQ L1 Food Preparation & Cooking: you study 7 of the units

519 (1FC1) Prepare and cook fish (Ch. 5, Part 2)

523 (1FPC5) Prepare and cook eggs (Ch. 5, Part 2)

524 (1FPC6) Prepare and cook pulses (Ch. 5, Part 2)

522 (1FPC4) Prepare and cook rice (Ch. 5, Part 2)

525 (1FPC7) Prepare and cook vegetable protein (Ch. 5, Part 2)

526 (1FPC8) Prepare and cook simple bread and dough products (Part 2)

527 (1FPC9) Prepare and cook grain (Ch. 5, Part 2)

603 (2GEN3) Maintain food safety when storing, preparing and cooking food (Ch. 7, 8, Part 2)

101 Introduction to the catering and hospitality industry (Ch. 1, 2)

103 Health and safety awareness for catering and hospitality (Ch. 3)

104 Introduction to healthier foods and special diets (Ch. 4)

105 Introduction to kitchen equipment (Ch. 5)

202 Food safety in catering (Ch. 8)

VRQ Diploma Level 1 in Professional Cookery: you study all 12 units

106 Introduction to personal workplace skills (Ch. 6)

112 Cold food preparation (Ch. 12)

107 Prepare and cook food by boiling, poaching and steaming (Part 2)

111 Regeneration of pre-prepared food (Ch. 7)

110 Prepare and cook food by deep frying and shallow frying (Part 2)

109 Prepare and cook food by baking, roasting and grilling (Part 2)

108 Prepare and cook food by stewing and braising (Part 2)

Recipe		Page	NVQ	VRQ	Boiling	Poaching	Steaming	Grilling	Braising	Stewing	Roasting	Baking	Shallow frying	Deep frying
Eggs	Boiled	177		x	x									
	Fried	176	x	x									x	
	Omelette	178		x									x	
	Poached	177	x	x		x								
	Red onion and sweetcorn frittata	179	x	x	x							x	x	
	Scrambled	174		x	x									
	Steamed with chicken and spring onions	181		x			x							
Pasta	Farfalle with chives and bacon	185		x	x									
	Green tagliatelle with sausage and cream	186	x	x	x								x	
	Macaroni bake	184		x	x			x					x	
	Penne with peas and cream	188	x	x	x									
	Penne with tomato sauce	184		x	x									
	Spaghetti with vegetable and meat sauce	182		x	x								x	
	Spirals with asparagus and peanut sauce	187	x	x	x								x	
	Tuna pasta bake	189	x	x	x							x	x	
Rice	Braised	192	x	x					x				x	
	Plain boiled	192		x	x									
	Plain steamed	108		x			x							
	Risotto	193	x	x	x								x	
	Risotto with lemon grass, capers and green olives	195	x	x	x								x	
Fish	Baked cod with a cheese and herb crust	201	x	x								x		
	Baked fish pie	202	x	x								x		
	Batter for frying	199	x	x										
	Coley on a mustard mash	204	x	x	x								x	
	Fish cakes	203	x	x										x
	Frying in batter	199	x	x										x
	Grilled sardines	120	x	x				x						
	Poached salmon	105		x		x								
	Salmon, spinach and potato bake	205	x	x								x	x	
	Shallow frying	198	x	x									x	
	Steamed gingered snapper	206	x	x			x						x	
	Steamed with garlic and spring onion	197		x			x							

Recipe		Page	NVQ	VRQ	Boiling	Poaching	Steaming	Grilling	Braising	Stewing	Roasting	Baking	Shallow frying	Deep frying
Lamb	Biryani	224	x	x	x							x	x	
	Braised shanks	219	x	x					x					
	Brown stew	216	x	x						x			x	
	Grilled chops	213	x	x				x						
	Grilled cutlets	212	x	x				x						
	Irish stew	218	x	x						x				
	Kashmiri lamb	225	x	x								x	x	
	Kebabs	214	x	x				x						
	Lamb and vegetable pie	222	x	x	x							x	x	
	Mint sauce	211	x	x	x									
	Roast rack	210	x	x							x			
	Shallow-fried cutlets	215	x	x									x	
	Shepherd's pie	220	x	x	x							x	x	
	Spicy chops	213	x	x				x						
	Tagine with prunes and almonds	223	x	x								x	x	
Beef	Beef olives	242		x						x				
	Boiled silverside, carrots and dumplings	239		x	x									
	Goulash	110		x						x				
	Grilled steak	237	x	x				x						
	Horseradish sauce	234	x	x										
	Low-temperature roasting	236		x							x			
	Pan-fried steak	238	x	x									x	
	Pan-to-oven roast	234		x							x		x	
	Steak pie	244		x	x							x	x	
	Steamed steak pudding	245		x	x		x							
	Traditional braised	241		x						x				
	Traditional roast	232		x							x			
	Yorkshire pudding	233	x	x								x		
Pork and bacon	Boiled bacon	256		x	x									
	Egg and crumbed escalopes	255	x	x									x	
	Grilled chops	252	x	x				x						
	Noisettes with spiced pineapple, served with steamed rice	253	x	x			x						x	
	Pease pudding	257		x	x									
	Roast loin with apple and onion sauce	249		x							x			

Recipe		Page	NVQ	VRQ	Boiling	Poaching	Steaming	Grilling	Braising	Stewing	Roasting	Baking	Shallow frying	Deep frying
									Skills					
Pork and bacon	Roast stuffed loin with a sage and onion stuffing	250		x							x			
	Sautéed medallions	121											x	
	Stir-fried fillet	252	x	x									x	
Poultry	Boiled or poached chicken	258	x	x	x			x				x	x	
	Breadcrumbed turkey escalopes with ginger and lemon grass	263	x	x									x	
	Chicken breasts with mango, peas and rice	265	x	x	x								x	
	Chicken Kiev	261	x	x										x
	Deep-fried chicken	124	x	x										x
	Jerk chicken	267	x	x								x	x	
	Sauté of chicken	260	x	x									x	
	Spiced chicken balti with quinoa	266	x	x	x								x	
	Turkey escalopes	262	x	x				x					x	
	Turkey fajita	264	x	x									x	
Vegetables and vegetarian food	Aloo gobi	286	x	x	x								x	
	Arlie potatoes	280	x	x								x		
	Aubergine and lentil curry	292					x						x	
	Baked jacket potatoes	278	x	x								x		
	Bean quesadillas	293	x	x								x	x	
	Bengali-style potatoes	282	x	x	x								x	
	Bergedil kentang	283	x	x	x								x	x
	Boiled/steamed broccoli	274		x	x		x	x						
	Boiled/steamed cabbage	273		x	x		x	x						
	Boiled/steamed cauliflower	274		x	x		x	x						
	Boiled/steamed potatoes	276		x	x		x	x						
	Boiled/steamed spinach	275		x	x		x	x						
	Braised bean curd	284					x						x	
	Braised mushrooms	112	x	x			x						x	
	Chickpea and vegetable protein curry	298	x				x						x	

Category	Recipe	Page	NVQ	VRQ	Boiling	Poaching	Steaming	Grilling	Braising	Stewing	Roasting	Baking	Shallow frying	Deep frying
Vegetables and vegetarian food	Chickpea stew	292		x	x								x	
	Chips	280	x	x										x
	Fried mixed vegetables	281	x	x	x								x	
	Grilled vegetable bake	291	x	x				x				x		
	Leek and mustard mash	282			x								x	
	Mashed potatoes	276		x	x		x	x						
	Mushrooms with a polenta crust	297	x		x									x
	Polenta	296			x									
	Red Dragon pie	295	x	x	x							x	x	
	Roasted beetroot	117		x							x			
	Roast potatoes	277		x							x			
	Sauté potatoes	277		x	x			x					x	
	Savoury potatoes	279	x	x								x		
	Vegetable casserole	287	x	x	x								x	
	Vegetable couscous	289		x	x								x	
	Vegetable pakoras	290	x	x	x									x
Pastry	Apple crumble	319	x	x								x		
	Baked rice pudding	114		x								x		
	Banana and coconut mini pancake	321		x									x	
	Banana loaf	323		x								x		
	Bread rolls	313	x	x								x		
	Bun dough	312	x	x								x		
	Crème caramel	325	x	x	x							x		
	Focaccia	310	x	x								x		
	Fruit buns	312	x	x								x		
	Fruit pies	302	x	x								x		
	Fruit salad	316	x	x										
	Fruit tartlets	305	x	x								x		
	Gluten-free bread	310	x	x								x		
	Pancakes	320	x	x									x	
	Pastry cream	304	x	x	x									
	Polenta and ricotta cake	324	x	x								x		
	Rice pudding with fruit and nuts	322		x								x		
	Scones	314	x	x								x		
	Semolina pudding	322		x	x									
	Simple white loaf	308	x	x								x		
	Sponge pudding	315		x			x							
	Winter smoothie	318	x	x										

Reasons to come to Booker the UK's biggest wholesaler

To find your nearest branch visit www.booker.co.uk

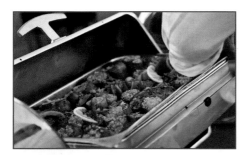

choice up

Huge range
The average branch carries over 10,000 lines in stock the whole time, with even more available to order.

New Lines
Our expert buyers are constantly sourcing great new lines for you. Look for the 'New Line shelf' cards in branch, every week.

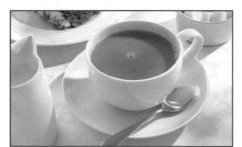

prices down

Catering Price check
Our catering price check service allows you to enter your current Brakes or 3663 prices and, with one click, instantly see if you can buy cheaper from Booker. Why not compare our prices for yourself by visiting www.booker.co.uk today!

Essentials - every day low price
We have lock down prices on a range of products that are essential to your business. From bread, milk, eggs and potatoes through to sugar, tuna, chips and peas we will give you a low price, every day to help you plan your menu and your budget.

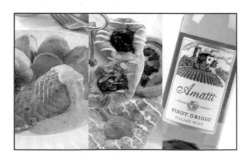

better service

Internet ordering
The easiest way to place your order with your branch is via our website. Simply log on to www.booker.co.uk, and register for online ordering. Its so simple - start today!

Free, 7 days a week, delivery service
All your fresh produce, frozen, wet and dry goods delivered to your door on the one vehicle - 7 days a week.

Acknowledgements

We are most grateful to the following for their assistance in preparing *Foundation Practical Cookery*:

Booker Ltd for its support for the book, and for supplying some of the photographs.

The staff at the Vineyard at Stockcross, especially Claire Haines, Simon McKenzie, Peter Eaton and Josh Johnson.

Harrison Catering for its assistance with some of the recipes.

Steve Thorpe, Phil Dobson, MaryJo Hoyne, Iain Middleton and Stephen Stackhouse for their expert advice and input.

Russums Catering Clothing and Equipment for supplying some of the photographs.

Steve Loughton, Managing Director, Enodis, for supplying some of the photographs.

Andrew Callaghan and Sarah Bailey for the photography.

Oliver Rouse for his assistance with the photography.

Pavol Nedved at Thames Valley University.

Adrian Moss of Instructional Design Ltd for producing and creating the videos for the *Foundation Practical Cookery* teacher resource.

Special thanks to Donald Russell Ltd for permission to use its photography and information taken from its *Meat Perfection* booklet. Donald Russell is a 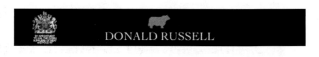 quality Scottish butcher, based in Aberdeenshire. For over three decades, Donald Russell has supplied the world's most demanding chefs and Michelin-starred restaurants with the finest grass-fed, traditionally matured beef and lamb, as well as pork, veal, poultry, game, fish and seafood. For more information, please visit www.donaldrussell.com.

About the contributors

Zamzani Abdul Wahab is a celebrity chef who has presented television programmes around the world and has published two books. He is Head of Special Projects at the School of Hospitality, Tourism and Culinary Arts, KDV College, Malaysia.

Jacqueline Parks is Head of Hospitality at Cardinal Wiseman School, Greenford, UK.

Patricia Paskins is a lecturer at The London School of Hospitality and Tourism, Thames Valley University, UK.

PART 1

THEORY

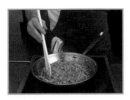 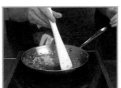 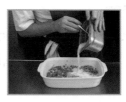 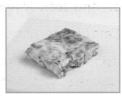

Contents list:

Introduction to the catering and hospitality industry

VRQ Unit 101 Introduction to the catering and hospitality industry

Learning outcomes:
- Demonstrate an awareness of the different sectors of the catering and hospitality industry
- Identify relevant qualifications, training and experience for employment within the catering and hospitality industry

The hospitality industry

Wherever there are groups of people there is likely to be some kind of hospitality provision, in other words somewhere where people can get food, drink and accommodation.

The hospitality industry in Britain employs around 1.7 million people and is growing all the time. It provides excellent opportunities for training and employment. Hotels, restaurants, bars, pubs and clubs are all part of what is known as the **commercial sector**. Businesses in the commercial sector need to make a profit so that they can survive.

Catering provided in places like hospitals, schools, colleges, prisons and the armed services also provides thousands of meals each day. These places are part of what is known as the **public sector**. Businesses in the public sector do not need to make a profit.

Types of hospitality and catering establishment*

Commercial catering

Hotels

Hotels provide accommodation in private bedrooms. Many also offer other services such as restaurants, bars and room service, as well as reception, porters and housekeepers. What a hotel offers will depend on the type of hotel it is and how many stars it has.

Hotels are rated from five-star down to one-star. A luxury hotel will have five stars while a more basic hotel will have one star. There are many international hotel chains, such as the Radisson group, in the five-star hotel market. There are also budget hotels, guesthouses and bed and breakfast accommodation.

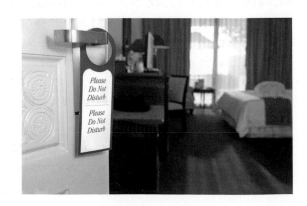

Please Do Not Disturb

Please Do Not Disturb

*Note: data in this section comes from the British Hospitality Association and Hospitality.net.

In the UK there are more hotel bedrooms in the mid-market three-star hotels than in any other category. Most hotels in this market are independent and privately owned, in other words they are not part of a chain of hotels.

Some hotels have speciality restaurants. For example, a restaurant may be run by a high-profile or 'celebrity' chef, or it may specialise in steaks, sushi or seafood.

To attract as many guests as possible, many hotels now offer even more services. These may include office and IT services (e.g. internet access, fax machines, a quiet area to work in), gym and sports facilities, swimming pool, spa, therapy treatments, hair and beauty treatments, and so on.

Country house hotels

Country house hotels are mostly in attractive old buildings, such as stately homes or manor houses, in tourist and rural areas. They normally have a reputation for good food and wine, and a high standard of service. They may also offer the additional services mentioned above.

Consortia

'Consortia' is the plural of 'consortium'. A consortium is a group of independent hotels that make an agreement to buy products and services together. For example, they might all pay a specialist company to do their marketing (advertising and so on).

Budget hotels

Budget hotels like motels and travel lodges are built near motorways, railway stations and airports. They are aimed at business people and tourists who need somewhere inexpensive to stay overnight. The rooms are reasonably priced and have tea and coffee making facilities. No other food or drink is included in the price. There are not many members of staff and there is no restaurant. However, usually there will be shops, cafés, restaurants or pubs close by. The growth and success of the budget hotel sector has been one of the biggest changes in the hospitality industry in recent years.

Guesthouses and bed and breakfasts

There are guesthouses and bed and breakfast establishments all over the UK. They are small, privately owned businesses. The owners usually live on the premises and let bedrooms to paying customers. Some guesthouses offer lunch and an evening meal as well as breakfast.

Clubs and casinos

People pay to become members of private clubs. Private clubs are usually run by managers appointed by club members. What most members want from a club in Britain, particularly in the fashionable areas of London, is good food and drink and informal service in the traditional English style.

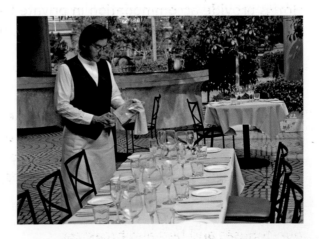

Most nightclubs and casinos are open to the public rather than to members only.

Restaurants

The restaurant sector has become the largest in the UK hospitality industry. It includes exclusive restaurants and fine-dining establishments, as well as a wide variety of mainstream restaurants, fast-food outlets, coffee shops and cafés.

Many restaurants specialise in regional or ethnic food styles, such as Asian and Oriental, Mexican and Caribbean, as well as a wide range of European-style foods. New restaurants and cooking styles are appearing and becoming more popular all the time.

Speciality restaurants

Moderately priced speciality restaurants are very popular these days. In order for them to succeed, the manager must understand what customers want and plan a menu that will attract enough customers to make a good profit.

Fast food

Many customers now want the option of popular foods at a reasonable price, with little or no waiting time. Fast-food establishments offer a limited menu that can be consumed on the premises or taken away. Menu items are quick to cook and have often been partly or fully prepared beforehand at a central production point.

Drive-ins (or drive-thrus)

Drive-ins are a relatively new idea in the UK. The concept came from America, and there are now many of them across the UK. The best-known are the 'drive-thrus' at McDonald's fast-food restaurants. Customers stay in their vehicles and drive up to a microphone where they place their order. As the car moves forwards in a queue, the order is prepared and is ready for the driver to pick up at the service window when they get there.

Delicatessens and salad bars

These offer a wide selection of salads and sandwich fillings to go in a variety of breads and rolls at a 'made to order' sandwich counter. The choice of breads might include panini, focaccia, pitta, baguette and tortilla wraps. Fresh salads, home-made soups, chilled foods and a hot 'chef's dish of the day' may also be available, along with ever-popular baked jacket potatoes with a good variety of fillings.

Chain catering organisations

There are many restaurant chains, coffee shops, chain stores and shops with restaurants in them. Many of these chains are spread over wide areas and, in some cases, overseas. These are usually well-known companies that advertise widely. They often serve morning coffee, lunches and teas, or may be in the style of snack bars and cafeterias.

Licensed house (pub) catering

Many pubs in the UK offer food.

There is a great variety of food available in pubs, from those that serve ham and cheese rolls to those that have exclusive à la carte restaurants. Pub catering can be divided into five categories:

1 luxury-type restaurants
2 gastro pubs that have well-qualified chefs who develop the menu according to their own specialities, making good use of local produce

3 speciality restaurants like steak bars, fish restaurants, carveries and theme restaurants

4 bar-food pubs where fork dishes are served from the bar counter and the food is eaten in the normal drinking areas rather than in a separate restaurant

5 bar-food pubs that just serve finger snacks such as rolls and sandwiches.

Food and leisure

Timeshare villas and apartments

A timeshare owner buys a particular amount of time (usually a few weeks) per year in a particular self-catering apartment, room or suite in a hotel or a leisure club. The arrangement may be for a period of years or indefinite. There will usually be a number of restaurants, bars and other leisure facilities within the same complex for timeshare owners to use.

Health clubs and spas

These are often luxury establishments or hotels where the client can have a number of specialist health treatments. They usually offer healthy food, therapies and activities that fit in with people's modern-day lifestyles, and their interest in being fit, healthy and contented.

Museums

In addition to displaying interesting exhibits, as you would expect them to, some museums also provide other services these days. For example, many museums have one or more cafés and restaurants for visitors.

Theme parks

Theme parks are now extremely popular venues for a family day out or even a full holiday. The larger theme parks include several different eating options, ranging from fast food to fine dining.

Holiday centres

Holiday centres around the UK provide leisure and hospitality facilities all together on a single site. They cater for families, single people and groups of people. Many holiday centres have invested large amounts of money to improve the quality of the holiday experience. They include a range of restaurants and food courts.

Historical buildings

Numerous historical buildings and places of interest have food outlets such as cafés and restaurants. Many in the UK specialise in light lunches and afternoon tea for the general public. Some are also used as venues to host large private or corporate events.

Visitor attractions

Places like Hampton Court, Kew Gardens and Poole Pottery can be categorised as visitor attractions. They will usually have refreshments outlets serving a variety of food and drinks. Some, like Kew Gardens, are also used to stage large theatrical events or concerts in the summer.

Farms

The tourism industry in the countryside is very important in the UK. Farmers understand this and have formed a national organisation called the Farm Holiday

Bureau. The farms that belong to this organisation usually offer bed and breakfast and holiday cottages.

Youth hostels

The Youth Hostels Association runs hostels in various locations in England and Wales. These establishments cater for single people, families and groups travelling on a limited budget. They mainly provide dormitory accommodation, but some also have a few private rooms. In some locations they include a number of sports and leisure facilities. Basic, wholesome meals are provided at a low cost in some hostels, and they all have a kitchen that can be used by visitors to store and prepare their own food.

Travel

Sea ferries

There are several ferry ports in the UK. Ferries leave from these every day, making a variety of sea crossings to Ireland and mainland Europe. As well as carrying passengers, many ferries also carry the passengers' cars and freight lorries. Most ferries have several shops, bars, cafés and lounges on board. Some also have very good restaurant and leisure facilities, fast-food restaurants and branded food outlets.

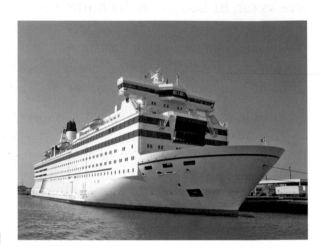

Cruise liners and other ships

Cruise ships are floating luxury hotels. The food provision on a large cruise liner is of a similar standard to the food provided in a five-star hotel. Many shipping companies are known for the excellence of their cuisine.

As cruising becomes more popular, cruise companies are getting more and bigger cruise liners. This means that there are excellent hospitality career opportunities. Many companies provide good training and promotion prospects, and the opportunity to travel all over the world. The caterers produce food and serve customers to a very high standard in extremely hygienic conditions. All these things mean that working on cruise liners can be an interesting and rewarding career.

Airline services

Airline catering is a specialist service. The catering companies are usually located at or near airports in this country and around the world. The meals provided vary from snacks and basic meals to luxury meals for first-class passengers. Menus are chosen carefully to make sure that the food can safely be chilled and then reheated on board the aircraft.

The price of some airline tickets includes a meal served at your seat. The budget airlines usually have an at-seat trolley service from which passengers can buy snacks and drinks.

At the airport

Airports offer a range of hospitality services catering for millions of people every year. They operate 24 hours a day, 365 days a year. Services include a wide variety of shops, along with bars, themed restaurants, speciality restaurants, coffee bars and food courts.

Roadside services

Roadside motoring services (often referred to as 'service stations') provide a variety of services for motorists. These include a variety of branded food outlets and often accommodation. The catering usually consists of food courts offering travellers a wide range of meals 24 hours a day, seven days a week. MOTO is an example of a company that provides these sorts of services nationwide.

Railway

Snacks can be bought in the buffet car on a train, and some train operators also offer a trolley service so that passengers can buy snacks without leaving their seats. Main meals are often served in a restaurant car. However, there is not much space in a restaurant car kitchen, and there is a lot of movement of the train, so it can be quite difficult to provide anything other than simple meals.

Two train services run by separate companies run through the Channel Tunnel. One is Euro Tunnel's Le Shuttle train, which transports drivers and their vehicles between Folkestone and Calais in 35 minutes. Passengers have to buy any food and drink for their journey before they board the train.

The other company, Eurostar, operates between London St Pancras and Paris or Brussels. This carries passengers only.

Public-sector catering

Public-sector organisations that need catering services include hospitals, universities, colleges, schools, prisons, the armed forces, police and ambulance services, local authorities and many more.

The aim of catering in hotels, restaurants and other areas of the leisure and travel industry (known as the private sector) is to make a profit. The aim of public-sector catering is to keep costs down by working efficiently. However, these days, the business of catering for public-sector organisations is tendered for. This means that different companies will compete to win a contract to provide the catering for these organisations.

For a variety of reasons, the types of menu in the public sector may be different from those in the private sector. For example, school children, hospital patients and soldiers have particular nutritional needs (they may need more energy from their food, or more of certain vitamins and minerals), so their menus should match their needs. Menus may also reflect the need to keep costs down. However, the standards of cooking in the public sector should be just as good as they are in the private sector.

Prisons

Catering in prisons may be carried out by contract caterers or by the Prison Service itself. The food is usually prepared by prison officers and inmates. The kitchens are also used to train inmates in food production. They can gain a recognised qualification to encourage them to find work when they are released.

In addition to catering facilities for the inmates, there are also staff catering facilities for all the personnel who work in a prison, such as administrative staff and prison officers.

The armed forces

Catering in the armed forces includes providing meals for staff in barracks, in the field and on ships. Catering for the armed forces is specialised, especially when they are in the field, and they have their own well-established cookery training programmes.

However, like every other part of the public sector, the forces need to keep costs down and increase efficiency.

The National Health Service

The scale of catering services in the NHS is enormous. Over 300 million meals are served each year in approximately 1200 hospitals. NHS Trusts must ensure that they get the best value for money within their catering budget.

Hospital caterers need to provide well-cooked, nutritious, appetising meals for hospital patients, and must maintain strict hygiene standards. All this helps the nursing staff to get patients well as soon as possible.

A well as providing nutritious meals for patients in hospital (many of whom need special diets), provision must also be made for out-patients (people who come into hospital for treatment and leave again the same day), visitors and staff. This service may be provided by the hospital catering team, but is sometimes allocated to commercial food outlets, or there may be a combination of in-house hospital catering and commercial catering.

The education sector school meals service

School meals play an important part in the lives of many children, often providing them with their only hot meal of the day.

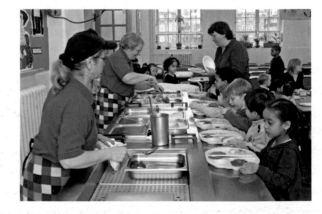

In 2006 the government announced new standards for school food. There are three parts to this, to be phased in by September 2009. Together they cover all food sold or served in schools: breakfast, lunch and after-school meals; tuck shops, vending machines, mid-morning break snacks, and anything sold or served at after-school clubs.

The three phases are as follows.

1 Phase 1 introduced interim food-based standards for school lunches, which all schools had to meet by September 2006.
2 Phase 2 brought in standards for school food other than lunch, which all schools had to meet by September 2007 (although schools were recommended to adopt these from September 2006).
3 Phase 3 introduced nutrient-based standards and the final food-based standards for school lunches. Primary schools had to meet these standards by September 2008 at the latest and secondary schools by September 2009 at the latest.

Use the eatwell plate to get the balance right. It shows how much of what you eat should come from each food group.

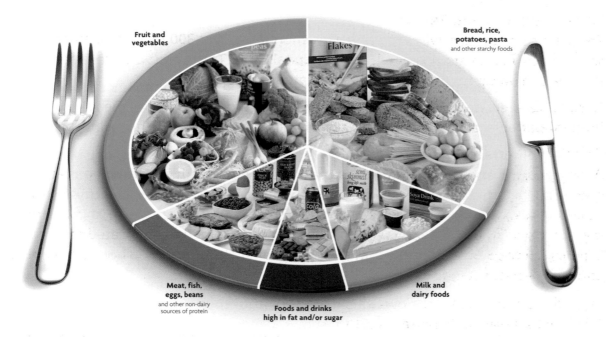

The eatwell plate

FOOD
STANDARDS
AGENCY
food.gov.uk

Use the eatwell plate to help you get the balance right. It shows how much of what you eat should come from each food group.

Fruit and vegetables

Bread, rice, potatoes, pasta and other starchy foods

Meat, fish, eggs, beans and other non-dairy sources of protein

Foods and drinks high in fat and/or sugar

Milk and dairy foods

The eatwell plate

Residential establishments

Residential establishments include schools, colleges, university halls of residence, nursing homes, homes for the elderly, children's homes and hostels, where all the meals are provided. It is very important to consider the nutritional balance of food served in these establishments. It should satisfy all the residents' nutritional needs, as the people eating these meals will probably have no other food provision. Many of these establishments cater for children, who may lead energetic lives and will probably be growing fast so have large appetites, so the food should be well prepared from good ingredients, and should be nutritious, varied and attractive.

Catering for business and industry

The provision of staff dining rooms and restaurants in industrial and business settings has provided employment for many catering workers outside traditional hotel and restaurant catering. Working conditions in these settings are often very good. Apart from the main task of providing meals, these services may also include retail shops, franchise outlets (see page 10) and vending machines. They will also include catering for meetings and conferences as well as for larger special functions.

In some cases a 24-hour, seven-days-a-week service is necessary, but usually the hours are more streamlined than in other areas of the hospitality industry. Food and drink is provided for all employees, often in high-quality restaurants and dining rooms. The catering departments in these organisations are keen to keep and develop their staff, so there is good potential for training and career development in this sector.

The contract food service sector

The contract food service sector, which has already been mentioned several times in relation to other sectors of the hospitality industry, is made up of companies that provide catering services to other organisations. This sector has grown a lot over recent years.

Contract food service management provides food for a wide variety of people, such as those at work in business and industry, those in schools, colleges and universities, private and public healthcare establishments, public and local authorities, and other non-profit-making outlets such as the armed forces, police or ambulance services.

It also includes more commercial areas, such as corporate hospitality events and the executive dining rooms of many corporations, special events, sporting fixtures and places of entertainment, and outlets such as leisure centres, museums, department stores, airports and railway stations. Some contractors also provide other support services such as housekeeping and maintenance, reception, security, laundry, bars and retail shops.

Outside catering

When events are held at venues where there is no catering available, or where the level of catering required is more than the normal caterers can manage, then a catering company may take over the management of the event. This type of function will include garden parties, agricultural shows, banquets, sporting fixtures such as football or rugby, and so on.

There is a lot of variety in this sort of outside catering work, but the standards are very high and people employed in this area need to be adaptable and creative. Sometimes specialist equipment will be required, especially for outdoor jobs, and employees need to be flexible as the work often involves a lot of travel, remote locations and outdoor venues.

Corporate hospitality

Corporate hospitality is hospitality provided by businesses, usually for their clients or potential clients. The purpose of corporate hospitality is to build business relationships and to raise awareness of the company. Corporate entertaining is also used as a way to thank or reward loyal customers.

Companies these days understand the importance of marketing through building relationships with clients and through the company's reputation. They are willing to spend large amounts of money to do this well.

Franchising

A franchise is an agreement where a person or group of people pay a fee and some set-up costs to use an established name or brand that is well known and is therefore likely to attract more customers than an unknown or start-up brand.

An example of this is where the contract caterer, Compass Group, buys a franchise in the Burger King brand from Burger King's owner. It pays a fee and a proportion of the turnover. The franchisor (the branded company franchise provider) will normally lay down strict guidelines or 'brand standards' that the franchisee (franchise user) has to meet. In this example these will affect things like which ingredients and raw materials are used and where they come from, as well as portion sizes and the general product and service.

Foundation and training for career progression

Staffing and organisation structure

Hospitality companies need to have a structure for their staff in order for the business to run efficiently and effectively. Different members of staff have different jobs and roles to perform as part of the team so that the business is successful.

In smaller organisations, some employees have to become multi-skilled so that they can carry out a variety of duties. Some managers may have to take on a supervisory role at certain times.

A hospitality team will consist of operational staff, supervisory staff, management staff and, in large organisations, senior management.

Operational staff

These are usually practical, hands-on staff. These will include the chefs de partie, (section chefs), commis chefs, waiters, apprentices, reception staff and accommodation staff.

Supervisory staff

Generally the supervisors work with the operational staff. They supervise the work. In some establishments the supervisors will be the manager for some of the operational staff.

A sous chef will have supervisory responsibilities, and a chef de partie will have both operational and supervisory responsibilities.

Management staff

- Managers have the responsibility of making sure that the operation runs smoothly and within the budget.
- They are accountable to the owners to make sure that the products and services on offer are what the customer expects and wants, and provide value for money.
- Managers may also be responsible for planning for the future.
- They will be required to make sure that all the health and safety policies are in place and that health and safety legislation is followed.
- In smaller establishments they may also act as the human resources manager.

A hotel will normally have a manager, assistant managers, accommodation manager, restaurant manager and reception manager. So in each section of the hotel there could be a manager with departmental responsibilities. A head chef is a manager.

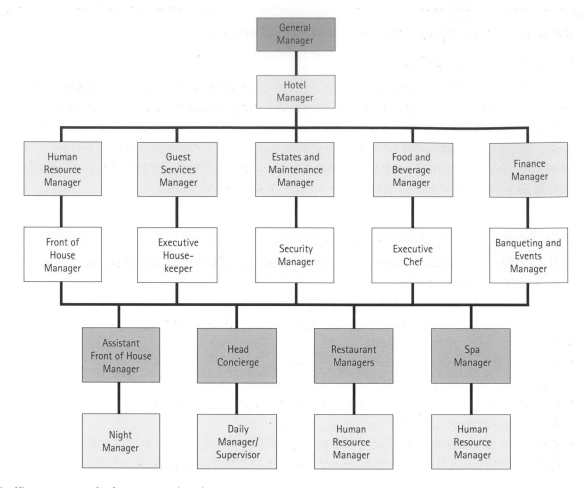

Staffing structure of a four-star spa hotel

Employment rights and responsibilities

People have rights in employment.

Employers must provide the employee with:

- a detailed job description
- a contract of employment that gives details of the job itself, working hours, the amount of annual holiday the employee will have and the notice period.

Employers must follow the relevant laws, such as employment law, health and safety law, and food safety law.

Employees must work in the way that has been agreed to in the contract and job description, and follow all the organisation's policies and practices.

What about qualifications?

Qualifications show that a person has studied a subject successfully. Achieving a qualification usually involves some sort of assessment, either in the form of examinations, coursework, observation by an assessor, or a combination of these things.

Qualifications inform employers of what you should be able to do. There are many different qualifications and that is why some employers ask job applicants to do a practical test, such as a trial day, before they have an interview.

Qualifications are important as they give you better career prospects and develop you

An example of a job description: Senior Sous Chef

Reporting to Head Chef

The Senior Sous Chef position reports to the Head Chef and is responsible for the day-to-day kitchen operation, overseeing the stores, preparation and production areas. The position involves supervising and managing the kitchen staff, with direct responsibility for rostering and scheduling production. In the absence of the Head Chef, the Senior Sous Chef will be required to take on the duties of the Head Chef and to attend Senior Management meetings in his/her absence.

Duties

- Monitor and check stores operation.
- Train new and existing staff in Health & Safety, HACCP (hazard analysis critical and control point), etc.
- Chair of the Kitchen Health and Safety Committee.
- Develop new menus and concepts together with Senior Management.
- Schedule and roster all kitchen staff.
- Maintain accurate records of staff absences.
- Maintain accurate kitchen records.
- Responsible for the overall cleanliness of the kitchen operation.
- Assist in the production of management reports.
- Establish an effective and efficient team.
- Assist with the overall establishment and monitoring of budgets.

Conditions

- Grade 3 management spine.
- Private health insurance.
- 5-day week.
- 20 days' holiday.
- Profit-share scheme after one year's service.

Personal specification: Senior Sous Chef

- Qualifications
  (i) Diplomas in Professional Cookery

- Experience
  (i) Five years' experience in four- and five-star hotel kitchens; restaurant and banqueting experience

- Skills
  (i) Proficiency in culinary arts
  (ii) Microsoft Excel, Access, Word
  (iii) Operation of inventory control software
  (iv) Written and oral communication skills
  (v) Team-building skills

- Knowledge
  - (i) Current legislation in Health & Safety
  - (ii) Food hygiene
  - (iii) HACCP
  - (iv) Risk assessment
  - (v) Production systems
  - (vi) Current technology

- Other attributes
  - (i) Honesty
  - (ii) Reliability
  - (iii) Attention to detail
  - (iv) Initiative
  - (v) Accuracy

- Essential
  - (i) Basic computer skills
  - (ii) High degree of culinary skills
  - (iii) Good communication skills
  - (iv) Supervisory and leadership skills

- Desirable
  - (i) Knowledge of employment law
  - (ii) Public relations profile

personally. They help to boost your confidence. There are a number of college-based courses that will help you to develop a range of skills such as numeracy, language and information technology.

Apprenticeships are a way to learn skills within a workplace while also getting a qualification. Apprenticeship can be through a day-release course at college or may be completely work-based.

It is important to understand that learning is for life. You must continue to learn and develop your skills. You can improve your knowledge by reading hospitality journals, books and food magazines. Find out how you learn best. Electronic learning (using CDs, DVDs and the internet) can help you to learn at your own pace, testing yourself when you are ready to be tested. Assessment will help you to understand what you have achieved and what you must do to improve. It provides the building blocks for further learning and achievement.

Activity

1 Name the two sectors of the hospitality and catering industry.

2 Name three types of establishment from each sector.

3 Name one job role from each establishment you have listed.

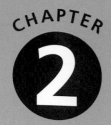

Teamwork

VRQ Unit 106 Introduction to personal workplace skills

Learning outcomes:
- Work effectively in a team
- Communicate with team members

NVQ 1GEN4 Contribute to effective teamwork

Teamwork in the hospitality industry

The hospitality and catering industry relies on teamwork. Lots of other industries do, too.

Great teams produce great results. Think of a great team. What has the team achieved? A winning football team is made up of good players, all working together and aiming to score goals!

Why is teamwork important?

All staff in a kitchen, restaurant or hotel have to work together to get things done. When you are working in hospitality you must:

A good team can do a great job

- understand that you are part of a team
- work with the rest of your team
- see yourself as part of the team
- understand what your team has to do.

Exactly who is in your team will vary from place to place. Different organisations are run in different ways.

Different kinds of team

The department head, or the person in charge, will set up teams in a department. This person should set an example of good teamwork for everyone else to follow.

- A **formal team** is when you work with a group of people in a formal section in the organisation (e.g. pastry section, sauce section).
- An **informal team** is organised to do a particular job (e.g. catering for a one-off event).

Team responsibilities

As members of the catering team, you and your teammates will have certain responsibilities. It is important to the organisation that you fulfil these responsibilities.

- Be loyal to your team leader (e.g. head chef, partie chef, manager or lecturer).
- Be punctual when reporting for duty.

- Be correctly dressed in a clean uniform.
- Be prepared to help other members of your team if the need arises.
- Be reliable.
- Work methodically.
- Share information and learn from each other.
- Communicate effectively.
- Motivate each other to learn new skills and techniques.

Good working relationships

It is important that you have good working relationships with other team members. You can do this by following these guidelines.

- Communicate sensibly and cheerfully at all times.
- Be willing to help others who may be in difficulties.
- Share your knowledge to help the team become stronger and more effective.

Helping team members

It is important to help team members in their work for the following reasons.

- Different members of the teams will have different strengths. Some members will be better at certain tasks than others, and vice versa.
- A good team member will be willing to help others and accept help if it is needed.

If team members help each other the team will feel stronger and happier, and so will work better.

When helping other team members:

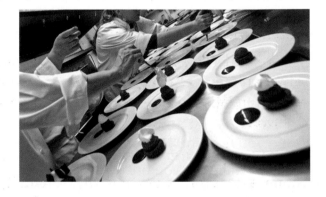

- always communicate in a helpful and friendly way
- offer help if you think you may know something that others do not
- offer help quietly, without making a fuss.

Do not:

- be patronising
- be rude or sarcastic if a member of your team is finding it difficult to do something that you are better at
- make rude or sarcastic comments about other people's efforts.

Bullying can damage team relationships. Read about bullying in Chapter 3.

An efficient team will communicate well with one another and will listen to what each team member has to say.

New team members

When somebody new joins your team, they need to know:

- the names of all the team members – introduce everybody
- where to find the lockers, changing room, washing facilities, laundry for uniforms, staff canteen and so on.

If you have experience of the job, tell the new team member about it.

It is important to share information with new team members:

- so that they feel welcome
- so that they feel that the team is friendly, relaxed and helpful.

Working well as a team

You can help your team to work well by behaving in an organised and respectful way.

- Show respect for all the members of your team.
- If you think you can help someone else then always offer to do so.
- Always be on time.
- Always dress correctly in a clean uniform.
- Take pride in being a chef, and always try to understand and learn more about what you are doing.

A team member who behaves badly can cause problems for the whole team.

- Do not show disrespect to other team members, or anyone you have contact with at work.
- Do not behave rowdily, especially in the changing room.
- Do not use unsuitable names for other people.
- Do not behave as if you are the most important person on the team.
- Do not dress in a dirty or untidy way.
- Do not neglect your personal cleanliness.

If there are problems in a team, working relationships can be upset. You should report problems to your **line manager** in writing. This is important because bad working relationships lead to tension and friction within the team, preventing good teamwork.

Forms of communication

Communication is essential in the hospitality industry, and it is important to communicate clearly. You can communicate face to face, by telephone or in writing. To work well and achieve the team's aims, team members must understand and communicate clearly with each other and people outside the team. Communication only happens when each person taking part understands what the other is saying.

Face to face

When you are speaking to someone you should look at them. Speak clearly, without shouting. Be patient if the person to whom you are speaking does not understand you. Repeat what you have said, trying to speak more clearly the second time.

Telephone

The telephone is one of the most common ways of communicating with people who are not in the same place as you.

- When you make a call, if the telephone is answered, say who you are and check that you are speaking to the correct person.
- If the call switches to an answer phone, wait for the beep before you speak. Give your name and say your message slowly and clearly – do not babble. If you need the person you are phoning to call you back, say your telephone number slowly and clearly.

- Speak clearly – if you have a long message to give someone it can help to write it down before you make the call.
- Think about your tone of voice. This is very important, as it will tell the other person how you are feeling.

Letter

Letters are another common form of communication in business.

- If you are not a skilled letter writer, it is a good idea to write a rough version first. This gives you the chance to check it and, if necessary, to ask someone else to check it for grammar, sense and spelling.
- When writing a letter, put your address and telephone number at the top right of the page and write the date beneath this.
- If you know the name of the person to whom you are writing then use it, e.g. *Dear Mr Brown*. If you do not know their name then write *Dear Sir or Madam*.
- When you have finished the letter, end it with *Yours sincerely* (or *Yours faithfully* if you do not know the name of the person you are writing to) followed by your signature. Print your name clearly beneath the signature.
- When addressing an envelope, ensure that you spell the person's name correctly and double-check the address, particularly the postcode. Do not forget to put a stamp on before posting.
- If you need a reply, it can be helpful to enclose a stamped envelope addressed back to you.

Email

Today many people communicate by email (electronic mail). You should treat email like any other method of communication, with respect. You should write clearly, politely and in the appropriate tone. Although it is a quick and easy way of communicating, you must remember always to be courteous and businesslike when emailing people at work. Try to avoid writing in capital letters as this can be seen as aggressive, as if you are shouting.

Activity

1 What does it mean to be a good team player? Name three aspects of a team player.

2 In a small group, discuss why good team players are important in hospitality.

3 Name a successful team in any field. Why are they successful? Could the features of that team be applied to a catering business?

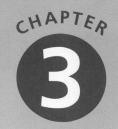
Health and safety awareness

VRQ Unit 103 Health and safety awareness for catering and hospitality

Learning outcomes:

- Demonstrate awareness of health and safety practices in the catering and hospitality workplace
- Identify hazards in the workplace
- Follow health and safety procedures

NVQ 501 (1GEN1) Maintain a safe, hygienic and secure working environment

Bullying and harassment

Bullying and harassment can be when someone constantly finds fault with and criticises someone else. It can seem quite trivial, but it can feel very unpleasant. For example, people may:

- refuse to acknowledge you and your achievements
- undermine you, your position and your potential
- ignore you and make you feel isolated and separated from your colleagues
- deliberately exclude you from what is going on at work
- humiliate, shout at and threaten you, often in front of others
- set you unrealistic tasks, which they keep changing.

Who is bullied?

Adults may be bullied by members of their family, by work colleagues or by neighbours.

People who are being bullied can feel scared, vulnerable and isolated. If you are aware of any bullying, of you or of someone else, you must report it so that it can be stopped. Nobody deserves to be bullied.

What is the difference between bullying and harassment?

Bullying tends to consist of many small incidents over a long period of time, whereas harassment may consist of one or more serious incidents. Harassment is the sort of unpleasant behaviour that creates an intimidating, hostile or offensive environment. This can take many forms and can happen for many reasons. For example, it may be related to age, sex, race, disability, religion, sexuality or any personal characteristic of an individual.

Injuries, accidents and disease

Common causes of accidents in kitchens

The following are some common causes of accidents in the kitchen:

- slipping on a slippery floor
- tripping over objects and falling
- lifting objects
- being exposed to hazards such as hot or dangerous substances, e.g. steam, oven cleaner
- being hit or hurt by moving objects, such as being cut by a knife when chopping
- walking into objects
- machines such as vegetable cutting machines, liquidisers, mincing machines
- fires and explosions
- electric shocks.

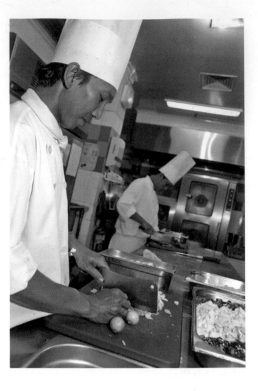

RIDDOR (Reporting Injuries, Diseases and Dangerous Occurrences) Act 1996

The law says that all work-related accidents, diseases and dangerous occurrences must be recorded (written down) and reported. Employers must inform the Incident Contact Centre, Caerphilly Business Park, Caerphilly CF83 3GG.

These are examples of injuries that must be reported:

- fractures (apart from fractures to fingers, thumbs or toes)
- eye injuries from chemicals getting into the eye, a hot metal burn to the eye or any penetration of the eye
- any injury from electric shock or burning that leads to unconsciousness or the need to resuscitate the person or send them to hospital for more than 24 hours
- unconsciousness caused by exposure to a harmful substance or biological agents (e.g. cleaning products and solvents)
- unconsciousness or illness requiring medical treatment caused by inhaling a harmful substance or absorbing it through the skin (e.g. breathing in poisonous carbon monoxide leaking from a gas appliance)
- illness requiring medical treatment caused by a biological agent or its toxins or infected material (e.g. harmful bacteria used in laboratories).

Examples of reportable diseases:

- dermatitis
- asthma
- hepatitis
- tuberculosis.

Control of hazardous substances

The Control of Substances Hazardous to Health (COSHH) regulations state that an employer must not carry on any work that might expose employees to any substances that are hazardous to health, unless the employer has assessed the risks of this work to employees.

Hazardous substances in catering

In catering establishments there are many chemicals and substances used for cleaning that can be harmful if not used correctly.

In the kitchen:

- cleaning chemicals
- chemicals such as detergents, sanitisers, descalers and pest control substances.

In the restaurant:

- cleaning chemicals
- polishes
- methylated spirits.

In the bar:

- beer-line cleaner
- glass-washing detergent
- sanitisers.

Other rooms:

- cleaning chemicals.

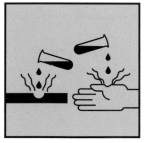

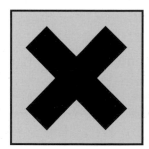
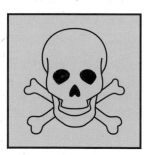

| Corrosive | Flammable | Harmful | Toxic |

Symbols to show hazardous substances

Substances that are dangerous to health are labelled as very toxic, toxic, harmful, irritant or corrosive.

People using these chemical substances must be trained to use them. They must also wear protective clothing such as goggles, gloves and face masks. Hazardous substances can enter the body through the skin, the eyes, the nose (by inhaling) and the mouth (by swallowing).

Ways to prevent an accident

COSHH says that the employer has to assess the risk from chemicals and decide what precautions are needed. The employer should make sure that measures are in place to control the use of chemical substances and monitor their use. If chemical substances are used you should:

- inform, instruct and train all staff in their use and safety

- always follow the manufacturer's instructions
- always store them in their original containers, away from heat
- keep the lids tightly closed
- not expose them to heat or to naked flames
- read all the labels carefully
- never mix chemicals
- know the first-aid procedure
- get rid of empty containers immediately
- get rid of waste chemical solutions safely
- wear safety equipment and clothing.

Identifying hazards in the workplace

The Health & Safety at Work Act covers all full-time and part-time workers and unpaid workers. The Health & Safety Executive (HSE) is responsible for enforcing health and safety in the workplace.

When we assess health and safety we talk about hazards. A hazard is anything that can cause harm, such as:

- extremes of cold and heat
- uneven floors
- excessive noise
- chemicals
- electricity
- working using ladders
- moving parts and machinery
- dust and fumes.

Risk

Risk is the chance of somebody being harmed by the hazard. There may be a high risk or a low risk of harm.

> *Example*
>
> Using a liquidiser is a hazard. What is the likelihood of it causing harm?
>
> If it is overfilled, the contents can force the lid off. If the contents are hot, they may burst into the air and hit the chef, which may cause a burn.
>
> This risk is medium.

Here are five steps to assessing risk.

1 Look for hazards, i.e. the things that can cause harm.
2 Identify who could be harmed and how.
3 Work out the risks and decide if the existing precautions are good enough or whether more should be done to prevent any harm being caused.
4 Write down what the hazard is and what the risk is, and keep this as a record.
5 Re-check the hazard and the risk at regular intervals and go back and change the risk assessment (the written record) if necessary.

Safety in the workplace

Avoiding accidents

There are lots of precautions that can be taken to avoid accidents happening in catering premises.

- The main type of accident is people falling or tripping. Floors should be even, with no unexpected steps, and they should be kept dry. Clean up spillages immediately and use warning notices if a floor is slippery.
- Keep corridors and walkways clear so that people do not trip over objects that are in the way.
- There should be adequate lighting so that people can see clearly where they are going.
- There should be adequate ventilation so that any excess heat and fumes can escape.
- Kitchens should not be overcrowded. There should be enough space for people to move around without bumping and pushing into one another.
- Follow the rules and working practices.
  - Always work in an organised way.
  - Clean up as you go.
- Follow the flow of traffic in the kitchen.
  - People should flow through the preparation area to the service area without backtracking or crossing over, so that they do not bump into each other.
  - Food should flow through the preparation area to the service area. Raw food should never go into the area where there is cooked food.
  - Equipment should flow through the preparation area to the service area. Dirty equipment should not come into contact with or get mixed up with clean equipment.

Manual handling

Picking up and carrying heavy or difficult loads can lead to accidents if it is not done properly. Handling loads wrongly is the main cause of back problems in the workplace. The safest way to lift objects is to bend your knees rather than your back. It is also better if two people lift the object together, rather than one person trying to do it on their own. This will help to prevent straining and damaging your back.

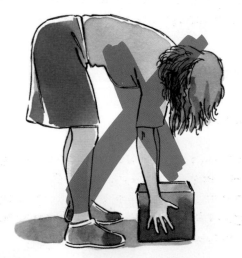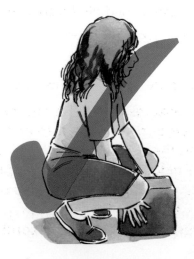

How to lift correctly

Handling checklist
- When you move goods on trolleys, trucks or other wheeled vehicles:
  - load them carefully
  - do not overload them
  - load them in a way that allows you to see where you are going.
- In stores, stack heavy items at the bottom.
- If steps are needed to reach higher items, use them with care.
- Take particular care when moving large pots of liquid, especially if the liquid is hot. Do not fill them to the brim.
- Use a warning sign to let people know if equipment handles, lids and so on might be hot. This is traditionally done by sprinkling a small amount of flour, or something similar, onto the part of the equipment that might be hot.
- Take extra care when removing a tray from the oven or salamander. You do not want the tray to burn you or someone else.

Safety signs

We use safety signs to control a hazard. They should not replace other methods of controlling risks.

Yellow signs

These are warning signs to alert people to various dangers, such as slippery floors, hot oil or hot water. They also warn people about hazards such as corrosive material.

A yellow warning sign

Blue signs

These signs inform people about precautions they must take. They tell people how to progress safely through a certain area. They must be used whenever special precautions need to be taken, such as wearing protective clothing.

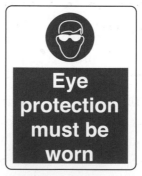
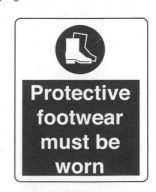

Blue information signs

Red signs

Red signs tell people that they should not enter. They are used to stop people from doing certain tasks in a hazardous area. Red signs are also used for fire-fighting equipment.

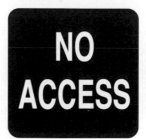
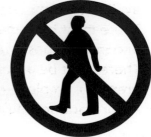

A red warning sign

Green signs

These are route signs designed to show people where fire exits and emergency exits are. Green is also used for first aid equipment.

Personal protective equipment

According to the Personal Protective Equipment (PPE) at Work Regulations 1992, employees must wear personal protective clothing and equipment (e.g. safety shoes, eye protection such as goggles) for certain things. For example, chefs must wear chefs' whites.

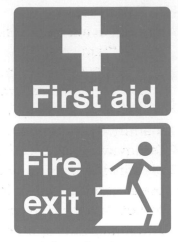

Green information signs

Electricity

Great care must be taken when dealing with electricity. If a person comes into direct contact with electricity the consequences can be very serious and sometimes fatal. If a person has an electric shock, switch off the current. If this is not possible, free the person using something that is dry and will insulate you from the electricity, such as a cloth, or something made of wood or rubber. You must take care not to use your bare hands otherwise the electric shock may be transmitted to you. If the person has stopped breathing, send for an ambulance. If you have been trained how to, you can give artificial respiration.

In an emergency:

- switch off the current
- raise the alarm
- call for a doctor/first aid help.

Fire safety

The Regulatory Fire Safety Order 2005 emphasises that fires should be prevented. It says that fire safety is the responsibility of the occupant of premises and the people who might be affected by fire, so in catering this will usually be the employer (the occupant) and the employees (who will be affected by fire).

Fire precautions

Below are some guidelines for good practice.

- Remove all hazards, or reduce them as much as possible.
- Make sure that everyone is protected from the risk of fire and the likelihood of a fire spreading.
- Make sure that all escape routes are safe and used effectively, in other words they are signposted, easy to access and people know where they are.
- Some way of fighting fires (e.g. a fire extinguisher or fire blanket) must be available on the premises.
- There must be some way of detecting a fire on the premises (e.g. smoke alarms) and instructions as to what to do in case of fire.
- There must be arrangements in place for what to do if a fire breaks out on the premises. Employees must be trained in what to do in the event of a fire.
- All precautions provided must be installed and maintained by a competent person.

Fire risk assessment

A fire risk assessment will:

- help to find out how likely it is that a fire might happen
- help to highlight the dangers from fire in the workplace.

There are five steps to complete for a fire risk assessment.

1 Identify the potential fire hazards in the workplace.
2 Decide who will be in danger in the event of a fire, e.g. employees, visitors.
3 Identify the risks caused by the hazards. Decide whether the existing fire precautions are adequate or whether more needs to be done, for example to remove a hazard to control the risk.
4 The things that are found out and changes that are made in steps 1 to 3 should be written down and kept on record, and all staff should be informed of them.
5 The risk assessment should be reviewed regularly to check that it is up to date. If things change it should be revised when necessary.

The fire triangle

For a fire to start, three things are needed:

1 a source of heat (ignition)
2 fuel
3 oxygen.

If any one of these three things is missing a fire cannot start. So, taking precautions to avoid the three coming together will reduce the chances of a fire starting.

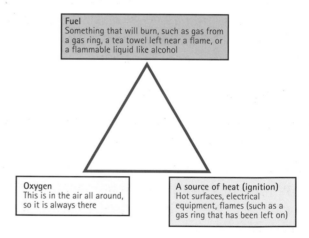

The fire triangle

Fuel
Something that will burn, such as gas from a gas ring, a tea towel left near a flame, or a flammable liquid like alcohol

Oxygen
This is in the air all around, so it is always there

A source of heat (ignition)
Hot surfaces, electrical equipment, flames (such as a gas ring that has been left on)

Fire detection and fire warning

There needs to be an effective way of detecting a fire and warning people about it quickly enough to allow them to escape before the fire spreads too far.

In small workplaces, such as small restaurants, a fire will be detected easily and quickly and is unlikely to cut off the escape routes. In this case, if people can see the exits clearly, shouting 'FIRE!' may be all that is necessary.

In larger establishments fire warning systems are needed. Manually operated call points are likely to be the least that is needed. These are the type of fire alarm where you break glass to set off the alarm (as seen on the wall in schools, etc.).

Fire-fighting equipment

Portable fire extinguishers enable people to tackle a fire in its early stages. People should be trained to use the extinguishers and should use them only if they can do so without putting themselves in danger.

Fires are classified in accordance with British Standard EN2 as follows.

- Class A – fires involving solid materials where combustion (burning) normally forms glowing embers, e.g. wood.
- Class B – fires involving liquids (e.g. methylated spirits) or liquefiable solids (e.g. any a kind of flammable gel used under a burner).

- Class C – fires involving gases.
- Class D – fires involving metals.
- Class F – fires involving cooking oils or fats.

There are different types of fire extinguishers that are suitable for different types of fire. Portable extinguishers all contain a substance that will put out a fire. The substance will vary, but whatever it is it will be forced out of the extinguisher under pressure. Generally, portable fire extinguishers contain one of the following five substances (extinguishing mediums):

1 water
2 foam
3 powder
4 carbon dioxide
5 vaporising liquids.

The most useful form of general-purpose fire-fighting equipment is the water-type extinguisher or hose reel. Areas of special risk, such as kitchens where oil, fats and electrical equipment are used, may need other types of extinguisher such as carbon dioxide or dry powder. Your local fire authority will be able to advise you on everything to do with fire safety.

Security in catering

Security in catering premises is a major concern these days. The main security risks in the hotel and catering industry are:

- theft – where customers' property, employers' property (particularly food, drink and equipment) or employees' property is stolen
- burglary – where the burglar comes on to the premises (trespasses) and steals property
- robbery – theft with assault
- fraud – e.g. stolen credit cards
- assault – fights between customers; assaults on staff by customers
- vandalism – damage to property caused by customers, intruders or employees
- arson – setting fire to the property
- undesirables – having people such as drug traffickers and prostitutes on the premises
- terrorism – bombs, telephone bomb threats.

The Health & Safety at Work Regulations now require employers to conduct a risk assessment regarding the safety of staff in the catering business. Preventing crime is better than having to deal with it once it has happened. Here are some ideas for helping to prevent crime.

- The best way to prevent theft is to stop the thief entering the premises in the first place. Everyone who comes in should be asked to sign in at reception and, if they are a legitimate visitor, be given a security badge.
- All contract workers should be registered and given security badges, and they may be restricted to working in certain areas.
- There should also be a good security system at the back door, where everyone delivering goods has to report to the security officer.

- All establishments should try to reduce temptation for criminals, for example by reducing the amount of cash that is handled.
- Staff who handle money should be trained in simple anti-fraud measures such as checking bank notes, checking signatures on plastic cards and so on.
- It is impossible to remove all temptation, so equipment (e.g. computers, fax machines, photocopiers) should be marked with some sort of security tag or identification.
- It is important to lock doors and windows.
- Good lighting is also important for security reasons – criminals are less likely to come on to the premises at night if people can see them easily.
- Closed-circuit television (CCTV) cameras are also used as a deterrent against crime.
- With regard to staff, the first step is to appoint honest staff by checking their references from previous employers.
- Some companies write into employee contracts the 'right to search'. This means that from time to time the employer can carry out searches of the employees' lockers, bags and so on. This discourages employees from stealing. It is not legal to force a person to be searched even if they have signed a contract about it, but if they refuse they may be breaking their employment contract.

Activity

1 In a small group, discuss the benefits for a catering establishment of having good health and safety procedures.

2 What risk is created by each of these incidents?
   - Cooking oil spilled on the kitchen floor.
   - A chef not wearing protective clothing.
   - Using a deep fat fryer.
   - Poor ventilation in the kitchen.
   - Using chemical cleaning products.

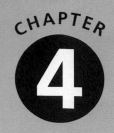

Introduction to healthier foods and special diets

VRQ Unit 104 Introduction to healthier foods and special diets

Learning outcomes:
- Demonstrate awareness of healthier food
- Identify the need for special diets

The importance of a healthy diet

There are no bad foods, only bad diets. It is important that everyone – children, adolescents and adults – eats a balanced diet to improve their health.

There is no such thing as a perfect food that gives you everything you need. No single food provides all the nutrients essential to keep us healthy. Different foods have different nutritional contents (in other words, they are good for us in different ways). So we need to eat a variety of foods to give us all the nutrients we need for a healthy diet. A balanced diet also makes our mealtimes more interesting.

Nutrients in foods help our bodies to do everyday things like moving, growing and seeing. They also help our bodies to heal themselves if they are injured, and a balanced diet can help to prevent illness and disease. In ancient times, many foods (e.g. olive oil, pomegranates and spices such as ginger) were used for their healing properties.

The main nutrients are:

- carbohydrates
- protein
- fats
- vitamins
- minerals
- water.

We will now look at each of these in more detail to find out what they do and which foods they are in.

Carbohydrates

We need carbohydrates for energy. They are made by plants and then either used by the plants as energy, or eaten by animals and humans for energy or as dietary fibre.

There are three main types of carbohydrate:

- sugars
- starches
- fibre.

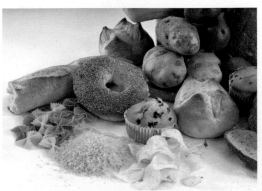

These foods are high in carbohydrates

Sugars

Sugars are the simplest form of carbohydrate. When carbohydrates are digested they turn into sugars.

There are several types of sugar:

- glucose – found in the blood of animals and in fruit and honey
- fructose – found in fruit, honey and cane sugar
- sucrose – found in beet and cane sugar
- lactose – found in milk
- maltose – found in cereal grains and used in beer making.

Types of carbohydrate

Starches

Starches break down into sugars. Starches are present in many foods, such as:

- pasta, e.g. macaroni, spaghetti, vermicelli
- cereals, e.g. cornflakes, shredded wheat
- cakes, biscuits, bread (cooked starch)
- whole grains, e.g. rice, barley, tapioca
- powdered grains, e.g. flour, cornflour, ground rice, arrowroot
- vegetables, e.g. potatoes, parsnips, peas, beans
- unripe fruit, e.g. bananas, apples, cooking pears.

Fibre

Dietary fibre is a very important form of starch. Unlike other carbohydrates, dietary fibre cannot be digested and does not provide energy to the body. However, dietary fibre is essential for a balanced diet because it:

- helps to remove waste and toxins from the body, and maintain bowel action
- helps to control the digestion and processing of nutrients
- adds bulk to the diet, helping us to stop feeling hungry; it is used in many slimming foods.

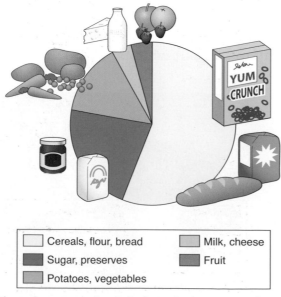

The main sources of carbohydrates in the average diet

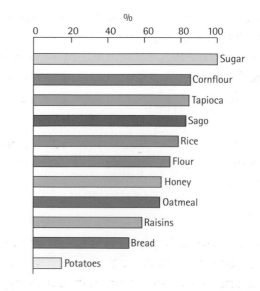

The percentage of carbohydrate in some foods

Fibre is found in:

- fruits and vegetables
- wholemeal and granary bread
- wholegrain cereals
- wholemeal pasta
- wholegrain rice
- pulses (peas and beans) and lentils.

Proteins

Protein is an essential part of all living things. Every day our bodies carry out millions of tasks (bodily functions) to stay alive. We need protein so that our bodies can grow and repair themselves.

There are two kinds of protein:

1 animal protein
2 vegetable protein.

The lifespan of the cells in our bodies varies from a week to a few months. As the cells die they need to be replaced. We need protein for our cells to repair and for new ones to grow.

We also use protein for energy. Any protein that is not used up in repairing and growing cells is converted into carbohydrate or fat.

What is protein?

Protein is made up of chemicals known as amino acids. There are 20 types of amino acid. The protein in cheese is different from the protein in meat because the amino acids are different. Ideally our bodies need both animal and vegetable protein so that we get all the amino acids we need: eight are essential for adults and nine for children.

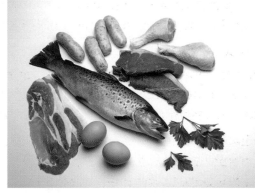

These foods are high in protein

- Animal protein is found in meat, game, poultry, fish, eggs, milk and cheese.
- Vegetable protein is found in vegetable seeds, pulses, peas, beans, nuts and wheat, and in special vegetarian products such as Quorn.

For detailed nutritional information about different foods, refer to *The Theory of Catering*.

Fats

Fats are naturally present in many foods and are an essential part of our diet. The main functions of fat are to protect the body, keep it warm and provide energy. Fats form an

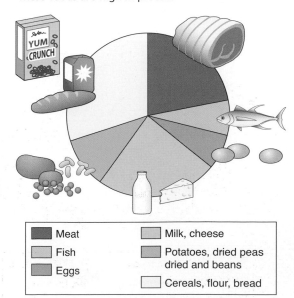

■	Meat	■	Milk, cheese
□	Fish	■	Potatoes, dried peas dried and beans
■	Eggs	□	Cereals, flour, bread

The main sources of protein in the average diet

insulating layer under the skin, and this helps to protect the vital organs and to keep the body warm. Fat is also needed to build cell membranes in the body.

Some fats are solid at room temperature and others, usually called oils, are liquid at room temperature. Hard fats are mainly animal fats.

- Animal fats are butter, dripping (beef), suet, lard (pork), cheese, cream, bacon, meat fat, oily fish.
- Vegetable fats are margarine, cooking oils, nut oils, soya bean oils.

Too much fat is bad for us. It can lead to:

- being overweight (obesity)
- high levels of cholesterol, which can clog the heart's blood vessels (arteries)
- heart disease
- bad breath (halitosis)
- type 2 diabetes (the other type of diabetes, type 1, is something people are born with and is not caused by eating too much fat).

There are two types of fats:

1 saturated fat

2 unsaturated fat.

A diet high in saturated fat is thought to increase the risk of heart disease. The table below shows the percentage of saturated fat in an average diet.

Type of food	% saturated fat
Milk, cheese, cream	16.0
Meat and meat products *This splits down into:*	25.2
Beef	4.1
Lamb	3.5
Pork, bacon and ham	5.8
Sausage	2.7
Other meat products (e.g. burgers, faggots, pâté)	9.1
Other oils and fats (e.g. olive oil, margarine, sunflower oil)	30.0
Other sources, including eggs, fish, poultry	7.4
Biscuits and cakes	11.4

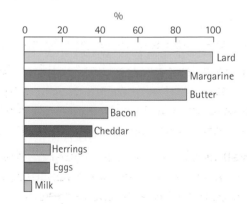

The percentage of fat in some foods

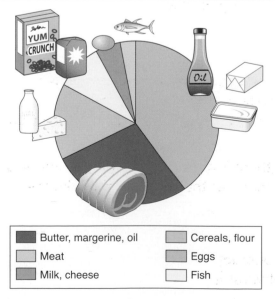

Butter, margerine, oil   Cereals, flour

Meat   Eggs

Milk, cheese   Fish

The main sources of fat in the average diet

Vitamins

Vitamins are chemicals that are vital for life. They are found in small amounts in many foods. If your diet is deficient in any vitamins, you can become ill or unhealthy. Vitamins help with many of our bodily functions, such as growth and protection from disease.

Vitamin A

Vitamin A:

- helps children to grow
- helps the body to resist infection
- helps prevent night blindness (difficulty seeing in dark areas)

Vitamin A is found in fatty foods. Dark green vegetables are a good source of vitamin A.

Other sources of vitamin A are:

- halibut liver oil
- milk
- butter
- watercress
- cod liver oil
- herrings
- kidneys
- carrots
- liver
- spinach
- margarine
- tomatoes
- cheese
- apricots
- eggs.

Fish liver oils have the most vitamin A.

Vitamin D

Vitamin D:

- controls the way our bodies use calcium (a mineral that you will read about on page 35)
- is necessary for healthy bones and teeth.

An important source of vitamin D is the action of sunlight on skin. Other sources are fish liver oils, oily fish, egg yolk, margarine and dairy produce.

Vitamin B

There are two main types of vitamin B.

1 Thiamin, also known as B1 – this helps our bodies to produce energy, and is necessary for our brain, heart and nervous system to function properly.
2 Riboflavin, also known as B2 – this helps with growth, and helps us to have healthy skin, nails and hair, among other things.

As well as these two main types of vitamin B there is a third, niacin or nicotinic acid. This is vital for normal brain function, and it improves the health of the skin, the circulation and the digestive system.

Vitamin B:

- helps to keep the nervous system in good condition
- enables the body to get energy from carbohydrates
- encourages the body to grow.

When you cook food the vitamin B in it can be lost. It is important to learn how to preserve vitamin B when you cook foods. You will learn about this as you study cookery in more depth.

The table below shows sources of vitamin B.

Thiamin (B1)	Riboflavin (B2)	Nicotinic acid
Yeast	Yeast	Meat extract
Bacon	Liver	Brewers' yeast
Oatmeal	Meat extract	Liver
Peas	Cheese	Kidney
Wholemeal bread	Egg	Beef

Vitamin C (also called ascorbic acid)
Vitamin C:

- is need for children to grow
- helps cuts and broken bones to heal
- prevents gum and mouth infections.

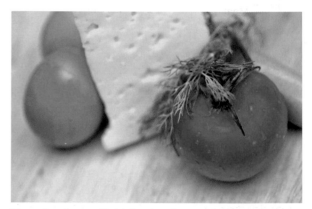

These foods are all rich in vitamins

When you cook food the vitamin C in it can be lost. It is important to learn how to preserve vitamin C when you cook foods; an important source of vitamin C in our diet is potatoes. You will learn about this as you study cookery in more depth.

Sources of vitamin C are:

- blackcurrants
- green vegetables
- lemons
- grapefruit
- bananas
- potatoes
- strawberries
- oranges
- tomatoes
- fruit juices.

Minerals

There are 19 minerals in total, most of which our bodies need, in very small quantities, to function properly.

- We need minerals to build our bones and teeth.
- Minerals help us to carry out bodily functions.
- Minerals help to control the levels of fluids in our bodies.

We will now look at a few of the most important minerals for our bodies.

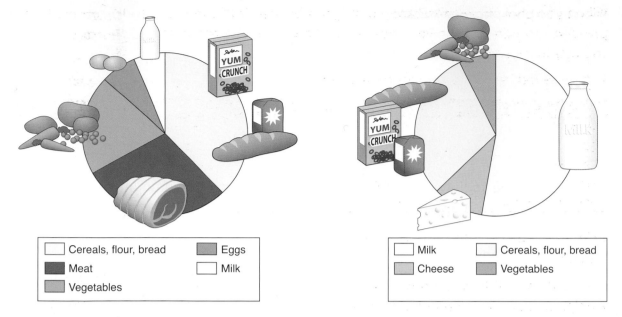

	Cereals, flour, bread		Eggs
	Meat		Milk
	Vegetables		

	Milk		Cereals, flour, bread
	Cheese		Vegetables

The main sources of calcium and iron in the average diet

Calcium

We need calcium to:

- build bones and teeth
- help our blood to clot
- help our muscles to work.

In order for our bodies to use calcium effectively they also need vitamin D. Sources of calcium are:

- milk and milk products
- green vegetables
- the bones of tinned oily fish (e.g. sardines)
- drinking water
- wholemeal bread, and white bread if calcium has been added.

Iron

We need iron to build haemoglobin, which is a substance in our blood that transports oxygen and carbon dioxide around the body.

Sources of iron include:

- lean meat
- wholemeal flour
- offal (animals' internal organs, such as the heart, liver and kidneys)
- green vegetables
- egg yolk
- fish.

Our bodies absorb iron more easily from meat and offal. Iron is also absorbed better if vitamin C is present.

Phosphorus

We need phosphorus to:

- build bones and teeth (together with calcium and vitamin D)
- control the structure of our brain cells.

Sources of phosphorous include:

- liver
- bread
- cheese
- eggs
- kidney
- fish.

Sodium

We need to have sodium in all our body fluids. It regulates the amount of water we have in our bodies. It also helps with the functioning of our muscles and nerves.

If we eat too much salt our bodies can get rid of some of it in our urine. Our kidneys control how much salt we get rid of in this way. We also lose sodium when we sweat, but our bodies cannot control how much salt we lose in this way.

Sodium is found in salt (sodium chloride).

Many foods:

- are cooked with salt, or
- have salt added to them (e.g. bacon and cheese), or
- already contain salt (e.g. meat, eggs, fish).

Too much sodium can cause hypertension (high blood pressure) and can increase the risk of a stroke. It is recommended that we do not eat more than 6 g of salt per day. Our bodies only need 4.1 g.

Iodine

We need iodine so that our thyroid gland can function properly. The thyroid gland produces hormones that control our growth. If it is not working properly it can make us underweight or overweight.

Sources of iodine include:

- sea foods
- iodised salt
- drinking water obtained near the sea
- vegetables grown near the sea.

Water

Water is vital to life. Without it we cannot survive for very long. We lose water from our bodies through urine and sweat, and we need to replace it regularly to prevent dehydration. It is recommended that we drink eight glasses of water a day.

Our organs require water to function properly.

- Water regulates our body temperature – when we sweat the water evaporates from our skin and cools us down.
- Water helps to remove waste products from our bodies. If these waste products are not removed they can release poisons, which can damage our organs or make us ill.
- We need water to help our bodies absorb nutrients, vitamins and minerals, and to help our digestive system.
- Water acts as a lubricant, helping our eyes and joints to work and stay healthy.

Sources of water are:

- drinks of all kinds
- foods such as fruits, vegetables, meat, eggs
- fibre.

As you have already read, fibre cannot be digested, but we need it to remove waste from our bodies.

Healthy eating

If you eat a healthy diet you will reduce the risk of a number of diseases, including stroke, heart disease, diabetes and some cancers.

The best way to stay fit and healthy is to eat a diet high in fruit, vegetables, whole grains and plant-based foods like beans and lentils, but low in fat, sugar and salt.

Fruit and vegetables

Fruit and vegetables contain valuable vitamins, minerals, fibre and folate acid, which help to protect us from illness. They also contain substances called phytochemicals, which are antioxidants. Antioxidants help to protect the body's cells from damage.

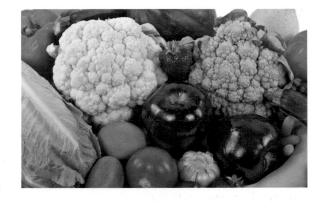

- There are some vegetables and fruits that protect us particularly well against strokes because they have such high levels of antioxidants. The vegetables include cauliflower, cabbage, broccoli and Brussels sprouts. The fruits include blackcurrants, oranges, kiwi fruit, and red and yellow peppers.
- The fibre found in fruit and vegetables plays an important role in preventing a stroke too. It also helps to lower cholesterol and maintain a healthy digestive system.
- Folate or folic acid is found in dark green vegetables like broccoli and spinach. This also helps to protect us against strokes.
- Potassium is another essential mineral, like sodium, that we need to balance the fluids in our bodies. It is also important in keeping our heart rate normal, and helps our nerves and muscles to function. It is found in bananas, avocados, citrus fruits and green, leafy vegetables.

Ideally you should aim to eat at least five portions of fruit and vegetables a day, e.g. one apple, one banana, two plums, a heaped tablespoon of dried fruit like raisins (15 g), or three broccoli or cauliflower florets.

The nutrient content of different foods

The table on the next page shows the main functions of different nutrients.

Energy	Growth and repair	Regulation of body processes
Carbohydrates	Proteins	Vitamins
Fats	Minerals	Minerals
Proteins	Water	Water

The effects of too much of some nutrients in the diet

The table below shows the effects of having too much of some nutrients in your diet.

Nutrient	Effect of excess in diet
Fat	Obesity Heart disease and heart attacks High blood pressure
Carbohydrate	Obesity Tooth decay Diabetes caused by too much sugar
Salt	High blood pressure and stroke

Special diets

There are various reasons why people may follow a particular type of diet.

Groups with special dietary requirements

There are certain groups of people in the population who have special nutritional needs. You may have different needs at different points in your life – for example, if you change your lifestyle or occupation and when you grow older.

Pregnant and breast-feeding women

Pregnant and breast-feeding women should avoid soft mould-ripened cheese, pâté, raw eggs, undercooked meat, poultry and fish, liver and alcohol.

Children and teenagers

As children grow their nutritional requirements change. Children need a varied and balanced diet rich in protein.

Teenagers need to have a good, nutritionally balanced diet. Girls need to make sure that they are getting enough iron in their diet to help with the effects of puberty.

Vegetarians

Most vegetarians choose to eat this way because they believe it is more healthy or because they do not agree with eating animals. It is not usually for a medical reason. Vegetarians have a lower risk of heart disease, stroke, diabetes, gallstones, kidney stones and colon cancer than people who eat meat. They are also less likely to be overweight or have raised cholesterol levels.

The elderly

As we get older our bodies start to slow down and our appetite will get smaller. However, elderly people still need a nutritionally balanced diet to stay healthy.

People who are ill

People who are ill, at home or in hospital, need balanced meals with plenty of the nutrients they need to help them recover. Good nutritional food is part of the healing process. In the days of Florence Nightingale, hospital wards were closed for two hours a day while patients ate their nutritious meals. No doctor was allowed in the wards at mealtimes. Florence Nightingale saw food as medicine.

Other reasons for special diets

Many people require special diets for various reasons, such as:

- religious beliefs
- health (diabetes, obesity, heart disease)
- allergies.

Allergies and intolerances

Some people may be intolerant of or allergic to some types of food, so caterers must tell customers what is in the dishes on the menu.

Food allergies are a type of intolerance where the body's immune system sees harmless food as harmful and this causes an allergic reaction. Food allergies can cause something called anaphylactic shock, which makes the throat and mouth swell so that it is difficult to swallow or breathe. They can also cause nausea, vomiting and unconsciousness. Some allergic reactions can be fatal.

Foods that sometimes cause an allergic reaction include:

- milk
- dairy products
- fish
- shellfish
- eggs
- nuts (particularly peanuts, cashew nuts, pecans, Brazil nuts, walnuts).

Diets for specific benefits

Different types of diet have different benefits. You can choose foods that will keep your heart healthy, detoxify your liver or boost your energy and concentration.

Activity

1 Name three groups of people who need special diets.

2 Choose a recipe from this book that you think is not very healthy.
   How would you adapt the recipe to make it healthier? Try making your adapted version.

Introduction to kitchen equipment

VRQ Unit 105 Introduction to kitchen equipment

Learning outcomes:

- Use large and small items of equipment and utensils
- Using knives and cutting equipment

NVQ 519 1FC1   Prepare and cook fish
NVQ 520 1FPC2 Prepare and cook meat and poultry
NVQ 521 1FPC3 Prepare and cook pasta
NVQ 522 1FPC4 Prepare and cook rice
NVQ 523 1FPC5 Prepare and cook eggs
NVQ 524 1FPC6 Prepare and cook pulses
NVQ 525 1FPC7 Prepare and cook vegetable protein
NVQ 527 1FPC9 Prepare and cook grain

Types of kitchen equipment

Kitchen equipment can be divided into three categories:

1 large equipment, e.g. ranges, steamers, boiling pans, fish fryers, sinks, tables
2 mechanical equipment, e.g. peelers, mincers, mixers, refrigerators, dishwashers
3 small equipment, e.g. knives, spoons.

Large equipment

General care and cleanliness tips

- Thoroughly wash equipment with hot detergent and water after use. Rinse with hot water and then dry.
- Moving parts of large-scale equipment should be greased occasionally. Report any faults with large equipment.
- Wear appropriate protective clothing when using chemicals to clean equipment.
- Always allow the equipment to cool before you clean it.

Ranges and ovens

A range is a collection of equipment together, usually stoves and ovens. There is a large variety of ranges available, fuelled by gas, electricity, microwave or microwave plus convection. Some have grills and wok cookers built in.

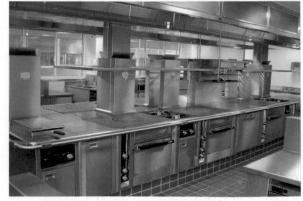

A central cooking range

⚠ Safety and cleaning

- Turning on ovens unnecessarily, or too early, wastes fuel, which is expensive.

- With gas ovens, it is very important to light the gas once it is turned on.
- Gas ovens and ranges must be fitted with a flame failure device. This switches off the gas if the flame blows out, to prevent explosion.
- Allow the equipment to cool before cleaning. Then scrub it down and wipe it clean. Apply a little oil to the surface of solid tops.

Convection ovens (fan-assisted ovens)

These are ovens with a built-in fan, which produces a current of hot air that moves around the inside of the oven. This creates a more even temperature in the oven, so they are very good for baking and roasting. Because they are more efficient, cooking temperatures can be lowered. For example, something that would have to be cooked at 200°C in a normal oven might cook at 180°C in a convection oven.

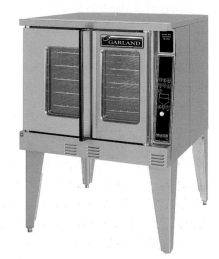
A convection oven

⚠ Safety and cleaning

- Take care when loading and unloading hot food.
- Allow the equipment to cool before cleaning, and wear protective clothing.

Combination ovens

These ovens are fuelled by gas or electricity. They have built-in computers that can be pre-programmed to cook something for exactly the right amount of time. They are also able to keep food at the correct temperature. They have brought about a revolution in baking, roasting and steaming.

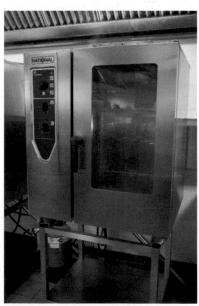

⚠ Safety and cleaning

- Take care when loading and removing trays of food. When using one as a steamer, make sure you release the steam gently before opening the door.
- Many modern models are self-cleaning, but they need to be checked regularly to make sure the cleaning programme is efficient.

A combination oven

Deck ovens

Deck ovens are also known as bakers' ovens. They have two, three or four tiers. They are usually fuelled by electricity but some are fuelled by gas.

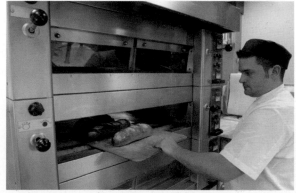

⚠ Safety and cleaning

Take great care when opening doors and moving items in and out of the oven, especially from the back of the oven. Special paddles known as 'peels' are used to move the trays of items around in the oven.

A deck oven

Microwave ovens

Microwave ovens use high-frequency power. They use the same sort of energy as that which carries television signals, but at a much higher frequency (i.e. much faster). The energy waves disturb the molecules or particles in the food and move them. This causes friction, which heats the food. Microwave ovens can cook food much more quickly than conventional ovens. They are often used for reheating food.

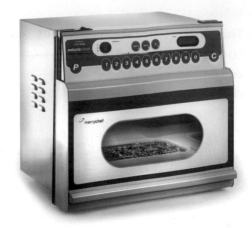

A microwave oven

⚠ Safety and cleaning

- If the door seal is damaged, do not use the oven. This should be reported to your employer or manager immediately. Microwave ovens should be inspected regularly.
- Metal containers should not be used in most microwaves as the energy waves will bounce off the metal surfaces. Some microwave ovens are fitted with metal reflectors so that metal containers can be used.
- Clean up any spillages immediately with appropriate cleaning materials. Hot, mild detergent water is usually sufficient.

Combination convection and microwave ovens

This type of oven combines hot-air convection and microwave energy. These can be used separately but are normally used together. This speeds up the cooking time of the food and at the same time gives it a good colour and texture.

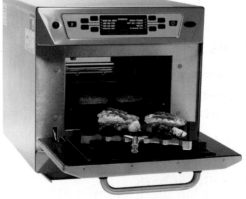

⚠ Safety and cleaning

- Metal pans can be used in this type of oven.
- Some of these ovens are self-cleaning. If you clean one manually, allow it to cool before cleaning, and wear appropriate protective clothing.

Hobs

A combination convection and microwave oven

Induction hobs

The burners on induction hobs are called induction coils. The coil will heat up only when a pan with a metal base is in direct contact with the hob. They work by magnetism, and it is the pan that actually heats the food, not the hob. When the pan is removed from the hob it turns off straight away. The hob will feel slightly warm after it is turned off, but it will not be too hot.

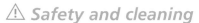

⚠ Safety and cleaning

- This type of hob is much safer than a conventional hob because it stays relatively cool even when cooking. There is very little chance of burning from direct contact with the hob.
- Induction hobs are very easy to clean and usually require only a wipe down with mild detergent water.

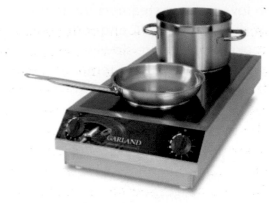

An induction hob

Halogen hobs

These hobs run on electricity. They are smooth ceramic surfaces with several controlled heat zones. Tungsten halogen lamps under the ceramic glass surface heat each zone. When the hob is switched on, most of the heat is passed directly into the base of the cooking pan as infra-red light.

⚠ Safety and cleaning

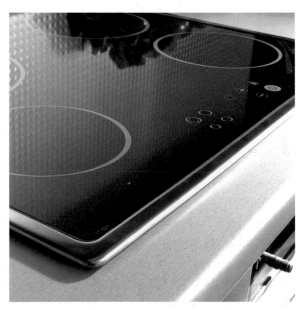

- Take care when working over heated surfaces.
- Carefully wipe up all spillages with a damp cloth. Clean with mild detergent water, then rinse and dry.

Steamers

There are three types of steaming ovens:

A halogen hob

1 atmospheric
2 pressure
3 dual.

In addition, combination ovens can be used to combine steaming and conventional oven cooking to get the benefits of both.

Atmospheric

An atmospheric steamer operates at normal atmospheric pressure (the same pressure as outside the steamer), creating steam at just above 100°C. These are often just normal saucepans with a metal basket in them.

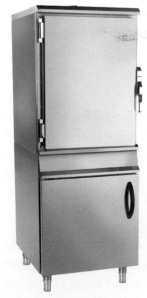

Pressure steamers

Pressure steaming is a good way to cook delicate food and foods cooked in a pouch.

Some pressure steamers cook at high pressure and some at low pressure.

An atmospheric steamer

In low-pressure steamers the temperature of the steam is 70°C and so food is cooked much more slowly. In high-pressure steamers the temperature of the steam is 120°C and so food is cooked faster.

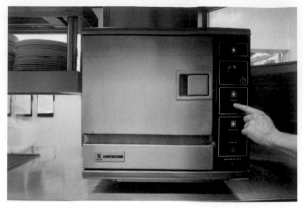

A pressure steamer

Dual steamers

These can switch between low pressure and high pressure. At low pressure they cook in the same way as pressure steamers. At high pressure the food is cooked more quickly than in atmospheric steamers and pressure steamers.

All steamers are available in a variety of sizes.

⚠ Safety and cleaning

- The main safety hazard associated with steamers is scalding. Take care when opening steamer doors: open the door slowly to allow the steam to escape gradually from the oven, then carefully remove the food items.
- Steamers have to be cleaned regularly. The inside of the steamer, trays and runners should be washed in hot detergent water, then rinsed and dried. Door controls should be lightly greased occasionally and the door left slightly open to allow air to circulate when the steamer is not in use.
- If water is held in the steamer then it must be changed regularly. The water chamber should be drained and cleaned before fresh water is added.
- Before use, check that the steamer is clean and safe to use. Any faults must be reported immediately.

Large pans, boilers and fryers

Bratt pans

The Bratt pan is one of the most versatile pieces of equipment. It can be used for deep frying, shallow frying, boiling, stewing and braising.

⚠ Safety and cleaning

- Take special care when using the pan for deep fat frying. Be extra careful when tilting the pan to remove hot liquids. Tilt the pan slowly.
- Allow the pan to cool down before cleaning. Clean with hot detergent water, then rinse and dry.

Bratt pans and boilers

Boiling pans

There are many types of boiling pan available. They can be made from aluminium, stainless steel or other metal. They also come in different sizes and can hold 10, 15, 20, 30 or 40 litres. They are heated by gas or electricity. Steam-jacketed boilers are heated by steam and generally prevent food from burning.

Boilers are used for boiling and stewing large quantities of food such as stock, soup and custard. Many of them tilt so that the contents can be removed easily.

⚠ Safety and cleaning

- Take great care when tilting boilers to remove liquids. Do not overfill boilers.
- If a boiler is gas fired, the gas jets and pilot light should be inspected regularly to ensure that they are working correctly. If a pressure gauge and safety valve are fitted then these should also be checked.
- Boiling pans and their lids should be thoroughly cleaned with mild detergent water and rinsed well. The tilting apparatus should be greased occasionally and checked to see that it tilts easily.

Deep fat fryers

A deep fat fryer has a container with enough oil in it to cover the food. The oil is heated to very hot temperatures. A deep fat fryer has a cool zone, which is a chamber at the base of the cooking pan that collects the odd bits of food that come away from the food when it is being fried, such as breadcrumbs or batter from fish.

Some fryers are computerised. These can be programmed to heat the oil to the correct temperature and cook the food for the right amount of time. They are often used in fast-food chains like McDonald's. They are easy to use and produce good-quality food.

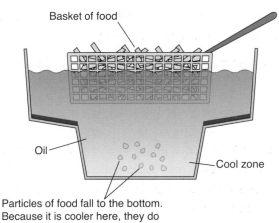

Basket of food

Oil

Cool zone

Particles of food fall to the bottom. Because it is cooler here, they do not burn and spoil the oil

The cool zone in a deep fat fryer

⚠ Safety and cleaning

- Deep fat fryers are possibly the most dangerous pieces of equipment in the kitchen. Many kitchen fires have been started through careless use of the deep fat fryer.
- Take care not to splash the oil when placing items of food in the fryer. Hot oil splashes can cause serious burns and eye injuries.
- When frying, remove all the food debris immediately and keep the oil as clean as possible.
- You will need to remove the oil to clean the fryer. Make sure the oil is cool before you remove it, and put suitable containers in place to drain the oil into. Replace the oil with clean oil.

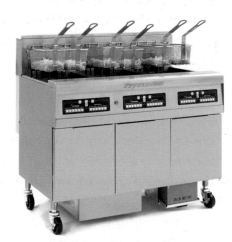

A deep fat fryer

Bain-marie

Bain-marie means 'water bath'. These are open wells of water for keeping food hot. They are available in many designs, some of which are built into hot cupboards and some into serving controls. There is a type that is fitted at the end of the working range or in the cooking range. They are heated by steam, gas or electricity.

⚠ Safety and cleaning

- It is important to never allow the bain-marie to run dry when the heat is turned on.
- Turn off the heat after use. Drain the water away and clean the bain-marie inside and out with hot detergent water. Then rinse it and dry it. If it has a drain-off tap, this should be closed.

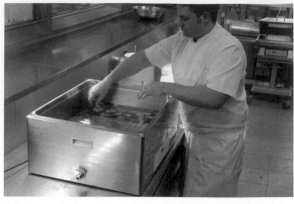

A bain-marie (modern water bath) being used to cook food in sealed pouches

Grills and griddles

Salamander

A salamander (also know as an over-heated grill) is heated from above by gas or electricity. Most salamanders have more than one set of heating elements or jets, and it is not always necessary to have them all fully turned on.

⚠ Safety and cleaning

- Take care when placing food under and removing food from the salamander.
- Salamanders have a tray to catch grease and food debris. This needs to be emptied and thoroughly cleaned with hot detergent water. Soda is very useful when removing grease. You should wear appropriate protective clothing.

Under-fired (under-heated) grills

The heat source for these is underneath the grill. They are used to cook food quickly, so they need to reach a high temperature. This type of grill makes criss-cross marks on the food, commonly known as quadrillage.

⚠ Safety and cleaning

- Take care when placing food on the grill and removing it. Use tongs to move the food around on the grill and to remove the food. Be extra careful when brushing the food with oil and do not allow the oil to drip on the flame.
- When the bars are cool, they should be removed and washed in hot water containing a grease solvent (detergent). They should then be rinsed, dried and replaced in the grill. If firebricks are used for lining the grill, take care with these as they break easily.

Contact grills

These are sometimes called double-sided grills or infragrills. They have two heating surfaces facing each other. The food is placed on one surface and is then covered by the second. These grills are electrically heated and cook certain foods, such as toast in a toaster, very quickly.

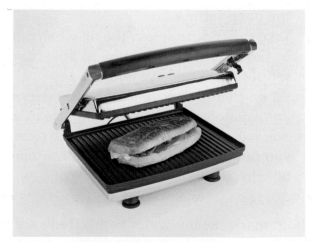

A contact grill

⚠ *Safety and cleaning*

Take great care when placing the food on or in the grill. Turn off the electricity when cleaning and avoid using water. Lightly scrape clean.

Fry plates or griddle plates

These are solid metal plates heated from below that are used for cooking individual portions of meat, hamburgers, eggs, bacon, etc. Before cooking on a griddle plate, apply a light coating of oil to the food and the griddle plate to prevent sticking.

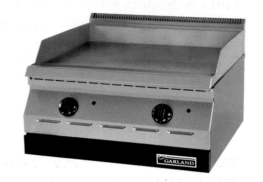

A griddle plate

⚠ *Safety and cleaning*

To clean griddle plates, warm them and scrape off any loose particles. Allow the plates to cool and then rub the metal with pumice stone or griddle stone, following the grain of the metal. Clean them with hot detergent water and rinse with clean hot water, then wipe dry. Finally, re-season (prove) the surface by lightly oiling with vegetable oil.

Roasting spits

These are large pieces of equipment used to roast meat. The meat is put on to a rod of metal (which is also known as a spit) above a flame or other heat source. The rod rotates so that the heat cooks the meat evenly.

⚠ *Safety and cleaning*

- Always wear protective clothing when spit roasting.
- When basting the joint being roasted, the basting action should always be away from you.
- When cleaning, remove excess food from the spit and scrape it down. Wash removable parts in hot detergent water, dry and then replace them on the spit.

Hot cupboards

Commonly referred to as a hotplate, a hot cupboard is used for heating plates and serving dishes, and for keeping food hot. You must make sure that the temperature in the hot cupboard is kept at a reasonable level (around 60–70°C) so that the food is not too hot or too cold. A thermostat can help in maintaining this temperature. Hot cupboards may be heated by gas, steam or electricity.

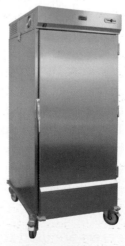

⚠ *Safety and cleaning*

Hot cupboards must be emptied and cleaned after each service.

A hot cupboard

Proving cabinet

Proving cabinets are for proving yeast products, such as dough. Proving means providing a warm and moist atmosphere that allows the yeast to grow, causing the dough to rise, usually to double its size. The most suitable temperature for this is 37°C. Proving cabinets are usually plumbed into the water supply. The heated to produce moist heat, and there is a drain to collect the excess water as the air cools.

⚠ Safety and cleaning

Keep all shelves clear and clean. Also clean the cabinet itself regularly and remove all food debris. Clean with hot detergent water, then rinse and dry.

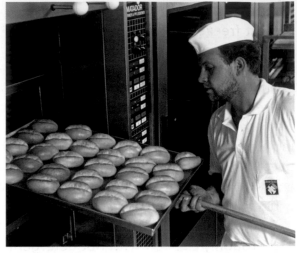

A proving cabinet

Other large equipment

Tables

In a professional kitchen, tables should be made from stainless steel.

Sinks

Sinks must be large enough to wash equipment or food items and there must be enough of them to cope with the amount of washing-up or food washing there is likely to be.

Storage racks

These should also be made from stainless steel. They should be tidied and wiped clean regularly.

Mechanical equipment

Refrigerators and chill rooms

Refrigerators and chill rooms keep food chilled at between 1°C and 5°C. These cold conditions slow down the growth of bacteria that make food go 'off'. They are used to store a whole range of products.

⚠ Safety and cleaning

- The way that food is stored in chill rooms and refrigerators is very important. There should not be cross-contamination between different foods, as this spreads bacteria. All food must be covered and labelled with its use-by date.
- The internal temperature of chill rooms and refrigerators must be checked at least twice a day. They must be tidied once a day and cleaned out once a week. Clean with hot water and suitable cleaning chemicals – diluted bicarbonate of soda is most suitable.

Freezers

Freezers are used to store food at between –18°C and –20°C. As in chill rooms, all food must be covered and date labelled. Food in the freezer does not last indefinitely, but the low temperature slows down the growth of bacteria and means that the food will last longer than if it was not frozen.

⚠ *Safety and cleaning*

- Most freezers today are frost-free, which means that they do not need to be defrosted.
- Tidy the freezer at least once a week and, depending on the freezer type, clean it out every three to six months. Clean it out with mild cleaning fluid, mild detergent or diluted bicarbonate of soda.

Other mechanical equipment

⚠ *Safety and cleaning*

- Take special care when cleaning electrical equipment. Turn off the power supply first.
- The parts of the machine that have been in touch with the food must be thoroughly cleaned with hot detergent water, then rinsed and dried. This prevents any cross-contamination from one food to another. This is especially important for ice cream machines, liquidisers, mixers and blenders.

Boilers

There is a range of boilers available. They produce large quantities of boiling water in a continuous flow, for making tea and coffee.

Chippers

Electric chipping machines are used for producing large quantities of chipped potatoes.

Dishwashers

Dishwashers are used for hygienic washing-up. They should use a good supply of hot water at a temperature of 60°C for general cleaning, followed by a sterilising rinse at 82°C for at least one minute. There are a number of dishwashing machines available. Size and efficiency will depend on the size of the establishment and the amount of washing-up that needs to be done.

Food mixers

These are labour-saving electrical devices used for many different tasks in the kitchen. They have a range of attachments for different jobs such as mincing, cutting, blending and mixing.

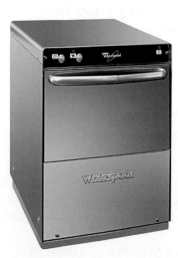 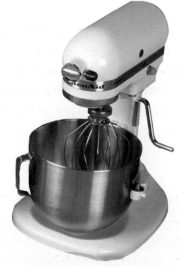 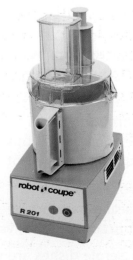

A dishwasher   A food mixer   A food processor

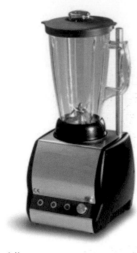

A liquidiser

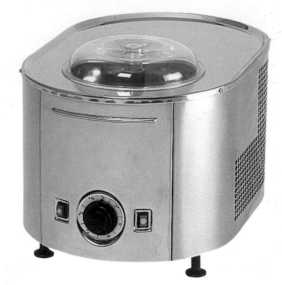

An ice cream machine

Food processing machines

These electrical machines are used for many jobs in the kitchen. They usually come with a range of blades for cutting, puréeing and mixing.

Food slicers

Electrical food slicers and gravity-feed slicers have very sharp cutting blades and must be operated with a safety guard. They are used for slicing meat so that every slice is the same thickness.

Liquidisers and blenders

These have high-speed motors attached to blades that blend and liquidise foods. They are operated by electricity.

Handheld liquidisers and stick blenders

These are used to liquidise foods quickly. They are operated by electricity.

Ice cream machines

Electric ice cream machines are used to make sorbets and ice creams.

Juicers

Electric juicers are used for making fruit and vegetable juices and smoothies.

Small equipment

Small equipment and utensils are made from a variety of materials such as non-stick coated metal, iron, steel, aluminium, wood and heat-proof plastic.

Care and cleanliness

Thoroughly wash equipment, pans and utensils with hot detergent and water after use. Rinse with hot water and then dry. Store pans upside-down on clean racks. Check that handles are not loose.

Cooking pans

Braising pans are deep pans with lids, usually these days made of stainless steel used for braising meats, vegetables and so on.

Casserole dishes are deep containers with lids. They are usually made of china and porcelain, and are used for stewing, braising and oven cooking.

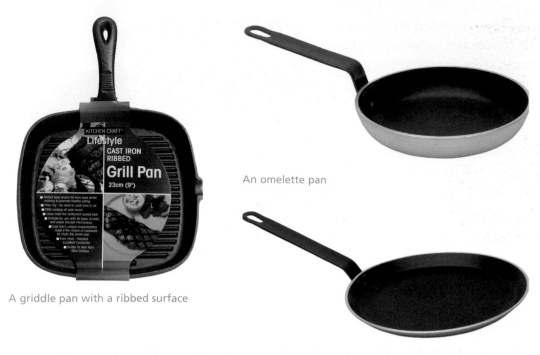

A griddle pan with a ribbed surface

An omelette pan

A pancake pan

Fish kettles are pans with lids, usually made of stainless steel. They are used for poaching whole fish.

Griddle pans have raised ribs to mark the food. The griddle lines (quadrillage) give the food a chargrilled effect. Modern griddle pans have a non-stick surface.

Non-stick frying pans are coated with a material such as Teflon, which prevents the food from sticking to them. They are used for shallow frying.

Omelette pans come in different sizes depending on the number of eggs you use – there are two-egg pans and three-egg pans. They are usually made from heavy black wrought iron.

Pancake pans are used for cooking individual pancakes. They are usually made from heavy black wrought iron, although pans made from other materials are also available.

Roasting trays are metal trays, usually made of stainless steel. They have deep sides and are used for roasting food such as meat and vegetables.

Saucepans come in various sizes and are made in a variety of materials, such as stainless steel or a mixture of metals such as stainless steel with an aluminium layer and a thick copper coil. Saucepans are used for a variety of cooking, such as boiling, poaching and stewing. They can also be used for steaming, when they will have a metal basket with holes in that can be placed in the pan above the water. The food to be steamed is placed in the basket.

Sauté pans are shallow, straight-sided pans made from stainless steel or a mixture of metals. They are used for shallow frying when a sauce is made after the food is fried. They may also be used for poaching, especially for shallow-poached fish.

Sauteuses are shallow, slant-sided pans made from stainless steel or a mixture of metals. They are used for similar types of cooking to a sauté pan, but are more likely to be used for reducing stocks and making sauces.

51

Woks are shallow, rounded frying pans used for stir-frying and oriental cookery. They are made from material that can conduct heat quickly. Thick copper-core stainless steel is the most effective.

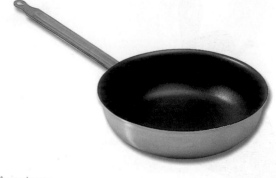

A sauteuse

Utensils

Baking sheets are made in various sizes from black wrought steel. They are used for baking and pastry work.

Baking tins (sometimes called **cake tins**) are used for baking cakes, bread and sponges. The mixture is placed in the tin before cooking.

Baking trays are similar to baking sheets. They are used to place items on for baking.

Balloon whisks are lightweight wired whisks used for whisking and beating air into products, e.g. whisking egg whites.

Bowls come in various sizes and can be stainless steel or plastic. They are used for a variety of purposes, such as mixing, blending and storing food.

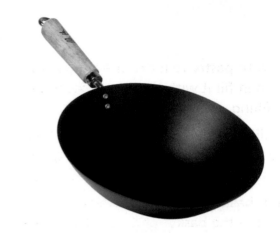

A wok

Chinois literally translated from the French means 'Chinaman's hat'. This is a very fine-mesh conical (V-shaped) strainer used for passing delicate soups and sauces. They are made from stainless steel.

Colanders are available in a variety of sizes and usually made from stainless steel. They are used for draining liquids.

Conical strainers are usually stainless steel with large mesh. They are used for general straining and passing of liquids, soups and sauces.

Cooling racks are made from stainless steel mesh and are usually rectangular. Baked items are placed on cooling racks to cool. The mesh allows air to circulate, which enables the items to cool quickly.

Corers are used to remove the fibrous core from fruits such as apples, pineapples and pears. They have a rounded blade, which you push down into the centre of the fruit to cut through the fruit around the core. The core stays tightly inside the corer and is removed from the fruit when you pull it out.

Deep frying trays are trays placed next to the deep fat fryer to place frying baskets on once they have been lifted from the oil.

Flan rings are used to make flan cases and flans. You line the flan

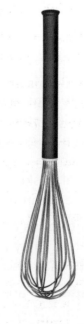

A balloon whisk

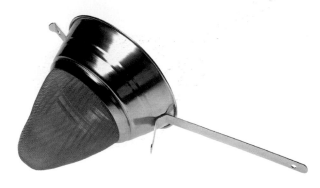

A chinois

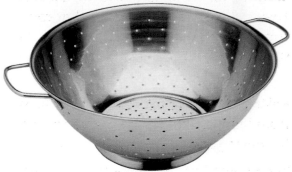

A colander

ring with pastry to make the pastry case, and then fill it with the flan mixture or tart filling.

Fish slices are made from stainless steel. They are used for lifting and sliding food on and off trays or serving dishes.

Frying baskets are wire baskets. Food is placed in the basket and then the basket is lowered into the hot oil of a deep fat fryer.

Graters are made from stainless steel. They come in various sizes and are used to shred and grate food such as cheese,

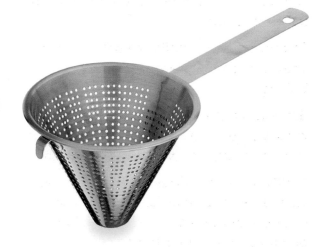

A conical strainer

the zest of citrus fruits and vegetables. Graters usually have a choice of grating edges: fine, medium or large.

Kitchen scissors are used for a number of purposes in the kitchen. Fish scissors are used for cutting the fins from fish. Poultry scissors are used to portion poultry.

Ladles come in various sizes. They are large, scoop-shaped spoons used to add liquids to cooking pots, and to serve sauces, soups and stews.

Mandolins are specialist pieces of equipment used for slicing vegetables. The blade is made from stainless steel and is adjustable to different widths, for thick or thin slices of food. They are usually used to slice vegetables such as potatoes, courgettes, cucumbers and carrots. The blade is particularly sharp, so you should be very careful when using one. Modern mandolins have a safety guard built in to them.

Mashers can be manual or electric and are used for mashing vegetables.

Measuring jugs are available in a variety of sizes. They can be made from stainless steel, glass or plastic. They are used for measuring liquids.

Moulds come in many shapes and sizes. They are used for shaping and moulding food for presentation. Moulds are very difficult to clean – you must make sure that all food debris is removed and that the mould is cleaned properly to prevent cross-contamination. Moulds are used for shaping tartlets, mousses, custards and blancmange.

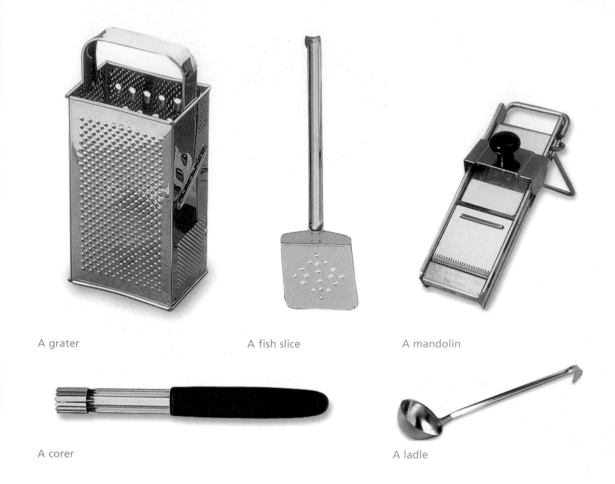

A grater

A fish slice

A mandolin

A corer

A ladle

Peelers are used for peeling certain vegetables and fruit.

Rolling pins are used for rolling pastry manually. Today they are usually made from plastic, although wooden ones are still available.

Sauce whisks are heavy wired whisks used for mixing and whisking sauces.

Sieves are made from plastic with nylon. They are available in various sizes and also in various mesh sizes. They are used for mashing, purées and draining. For mashing and purées, the food is pushed through the sieve using an instrument called a mushroom.

Skimming spoons are made from stainless steel and have holes in them. They are used for skimming and draining. Skimming is removing fat and other unwanted substances from the top of liquids, such as stocks and soups.

Spiders are made from stainless steel. They are used for removing food from containers, saucepans, water etc. They are also used for deep fat frying to remove food from a fryer.

Spoons come in variety of sizes for serving and moving food to and from containers. They are made from stainless steel.

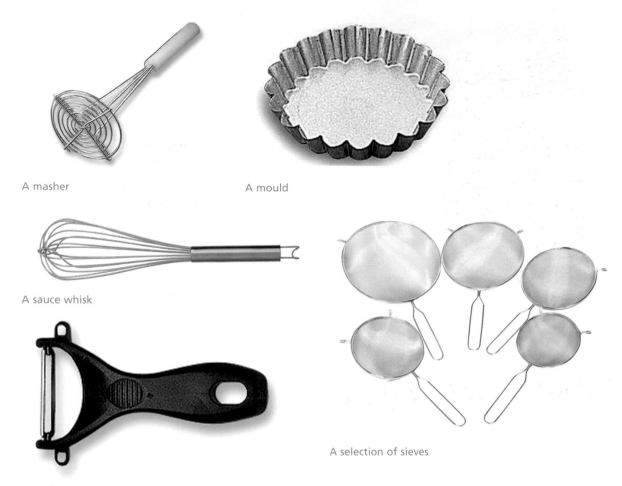

A masher

A mould

A sauce whisk

A peeler

A selection of sieves

Cutting boards

These are important items of kitchen equipment used for chopping and slicing food on. The most popular boards these days are made from polyethylene or plastic. Different boards should be used for different foods, to avoid cross-contamination. The accepted UK system is:

- yellow for cooked meats
- red for raw meats
- white for bread or dairy products
- blue for raw fish
- green for fruit and salads
- brown for raw vegetables.

As with all kitchen equipment and utensils, clean boards thoroughly with hot detergent water, then rinse and dry.

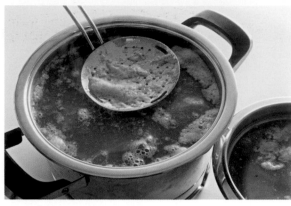

A skimming spoon

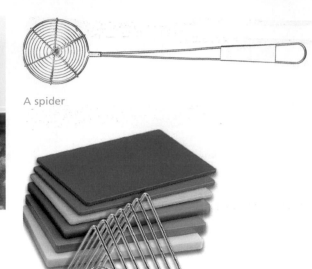

A spider

Chopping boards in different colours

Knives

The professional chef will use a whole range of knives in the kitchen.

The most common kitchen knives

Boning knives are short-bladed knives used for boning meat. The blade is strong and rigid, with a pointed end. The inflexible blade allows the chef to get close to the bones and cut away the meat.

Butchers' saws are commonly used in butchery to saw through bones.

Carving knives and forks – a French carving knife has a long, thin blade and is known as a tranchard. A carving fork is two-pronged. It is strong enough to support meats for carving, and to lift them to and from containers.

Chopping knives are used for a variety of jobs, such as chopping, cutting, slicing, shredding vegetables, meat, fruit, etc.

Filleting knives are used for filleting fish (removing the meat from the bones). They

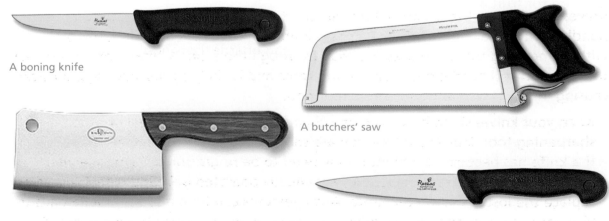

A boning knife

A meat cleaver

A butchers' saw

A filleting knife

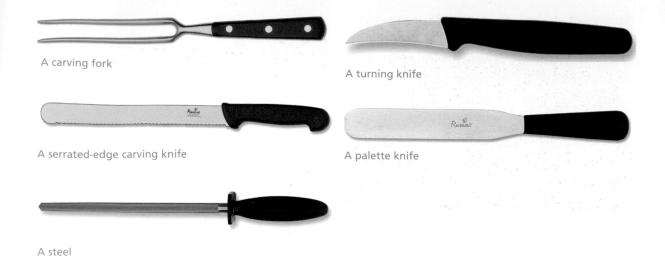

A carving fork

A turning knife

A serrated-edge carving knife

A palette knife

A steel

have a very flexible blade, which allows the chef to move the knife easily around the bone structure of fish.

Meat cleavers are also known as choppers and are usually used for chopping bones.

An **office knife** or **paring knife** is a small multi-purpose vegetable knife. It is used for topping and tailing vegetables, and for peeling certain fruits and vegetables.

A **palette knife** is a flat knife used for lifting and scraping, turning and spreading. It is a very useful knife when making a pastry section.

Serrated-edge carving knives are used for slicing foods. They have a long, thick serrated blade, which is used in a sawing action. These knives are not sharpened in the kitchen but have to be sent to a specialist company to be sharpened.

Steels are used for sharpening knives. They are cylindrical pieces of steel with a handle at one end. To sharpen a knife, run the knife at an angle along the steel edge.

A **turning knife** is a small curved-bladed knife used for shaping vegetables in a variety of ways.

Safety with knives

Knives are essential tools for all chefs, but they can cause serious injury to the user or to someone else if used wrongly or carelessly. Knives that are looked after and treated with care will give good service and will be less likely to cause injury.

Knives that are kept sharp are safer than blunt knives, provided that they are handled with care. This is because a sharp knife will cut efficiently and cleanly without needing too much pressure to cut through the food. A blunt knife is less easy to control. It will need more pressure and force and is likely to slip sideways, possibly causing injury as well as poorly prepared food.

- Keep your knives sharp by sharpening them frequently with a steel or other sharpening tool. Make sure that you are shown how to do this safely.
- If a knife has become very blunt it may need to be re-ground by someone who specialises in doing this. An electric or manually operated grinding wheel is used to replace the lost 'edge' on the knife. Arrangements can be made for mobile units to visit your premises to re-grind knives, or they can be sent away to be re-ground.

However, all knives can be dangerous if they are not used properly; if wrongly used they can cause serious injury as well as minor cuts. By following a few simple rules you should be able to avoid serious injury from knives and keep accidental cuts to an absolute minimum. Use your knives correctly at all times.

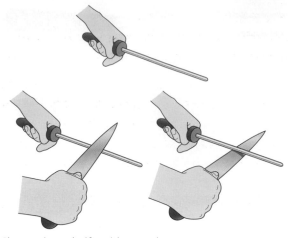

- Generally, you should hold a cook's knife with your fingers around the handle (thumb and index fingers on opposite sides) and well clear of the blade edge. This will sometimes vary, depending on the size and design of the knife, and the task you are carrying out.
- Grasp the knife firmly for full control.
- Always make sure that the fingers and thumb of the hand not holding the knife are well tucked in to avoid cutting them.

Sharpening a knife with a steel

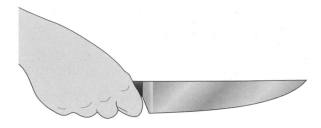

Good practice with knives

⚠ Knife safety

Here are some rules that will help you to stay safe when using knives.

- If carrying a knife in the kitchen, hold it to your side of your body with the blade pointing down and backwards. Never run while holding a knife.
- When handing a knife to someone else, offer them the handle while you hold the top (blunt edge) of the blade.
- Take great care to keep the blade away from you when cleaning or drying knives, and never run your finger along the blade edge.
- Do not have more than one knife at a time on a chopping board. When not actually using a knife, place it at the side of the board with the blade pointing in. Never carry knives around on top of chopping boards because they could slide off.
- Do not let knives overhang the edge of the work surface; they could be knocked off or fall and cause injury. Never try to catch a falling knife; stand back until it reaches the floor.
- Never leave a knife on a surface with the blade pointing upwards. You or someone else could put their hand down on the blade of the knife.
- Never place knives in washing-up water; the blade will not be visible so someone could put their hands in the water and cut themselves.
- Keep the handle of the knife clean and dry. If the handle is greasy or wet it could slip in your hands during use.
- Keep knives visible, i.e. not under vegetable peelings or a dishcloth.
- Store knives carefully, preferably in a box or carrying case with compartments to keep the knives separate and easy to find. Do not just throw knives loosely into a drawer or locker.

⚠ *Knives and food safety*

A knife can very easily transfer harmful bacteria from one place to another, becoming a 'vehicle' of contamination. Follow a few simple rules to avoid this.

- Wash and dry knives thoroughly between tasks.
- Do not use the same cloth to clean knives between tasks, especially when you are preparing raw or high-risk foods.
- If you have used a knife on raw meat or poultry, be sure to disinfect it before you use it for another task. Detergents remove the grease, but disinfectants kill harmful bacteria.
- When you have finished working with a knife, wash it thoroughly with hot detergent water, then rinse it, dry it and put it away. Bacteria will multiply on dirty or wet knives.

Activity

1 What equipment do you need to make each of these dishes?
- Poached eggs
- Roast beef
- Puréed vegetable soup

2 Which knife would you use for each of these tasks?
- Cutting vegetables into julienne
- Peeling potatoes
- Boning a joint of meat
- Finely chopping some fresh herbs

Examples of cooking methods associated with types of equipment

Cooking method	Large equipment	Small equipment
Baking	Ovens: • combination oven • bakers' oven • convection oven	Baking trays and sheets Baking tins Flan rings Moulds
Boiling	Large boiling pans Steam-jacketed boilers Bratt pans Hobs (stoves)	Saucepans
Braising	Various ovens, including Bratt pans	Braising pans Casserole dishes
Deep frying	Deep fat fryers: • thermostat-controlled cool-zone fryers • pressure fryers • computerised fryers	Frying baskets Spiders Trays
Grilling	Over-heat grills (salamanders) Under-heat grills (barbecuing) Between-heat (contact) grills (toasting)	Grill trays Grill pans
Poaching	Ovens: • combination ovens • Bratt pans Hobs (stoves)	Fish kettles Saucepans Sauté pans
Pot roasting	Ovens: • convection ovens • combination ovens	Casserole dishes Roasting trays
Roasting	Ovens: • convection ovens • combination ovens Roasting spits	Roasting
Shallow frying	Hobs (stoves)	Frying pans Griddle pans Omelette pans Pancake pans Wok pans Sauté pans Sauteuse
Steaming	Atmospheric steamers Pressure steamers Combination ovens	Saucepans with perforated insert
Stewing	Various ovens, including Bratt pans Hobs (stoves)	Casserole dishes Sauté pans Saucepans

Introduction to personal workplace skills

VRQ Unit 106 Introduction to personal workplace skills

Learning outcomes:
- Maintain personal appearance
- Demonstrate time management skills
- Work effectively in a team
- Deal effectively with customers

NVQ 501 (1GEN1) Maintain a safe, hygienic and secure working environment

NVQ 504 (1GEN4) Contribute to effective teamwork

Professional presentation and clothing

Being smart and wearing the correct clothing is an important part of working in the hospitality industry. All the clothing you wear at work must be smart, clean and in good repair. Your hair must be short or tied back neatly, and men should be clean-shaven or have a neat beard/moustache. You should always wear the correct uniform in the kitchen.

You must change your chefs' or cooks' uniform regularly – at least every day. Clean clothing is important to prevent the transfer of bacteria from dirty clothing to food. You should never wear the uniform outside the working premises, as this is unhygienic: bacteria from outside can be carried on the uniform into the kitchen and may cause harm.

Chefs' or cooks' jacket
These jackets are designed to protect the chef in the kitchen.

- They are usually made from cotton or polyester-cotton. The fabrics today are lightweight and comfortable.
- Your jacket must be comfortable and protect you from heat, burns and scalds.

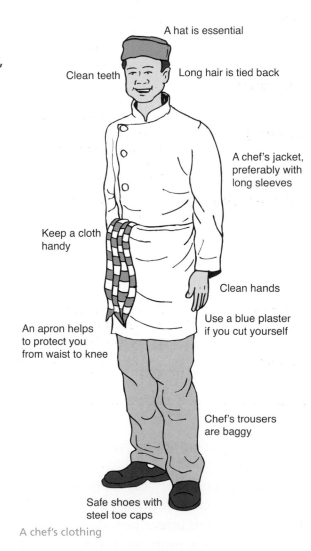

A hat is essential

Clean teeth

Long hair is tied back

A chef's jacket, preferably with long sleeves

Keep a cloth handy

Clean hands

An apron helps to protect you from waist to knee

Use a blue plaster if you cut yourself

Chef's trousers are baggy

Safe shoes with steel toe caps

A chef's clothing

- Your jacket should not be too tight. You should be able to move around in it comfortably.
- Another reason that it should not be too tight is so that if hot liquid is spilled on it, you can pull it away from your skin easily to prevent burning.
- It is safer to wear jackets with long sleeves as these protect your arms from splashed hot liquids or fats, although many chefs prefer the short-sleeved variety.

Chefs' or cooks' trousers

There are a number of different types of trousers available. Like jackets, they should be quite loose fitting so that they are comfortable and can be pulled away from the skin easily to prevent burning if hot liquid is spilled on them.

Chefs' or cooks' apron

Aprons also come in a variety of fabrics and styles. Your apron should come to just below your knees. Aprons are another important way of protecting chefs in the kitchen.

Chefs' or cooks' hat

The tall chefs' hat is called a toque. These show the status of the chef. In some establishments it used to be traditional for the head chef to wear a tall black chefs' hat. Today, skullcaps are used in many kitchens because they are more comfortable, easier to wash and cheaper. Sometimes, the status of the different chefs is shown by different-coloured skullcaps. You can also buy disposable skullcaps.

Chefs wear hats to prevent hair from falling into the food. In some establishments the chefs and cooks also wear a hairnet under their hats.

Neckties

Traditionally, kitchens have been very hot places and chefs have worn a necktie to mop sweat from their brow. Today, with improved ventilation systems and different styles of chefs' jackets, neckties are fast becoming a thing of the past.

Safety shoes

It is important that you wear safety shoes in the kitchen. There are many different varieties. They must be sturdy, with steel toecaps. Shoes should be the correct size and comfortable. You should not wear open-toed shoes or trainers in the kitchen.

Kitchen cloths

Chefs generally have a kitchen cloth as part of their uniform. This must be clean and dry. It is particularly important that it is dry when you handle hot items as the heat will come through a wet cloth and you may burn yourself.

You should have a clean kitchen cloth at the start of each new service period.

Personal hygiene

Personal hygiene is extremely important when handling food because bacteria can be transferred easily from humans to food.

- You must shower or bathe regularly to remove body odour, sweat, dirt and bacteria.
- Change your underwear daily and use antiperspirant deodorants.
- Wash your hands regularly with alcohol gel or liquid soap.
- Dry your hands under hot-air dryers or using disposable towels.
- When handling high-risk foods, wear disposable gloves and change these gloves for each task.

- Always cover any cuts with a blue waterproof dressing. People working in kitchens use blue dressings because they are easy to spot if they fall into food. If they are found in cooked food, the food should be thrown away.

There is more information about personal hygiene on page 81.

Hair
- You should wash your hair regularly and keep it tidy.
- It should be short or tied back.
- If you have long hair it must be covered with a hairnet.
- It is not a legal requirement for chefs to wear a hat, but ideally you should keep your hair covered.

Dental hygiene
It is important to look after your teeth and your mouth as part of your grooming.

- Clean your teeth at least twice a day and use a mouthwash.
- Try to visit your dentist regularly.
- Do not touch your mouth when handling food.

Tasting spoons
- Chefs have a habit of tasting food with their fingers. This is not good practice.
- Always use a clean tasting spoon. It is a good idea to keep your tasting spoons in a solution of Milton to sterilise them. Milton is a commercial product usually used to sterilise babies' bottles.
- Some establishments use disposable plastic spoons for tasting.

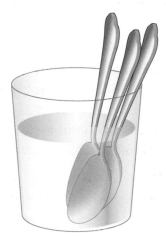

Tasting spoons in Milton, a chemical solution that completely destroys bacteria

Hands
Your hands are your most precious commodity and should be looked after.

- Wash your hands regularly, and always after visiting the toilet and before entering the kitchen.
- Bacteria are spread easily by dirty hands and nails, so wash your hands with anti-bacterial gel or liquid.
- Keep your nails short and clean. If necessary, scrub your nails with a nailbrush.
- Never wear nail varnish when preparing and serving food because it may chip off and fall into the food.

Smoking, eating and drinking
Smoking is now not allowed in any public areas. If you do smoke on a break, your hands will have touched your mouth, so it is essential to wash your hands again before returning to the kitchen and handling food. Establishments should discourage people from smoking as it is a major health hazard.

Eating and drinking should be discouraged during working times. Chefs and cooks should eat at regular set times and not snack or pick at food as this is unprofessional.

Being a good employee

You must always keep to the times and the conditions of your employment contract. This contract will be given to you before you start the job. If you do not work to your contract you could be disciplined or may lose your job.

Teamwork

Remember from Chapter 2 that, as a chef, you will need to be able to work as part of a team. The people in a team depend on each other to be successful. Your team will have targets and deadlines. To meet these there needs to be good communication and planning within the team. All members of the team have to understand what is expected of them and what deadlines and targets they have been set.

It is also important that you:

- do your job in a professional way
- are punctual for work
- inform your employer, ideally your line manager, if you are ill
- are reliable and courteous – other people depend on you; if one person is away, it puts pressure on the other members of staff and, in some cases, temporary staff may have to be employed as cover
- manage your time and deadlines well and are able to prioritise – food has to be served on time; breakfast, lunch and dinner must be ready when the customer is ready.

Understanding yourself

In order to be a good employee it is important that you try to understand yourself, for example:

- What are you capable of doing?
- What development do you need to help the team and yourself?
- What are your strengths?
- What are your weaknesses?
- Do you know when to ask for help?
- What training do you need? For example, would you like to improve your:
  - culinary skills
  - writing skills
  - IT skills
  - equipment skills?

Communication

In Chapter 2 we looked at the different forms of communication (e.g. face to face, email) and how successful communication can lead to a successful business. Communication is effective only if everyone involved understands what the message is and what is required of them.

A chef, particularly a head chef, is a leader. He or she has to build a team through communication. As the leader they have to motivate and develop the team. They have to encourage creativity and make the most of the skills and knowledge of their team members. Everyone in the team should be working towards the same goals and targets.

Listening

Listening is also an important part of effective communication. Learn to listen carefully and to understand facial expressions, gestures and body language.

Good listeners:

- avoid any distractions
- concentrate on what is being said
- think about what is being said
- show interest in the person speaking and do not look bored
- maintain eye contact with the person talking and acknowledge what is being said
- if necessary, ask sensible questions
- paraphrase, in other words clarify what has been said, in their own words.

Non-verbal communication

Communication can be non-verbal, in other words unspoken. Understand people's body language. Your body language includes:

- how you dress
- your posture
- how far you are from the other person
- your stance – how you sit or stand
- your facial expressions
- your movements and gestures
- your eye movements.

Body language can tell us what people really think or feel.

Think about how you approach people and what body language you use. Everyone uses body language, but it can mean different things in different cultures and to different people.

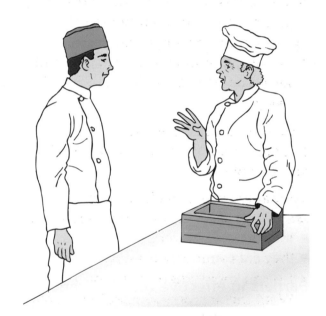

- **Eye contact** – In Western cultures, people make eye contact every now and then while speaking to someone. This shows that they are interested. People in the Middle East look very closely into the eyes of people they are talking to and do not look away. They do this to gauge what the other person wants and to check that they can trust them. However, in Japan direct eye contact is seen as an invasion of a person's privacy and an act of rudeness.
- **Smiling** – North Americans usually smile automatically when greeting other people, while people from other cultures may interpret this as insincere. Asian people smile less than Westerners, and in Korea it is considered inappropriate for adults to smile in public. For Koreans, a smile usually indicates embarrassment, and not pleasure.
- **Head shaking** – Although shaking your head from side to side is often used to mean 'no', even this simple gesture does not have a universal meaning! Bulgarians shake their head to mean yes, and people from southern India and Pakistan move their head from side to side to express a variety of meanings. Depending on context, it could mean 'you are welcome' or 'goodbye', it could mean that they are enjoying themselves, or it could be the equivalent of a shrug.

- **Posture** – In the Middle East, it is extremely offensive to point the bottom of your foot in another person's direction, so sitting cross-legged might be a bad idea!
- **Personal space** – The amount of personal space North Americans like to have is about the length of an arm. In other words, when they are talking to someone they like the other person to be an arm's length away. The French, Latin Americans and Arabs need less personal space, while Germans and Japanese need more. The amount of personal space someone feels comfortable with can also be influenced by their social status, gender, age and other factors.

Signs and meanings

Some gestures are open and positive. For example, leaning forwards with the palms of your hands open and facing upwards shows interest, acceptance and a welcoming attitude. On the other hand, leaning backwards, with your arms folded and head down might show that you are feeling closed, uninterested, defensive and negative, or rejected.

If someone uses plenty of gestures this may indicate that they are warm, enthusiastic and emotional. If someone does not use many gestures this may indicate that they are cold, reserved and logical.

However, a gesture does not necessarily reveal exactly what a person is thinking. For example, if someone has their arms folded this may mean that:

- they are being defensive about something
- they are cold
- they are comfortable.

How do you think this person feels?

Barriers to effective communication

There are some things that can make it difficult for people to communicate effectively:

- speaking unclearly
- speaking too quietly
- not speaking the same language – there are many different cultures and nationalities employed in the hospitality industry
- not understanding another person's accent
- speaking too fast
- using too much unfamiliar terminology and jargon
- having hearing difficulties – if someone is hard of hearing, speak clearly and slowly as they may be able to lip-read
- poor grammar and spelling in written communication – read through any letters or faxes you write to check for grammar and spelling mistakes; if possible write it on a computer and use the grammar and spellchecker.

Try to be confident, not shy, when you are communicating with other people. If your job involves a lot of speaking and making presentations then the organisation you work for may train you in these areas. Drama classes are an excellent way to develop your communication and confidence skills, especially if you are working front of house, e.g. as a receptionist, waiter or waitress.

Looking after customers

A hospitality business cannot exist without customers. Customers mean money, commonly known as revenue, so customer care and customer service are very important. The main job of people working in the hospitality industry is to look after customers' needs, wants and expectations. Every organisation must have good customer service if it is to be successful. Even if a hotel has wonderful, luxurious facilities in comfortable surroundings, the business is doomed to failure if the customer service does not match the environment and the expectations of the customers. The most successful businesses are those that are customer focused.

Attracting and keeping customers

Businesses work hard to attract customers and spend a great deal of money on market research, in other words finding out what customers need, want and expect. This helps them to attract new customers and to keep existing customers. For customers to be loyal to a business, the service they receive and experience they have must be good, or even excellent, all the time. A bad experience can put someone off for good, and they may even tell other people about their bad experience and put them off as well.

Good experiences make happy customers, who go away and tell other people about their positive experience. 'Word of mouth' marketing is one of the most powerful forms of promoting a business.

All staff, both front and back of house, must understand customers and the importance of satisfying them. Some companies ask employees to come to the establishment as a customer, to give them a real idea of what the customers experience.

Appreciating the customer

Customer service is a very important aspect of business these days. There are many training courses centred around customer service, yet it is often difficult to find good customer service. This is because people do not appreciate that service is just as important as the product (e.g. the food, the hotel room) being sold to the customer. Good service involves acknowledging the customer, understanding the customer and anticipating the customer's needs. All this should be done as politely and efficiently as possible.

How many times have you stood in a queue and been ignored? No one has come to apologise or acknowledge that you are waiting to be served. A simple apology for the wait is often all that is needed to satisfy the customer.

The starting point for all customer service is good manners: saying 'please', 'thank you' and 'I beg your pardon'; being pleasant to people; showing that you care about what they want and apologising for anything that has been unsatisfactory, like having to wait.

Communicating with customers

Communicating well with customers is the key to good customer service. Keep customers informed so that they know what is happening to their order or their request. Never ignore customers. Always show care and attention. Great customer service is making the customer feel well cared for and important.

- Concentrate on being a good listener. Keep good eye contact and show that you are interested.
- Always be confident. Work on your confidence levels if this is a problem. If you are shy and withdrawn you may find it useful to take drama lessons, as mentioned earlier. Customers want to be served by confident professionals. Look smart and behave like a professional.
- New staff should be trained to cope with a variety of situations. Inexperienced staff will require several weeks of training before they are ready to deal with customers directly.

To make a good impression on customers, and to help them feel relaxed and confident in the service:

- look professional
- look smart and well groomed
- walk in a positive way and do not shuffle your feet; walk upright with a straight back, and hold your head up
- smile
- be confident
- speak clearly
- listen to the customer
- be charming
- be well mannered
- be graceful
- always put the customer first.

Do not be content just to keep customers satisfied. Strive to make customers happy so that they will want to return.

Service experience

The 'service experience' is when the customer has received the service they expected – it lives up to their expectations. When the customer's expectations have not been fulfilled, and they are disappointed, this is a 'negative service experience'.

Happy customers are usually those who are pleased with the product or service and the price they paid for them. This means that they are likely to come back again (repeat business), which helps the business to be profitable.

Activity

1 Name four items of protective clothing worn in the kitchen. Say what each item does to protect you.

2 In a small group, discuss why it is important to be punctual for work in a catering business. What will happen if staff are late to work?

Regeneration of pre-prepared food

VRQ Unit 111 Regeneration of pre-prepared food

Learning outcomes:
- Identify pre-prepared foods that can be regenerated
- Regenerate pre-prepared foods

NVQ 501 (1GEN1) Maintain a safe, hygienic and secure working environment

NVQ 603 (2GEN3) Maintain food safety when storing, preparing and cooking food

Pre-prepared foods

The term 'pre-prepared food' could describe any food that has been prepared before it is actually needed. It could be a lasagne prepared in the morning then chilled ready to be reheated in the evening. However, the term is more likely to be used to describe an ever-increasing variety of foods produced by numerous companies that form a vast worldwide pre-prepared food industry.

Some products are bought ready made and are widely used throughout the hospitality and catering industries. These include such things as bread, cakes, biscuits, pastries and pies that would be time consuming to make and need specific skills. Generally, these products need no further processing, other than perhaps heating or portioning.

Other pre-prepared foods will have undergone one or more processes to make them last longer and to make them suitable for packaging and transporting.

Processes used in pre-prepared foods

We will now look at some of the processes used in pre-prepared foods.

Packaging fresh foods

Examples of fresh foods that are packaged include pre-prepared and washed salad items and vegetables. These are often packaged and sealed in 'modified atmosphere' packaging. This means that the air surrounding the food in the package will keep it fresh and in good condition for longer.

Salads can be bought washed and ready mixed; vegetables may be peeled, trimmed and even presented in traditional cuts (e.g. turned potatoes).

Pre-prepared chilled foods

The market in pre-prepared chilled foods is growing rapidly. It includes everything from pork pies through to complete meals produced in large quantities.

- Some products, like chilled desserts, are ready to eat.
- Others, such as prepared but uncooked pies, need to be cooked.
- There is a large industry involved in producing complete chilled meals. These meals need to be reheated carefully and thoroughly to ensure that they are safe to eat.

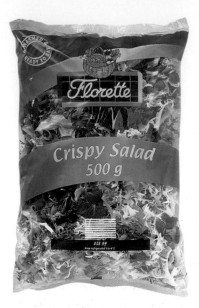

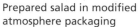

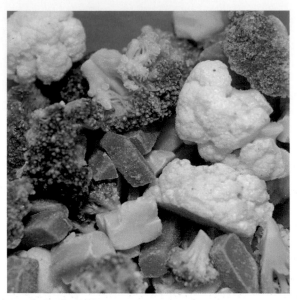

Prepared salad in modified
atmosphere packaging

Prepared vegetables

You should always follow carefully the instructions written on packaging, or ask for advice from your supervisor.

Frozen foods

There is a huge number and variety of frozen foods available to chefs. The industry that started with simple frozen peas and fish now produces thousands of items, including raw foods, ready-to-cook products, cooked items and complex desserts.

Bought frozen foods will have full instructions on the packaging for how to regenerate the contents. It is important to read and follow these instructions carefully.

- It is essential to fully defrost items such as joints of meat or a chicken before cooking them. If you do not defrost these items properly they may cause food poisoning.
- Small or thin food items like breaded scampi or pizza can usually be cooked directly from frozen and this often gives the best results.
- There are some products that just need to be defrosted before serving, like gateaux, mousses and flans.
- Others are meant to be served frozen, such as sorbet or ice cream cake. Again, be sure to follow the instructions on the packaging and ask for advice from a supervisor if you are unsure.

Some items will be produced 'in-house' (made on the premises from fresh ingredients) and frozen for use at another time. Or, too much of an item may be made and, rather than waste what is left over, it is frozen. These foods will vary from one establishment to another, but items that are often frozen in-house include:

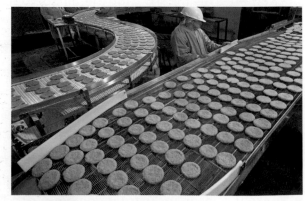

Commercial production of chilled meals

- soups
- sauces
- stocks
- stews
- pies and desserts.

Regeneration of these will vary from item to item, depending on what it is and how big it is. Most will need to be defrosted before use.

Dried food and mixes

These foods will last in the store cupboard for a long time – they have a long shelf life. This is because what normally causes food to deteriorate and go bad is moisture, and this has been removed from dried foods. They are available in three basic types:

1 foods that have part or all of the moisture dried out of them – these can be dried by mechanical processes like air tunnel drying, or they can be dried more naturally, say by drying in the sun; such foods include sun-dried tomatoes, dried fruits, dried mushrooms etc.
2 foods that have been processed to remove their natural moisture and produce a powder-like product, e.g. dried milk, stock and sauce mixes
3 a mixture of already dry ingredients to form a 'convenience mix' like scone mix, pastry mix or sponge mix; these will need a moist ingredient such as milk, eggs or water to be added to them to make them ready to use.

Canned foods

A process similar to canning was first invented as early as 1809 (to feed French armies during the Napoleonic wars), though the food was actually sealed in glass jars. A year later, an English scientist was the first to preserve food in tin cans.

We now have a very large selection of food available in cans; some in large cans for catering use. Most canned food is already cooked, so food such as soups and baked beans just need to be reheated. Sometimes canned food is used as part of another dish or as an ingredient (e.g. tinned tomatoes as part of a sauce or filling for a pie) and will be reheated during the cooking of the dish.

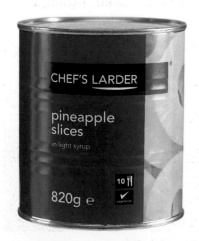

A modern can

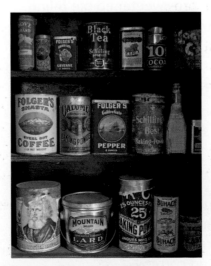

Early examples of canned food

Vacuum packaging

Vacuum packaging is now a popular way to store food. It protects the food by removing all the surrounding air, so the food stays good for longer. Some kitchens have the equipment necessary to vacuum pack on the premises, and many foods can be bought already vacuum packed in a plastic pouch.

Cooked, uncooked, processed or unprocessed food can all be vacuum packed, so the method of regeneration will depend on the food in the pack. However, many foods are cooked or reheated inside the vacuum pouch.

Part-baked products

The market for part-baked products has grown rapidly, and allows 'fresh' bread, rolls, Danish pastries and other baked goods to be served in premises where there may not be the space, time, equipment or skills available to make these items in the traditional way. As the name suggests, these are products that have been fully prepared and partly baked, then either vacuum packed or frozen.

Regeneration usually involves simply unwrapping the product, placing it on a baking tray and baking it in a finishing oven at the correct temperature for the required amount of time. You also have the option to apply other finishing methods, such as glazing or sprinkling with seeds and grains before baking. Products can be baked frequently in small batches so that hot, fresh bread or pastries are available as required.

Different establishments may want to do different amounts of pre-preparation, depending on the amount of time and labour they have available.

Say, for example, that apple pie is on the menu.

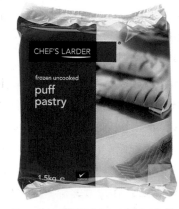

- Various sizes of apple pie could be bought already made. They might be: ready cooked or uncooked, chilled or frozen, individual, pre-portioned or whole.
- Or the apple pie cold be made in-house, in which case various kinds of pastry could be bought in ready made: fresh or frozen, rolled, unrolled or pre-cut to shape; or a pastry mix could be used.
- Apples could be bought ready prepared: frozen, vacuum packed, canned or as a pre-sweetened pie filling.

Frozen puff pastry could save time

All the above would save time, skills and equipment at some stage in the process of making apple pie.

What about quality?

All the pre-prepared foods and products mentioned above have been through some sort of process. So how do these processes affect the food?

This depends on:

- the type of food
- the quality and freshness of the food before processing
- the kind of process carried out
- what additives and preservatives are used
- whether they are stored correctly
- how they are handled and regenerated.

It would be unrealistic to expect all pre-prepared products to be as good as the fresh equivalent. The processing may change the texture, colour and flavour of the food. To make this less noticeable, additives are sometimes used to enhance the food and to make it look and taste more like the non-processed version. Preservatives may also be used to extend the life of the product and prevent deterioration.

Some processes also reduce the nutritional value of food – the vitamins and minerals that are naturally present in the food may be lost.

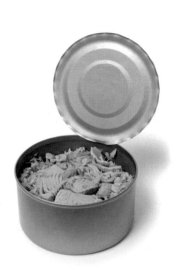

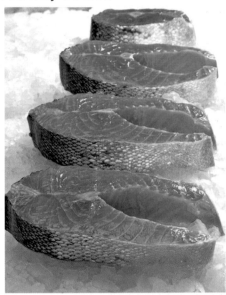

Canned salmon and fresh salmon

Demand for pre-prepared food

Why is there such a demand for pre-prepared food? Modern lifestyles and work patterns mean that many people want 'faster' food both at home and when they eat out.

There is now a huge selection of pre-prepared foods that require different levels of preparation from the consumer.

- Some people may want an instant hot meal, in which case they can buy an entire meal that just needs reheating in the microwave.
- Others may want to use fresh meat or fish but to cook it in a pre-prepared sauce.
- Others may decide to buy a chilled, pre-prepared pasta dish that just needs to be reheated in the oven, and serve this with fresh vegetables or salad.

The possible combinations are almost endless ...

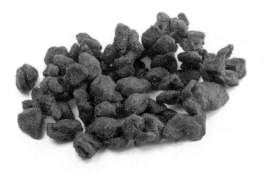

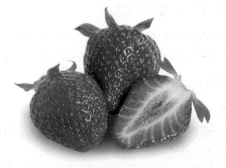

Freeze-dried strawberries and fresh strawberries

Some advantages of pre-prepared food

- Some seasonal foods are now available all year round because they can be pre-prepared and stored.
- Pre-prepared foods may last longer, with later 'use by' or 'best before' dates than fresh foods.
- Less waste will be produced when making meals from pre-prepared foods.
- Using pre-prepared food may mean that there is less raw and high-risk food in the same kitchen or production area. Many of the health and safety procedures will already have been carried out by someone else.

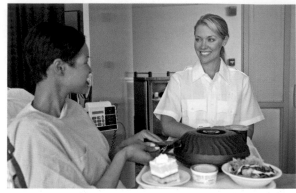

A hospital meal

- Pre-prepared meals are consistent because they come in a standard and size and are produced using very precise and strict procedures.
- Large numbers of people can be served at the same time, for example in hospitals or on an aircraft.

Some disadvantages of pre-prepared food

- Processing may change the texture, flavour and colour of the food. This could result in a lower-quality product being served to the customer.
- Processed foods are not suitable for all dishes or recipes. Some recipes may need to be adapted to use processed foods.
- Soft fruits do not regenerate well after freezing – they lose texture, become very soft and the juices run. Canned fruits also have a different texture from fresh fruit. Frozen plums or strawberries might be used in a crumble or a compôte, but you would not serve strawberries that had been frozen as traditional strawberries and cream.
- The regeneration of pre-prepared foods needs to be done carefully and correctly. If they are not prepared correctly they can cause food poisoning. Staff must be thoroughly trained in how to do this.
- With pre-prepared meals it is more difficult for the consumer to 'measure' the types of food they are eating. Many people understand that they should eat five portions of fruit and vegetables each day and that they should eat more whole grain foods. However, it is difficult to know how much of these things is in a pre-prepared meal.
- More and more customers want fresh, locally produced foods. Businesses need to respond to this demand.
- There is concern that with so much pre-prepared food available people in the industry will stop learning how to cook properly and culinary skills will be lost.

How foods are regenerated

Dried foods (dehydrated)

Moisture has been removed from these foods so they will keep for longer. Regeneration will involve putting moisture back.

Product	Method of regeneration
Dried fruit	Usually eaten in its dried state but occasionally soaked before use according to dish/recipe requirements.
Rice, dried pasta, pulses	Two processes are needed in the regeneration: rehydration (taking back moisture) and cooking to the required degree.
Stock or sauce mixes, soup and stuffing mixes	Mixed with water (or stock or milk) and cooked according to specific instructions on packaging.
Bread, scone, pastry or cake mixes	Mixed with water, milk and/or eggs then cooked according to dish specifications and instructions on packaging.
Dried milk	Mixed with water according to instructions then used in recipes in the same way as fresh milk.

Frozen foods

Some (but not all) frozen foods will need to be defrosted before use. Generally, larger, more solid items will need defrosting and small, less dense items will not.

Product	Method of regeneration
Meat, poultry, raw fish	Unless very small (or instructions on packaging say otherwise), these will need to be defrosted. If possible use a separate fridge or defrosting cabinet to do this, or defrost at the bottom of a multi-use fridge. Place food in a deep tray away from other foods, cover with clingfilm and label. Do not cook until completely defrosted.
Small frozen items – breaded fish, burgers, pizza etc.	Because these are small or thin they will heat up quickly, so they can be thawed and cooked at the same time. You must use the correct temperatures, equipment and time – refer to the packaging.
Uncooked pastry goods, pies, pasties, dough products etc.	Most of these can be cooked from frozen. Follow the instructions on the packaging.
Vegetables	Most vegetables can be cooked from frozen, but with large quantities they may cook better if defrosted first.
Stews, soups, stocks, large pies	Best defrosted before cooking or reheating.
Cooked pastry items, desserts, gateaux and cakes, canapés etc.	Defrost fully before use.

Chilled foods

Chilled raw foods should be cooked to individual dish requirements.

Chilled ready-to-eat foods should be kept below 5°C until needed.

Product	Method of regeneration
Chilled cooked food (multi-portion)	Reheat thoroughly to a core temperature (temperature right in the middle) of at least 75°C (82°C in Scotland). Make sure that this temperature is maintained for at least two minutes. When holding for service, don't let the temperature fall below 63°C at any time.
Individual meals (ready cooked)	As above, or follow the manufacturer's instructions exactly.

Canned foods

Once a can has been opened, treat the food in the same way as fresh food, i.e. store it below 5°C or hold it at above 63°C. When storing opened canned food in the fridge, empty the food into a clean bowl, cover, label and date.

Canned foods have already been cooked in the canning process, but may undergo further cooking as part of another dish (e.g. curry, soup, pasta dish). The texture of canned food is the same as that of cooked food. It is fine to cook tomatoes again as part of a sauce, but take care not to overcook delicate items such as asparagus.

Some canned food (e.g. salmon or kidney beans) will need to be drained before use to get rid of the surrounding liquid.

Part-baked products

Part-baked products include bread, bread rolls, Danish pastries, croissants and brioche.

- Vacuum-packed items just need to be removed from the packaging and placed on baking trays.
- Frozen items can usually be cooked from frozen.
- Finishes such as glazing can be carried out as required.
- Bake at the temperature and for the time recommended on the packaging.
- Cool on wire racks where possible to help keep the product crisp.

Purchase, delivery and storage

- Use a reputable supplier who can ensure consistent quality.
- Check that foods are delivered at the correct temperature and in the required condition (fresh, no discolouration, no unpleasant smell, etc.).
- Check that the food is of the type, size and quality ordered.
- Check that the packaging is unbroken, dry and clean.
- Check that all items are properly labelled.
- Check the 'use by' and 'best before' dates.
- Transfer to temperature-controlled storage within 15 minutes of delivery.
- Store carefully to avoid breakage and split packaging, which may cause cross-contamination.

Regeneration, cooking and serving

- Thaw frozen food thoroughly.
- Protect food from contamination.
- Rehydrate correctly, mixing the correct amount of liquid with dry products.
- Heat (or cook) the food at the correct temperature for the right amount of time.
- Check cooking and hot holding temperatures with a temperature probe, and record these temperatures.
- Do not regenerate food too early (it will burn or become dry and unpalatable).
- Do not regenerate food too late (it could be under-heated, which could lead to food poisoning).
- Make sure that instructions for regenerating are clear, easy to understand and available to all staff.
- Check the flavours and seasoning of all dishes.
- Report problems with any items to a supervisor immediately.

Activity

1 Give three advantages of using pre-prepared foods.

2 What is the correct temperature for storing frozen food?

VRQ Unit 202 Food safety in catering

Learning outcomes:

- Behave as a responsible individual within food safety procedures
- Keep him/herself clean and hygienic
- Keep the working area clean and hygienic
- Receive and store food safely
- Prepare, cook, hold and serve food safely

NVQ 501 (1GEN1) Maintain a safe, hygienic and secure working environment
NVQ 603 (2GEN3) Maintain food safety when storing, preparing and cooking food
NVQ 603 (2GEN3) Maintain food safety when storing and cooking food
NVQ 603 (2GEN3) Maintain food safety when storing, preparing and cooking food
NVQ 501 (1GEN1) Maintain a safe, hygienic and secure working environment
NVQ 603 (2GEN3) Maintain food safety when storing, preparing and cooking food

The importance of food safety

What is food safety?

People who eat food prepared for them by others when they are away from home (e.g. in canteens or restaurants) expect it to be safe. Food safety means making sure that foods and drinks served to consumers are suitable, safe and wholesome. This involves all the processes, from selecting suppliers, to delivery of food, right through to serving the food.

Eating 'contaminated' food can cause food poisoning. Thousands of cases of food poisoning are reported each year in England and Wales. However, as many cases of food poisoning are not reported, no one really knows the actual number, but it is very high.

Why is food safety important?

Food poisoning can be an unpleasant illness for anyone, but it can be very serious or even fatal for some people. High-risk groups include:

- babies and the very young
- elderly people
- pregnant women
- those who are already unwell.

It is therefore essential to take great care to prevent food poisoning. In 2005, the Food Standards Agency made a commitment to reduce the number of reported cases of food poisoning by 20 per cent by 2010.

The main symptoms of food poisoning are:

- nausea
- vomiting

- diarrhoea
- fever
- dehydration.

How is food contaminated?

There are three main ways that food is contaminated.

1 **Bacteria** are all around us, in the environment, on raw food, on humans, animals, birds and insects. When bacteria multiply in food or use food to get into the human body they can make people ill.
2 **Chemicals** can sometimes get into food accidentally and can make the consumer ill. The kinds of chemical that may get into food include cleaning fluids, disinfectants, machine oil, insecticides and pesticides.
3 **Physical contamination** is caused when something gets into food that should not be there. This could be anything that a person should not eat, such as glass, pen tops, paperclips, blue plasters, hair and fingernails.

All these are potentially dangerous and great care must be taken to avoid any of them. However, the most dangerous of all is bacteria.

Bacteria and contamination

Not all bacteria are harmful. In fact, some are very useful and are used in foods and medicines. For example, the process of making milk into yoghurt uses bacteria, and so does making salami.

The bacteria that are harmful are called 'pathogenic bacteria' (or 'pathogens') and can cause food poisoning. Bacteria are so small that you would need to use a microscope to see them – you cannot taste them or smell them on food. This is why pathogenic bacteria are so dangerous – you cannot tell when they are in food. If they have the right conditions (i.e. food, warmth, moisture and time) they can multiply approximately every 20 minutes by dividing in half. This is called binary fission.

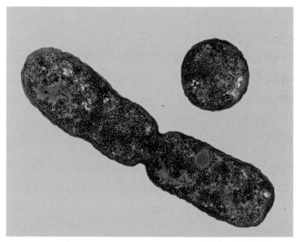

Bacteria multiplying by dividing in two (binary fission)

Pathogenic bacteria can act in different ways to cause food poisoning. Some produce toxins (poisons) that can survive boiling temperatures for half an hour or more. Some can produce spores to protect themselves from very high or low temperatures, or from chemicals such as disinfectant.

Some common food-poisoning bacteria

Salmonella

Pests such as rodents can carry salmonella, and it can also live and multiply in raw meat and poultry, eggs and shellfish. Animal products may contain salmonella if the animal was infected with it. Salmonella used to be the most common cause of food poisoning in the UK, but since measures were taken to reduce salmonella in chickens and in eggs, the number of cases of salmonella poisoning has dropped dramatically. Salmonella poisoning can also be passed on by humans, for example if someone with salmonella does not wash their hands properly after going to the toilet (they may be ill or they may be carrying salmonella but not show any signs of illness).

Staphylococcus aureus

The main source of this bacterium is the human body. It may be on the skin, hair and scalp, or in the nose and throat. Cuts, spots, burns and boils can also be a source of this organism. When *Staphylococcus* multiplies in food a toxin (poison) is produced that is very difficult to kill, even with boiling temperatures. To avoid food poisoning from this organism, food handlers need to maintain very high standards of personal hygiene. They should also tell their supervisor if they are ill, and not handle any food until the supervisor gives permission.

Clostridium perfringens

This is often present in raw meat, poultry and vegetables (also insects, soil, dust and sewage). It can also be passed on by humans, for example if they do not wash their hands properly after going to the toilet (it is present in human and animal faeces).

A number of incidents of *Clostridium perfringens* food poisoning have occurred when large amounts of meat have been heated up slowly before cooking, then allowed to cool slowly before reheating it and using it later. *Clostridium perfringens* can produce spores during this heating and cooling process. Spores are very resistant to any further cooking and allow bacteria to survive in conditions that would usually kill them.

Bacillus cereus

This is another organism that can produce spores; it can also produce toxins so can be very dangerous. It is often associated with cooking rice in large quantities, cooling it too slowly and then reheating it. The temperatures the rice is reheated at are not high enough to destroy spores and toxins. This organism has also been linked with other cereal crops, spices, soil and vegetables.

Clostridium botulinum

Fortunately this type of bacterial infection is rare in this country. Symptoms can be very serious and even fatal. Sources tend to be soil, vegetables and the intestines of fish.

Other bacteria

Some bacteria cause food-borne illnesses but do not multiply in food. Instead, they use food to get into the human gut (the digestive system) where they then multiply and cause a range of illnesses, some of them serious. These organisms include those listed below.

- *Campylobacter*, which now causes more food-related illness than any other organism. It is found in raw poultry and meat, sewage, animals, insects and birds.
- *E coli*, which is present in the intestines and faeces of animals and humans. It is also found in raw meat and can be present on raw vegetables.
- Listeria, which is of particular concern because it can multiply slowly at fridge temperatures (i.e. below 5°C). It has been linked with such chilled products as

unpasteurised cheeses, pâté and prepared salads, as well as cook/chill meals (ready-prepared meals, which are cooked and then chilled ready for reheating).

High-risk foods

Some foods pose a greater risk to food safety than others and are called high-risk foods. They are usually ready to eat, so would not need any cooking that would kill bacteria. They are moist, contain protein and need to be stored in the fridge.

High-risk foods include:

- soups, stocks, sauces, gravies
- eggs and egg products
- milk and milk products
- cooked meat and fish, and meat and fish products
- any foods that need to be handled or reheated.

Personal hygiene

Because humans are a source of food poisoning bacteria it is very important for all food handlers to take care with personal hygiene and to adopt good practices when working with food.

- Arrive at work clean (bathe or shower daily) and with clean hair.
- Wear approved, clean kitchen clothing and wear it only in the kitchen. This must completely cover any personal clothing.
- Keep your hair neatly contained in a suitable hat/hairnet.
- Keep your nails short and clean, and do not wear nail varnish or false nails.
- Do not wear jewellery or watches when handling food (a plain wedding band is permissible but could still trap bacteria).
- Avoided wearing cosmetics and strong perfumes.
- Smoking is not allowed in food preparation areas (ash, smoke and bacteria from touching the mouth area could get into food).
- Do not eat food or sweets or chew gum when handling food as this may also transfer bacteria to food.
- Cover any cuts, burns or grazes with a blue waterproof dressing, then wash your hands.
- Report any illness to the supervisor as soon as possible. For example, you should report diarrhoea and/or vomiting, infected cuts, burns or spots, bad cold or flu symptoms, or if you were ill while on holiday.

Hand washing

Hands are constantly in use in the kitchen and will be touching numerous materials, foods, surfaces and equipment. Contamination from hands can happen very easily and you must take care with hand washing to avoid this.

- A basin should be provided that is used only for hand washing.
- Wet your hands under warm running water.
- Apply liquid soap.
- Rub your hands together, and rub one hand with the fingers and thumbs of the other.
- Remember to include your fingertips, nails and wrists.
- Rinse off the soap under the warm running water.

- Dry your hands on a paper towel and use the paper towel to turn off the tap before throwing it away.
- If available, rub your hands with alcohol gel to kill any bacteria that are left.

You should always wash your hands:

- when you enter the kitchen, before starting work and handling any food
- after a break (particularly if you have used the toilet)
- between different tasks, but especially between handling raw and cooked food
- if you touch your hair, nose or mouth, or use a tissue for a sneeze or cough
- after you apply or change a dressing on a cut or burn
- after cleaning preparation areas, equipment or contaminated surfaces
- after handling kitchen waste, external food packaging, money or flowers.

Cross-contamination

Cross-contamination is the cause of a lot of food poisoning. It is when bacteria are transferred from contaminated food (usually raw food) to ready-to-eat food. Cross-contamination could be caused by:

- foods touching each other, e.g. raw and cooked meat
- raw meat or poultry dripping on to high-risk foods
- soil from dirty vegetables coming into contact with high-risk foods
- dirty cloths or dirty equipment
- equipment (e.g. chopping boards or knives) used with raw food and then used with cooked food
- hands touching raw food then cooked food and not washing hands between tasks.

Preventing cross-contamination

All the above can be avoided by having good working practices. For example, it is a good idea to have separate working areas and storage areas for raw and high-risk foods. If this is not possible, then they should be kept well away from each other, and the working areas should be thoroughly cleaned and disinfected between tasks.

Vegetables should be washed before preparation/peeling and again afterwards. Leafy vegetables may need to be washed in several changes of cold water to remove all the soil clinging to them.

Monitoring equipment

Colour-coded chopping boards are a good way to keep different types of food separate.

Worktops and chopping boards will come into contact with the food you prepare,

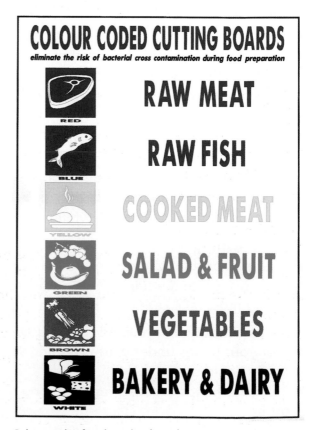

Colour codes for chopping boards

so need special attention. Make sure that chopping boards are in good condition – cracks and splits could harbour bacteria and this could be transferred to food.

As well as colour-coded chopping boards, some kitchens also provide colour-coded knives, cloths, cleaning equipment, storage trays, bowls and even staff uniforms to help prevent cross-contamination.

Cleaning and sanitising

Clean and sanitise worktops and chopping boards before working on them and do this again after use, paying particular attention when they have been used for raw foods. Chopping boards can be disinfected by putting them through a dishwasher with a high rinse temperature.

Small equipment, such as knives, bowls, spoons and tongs can also cause cross-contamination. It is important to wash them well, especially when they are used for a variety of food and for raw foods.

Cross-contamination and multiplication of bacteria

Here is an example of how quickly cross-contamination can spread bacteria.

Time		Number of bacteria
10.00	A chicken has been cooked to 75°C and left in the kitchen, uncovered, to cool. No bacteria have survived.	0
10.20	Chef uses a dirty cloth to transfer chicken to a plate	6000
10.40		12,000
10.40		24,000
11am		48,000
11.20		96,000
11.40		192,000
12 noon		384,000
12.20		768,000
12.40		1.5 million
1pm		3 million

From one careless action with a dirty cloth, 6000 bacteria (pathogens) have multiplied to 3 million in 2 hours 40 minutes. One million pathogens per gram of food is enough to cause food poisoning.

A clean kitchen

As a food handler it is your responsibility, along with those working with you, to keep food areas clean and hygienic at all times. Clean food areas play an essential part in the production of safe food, and the team must plan, record and check all cleaning as part of a 'cleaning schedule' (like the one shown on the next page). Clean premises, work areas and equipment are important to:

- control the bacteria that cause food poisoning
- reduce the possibility of physical and chemical contamination
- make accidents (e.g. slips on a greasy floor) less likely
- create a positive image for customers, visitors and employees
- comply with the law
- avoid attracting pests to the kitchen.

Room:			Main kitchen		
Item	Person responsible	Product	Method		Frequency
Walls, doors, woodwork	Cleaner	Easy degreaser	Solution strength: 2 cups per bucket of hot water Contact time: 5 minutes Apply with: Clean cloth or mop Rinse with: Clean water Dry: Air		Daily
Chopping boards and food prep surfaces	Chef	Easy sanitiser	1. Remove food debris 2. Wipe surface with clean damp cloth 3. Sprinkle on sanitiser wipe 4. Rinse cloth and wipe over surface 5. Allow to air dry		After use
Fridges	2nd chef	Easy sanitiser	1. Make up sanitiser solution (2 scoops/bucket) 2. Wipe all surfaces with solution 3. Rinse thoroughly with clean water 4. Allow to air dry		Weekly

An example of a cleaning schedule

Controlling bacteria

In the same way as you can limit cross-contamination, you can help to control the spread and growth of bacteria by having good working practices.

- Clean and tidy as you go and do not allow waste to build up. It is very difficult to keep untidy areas clean. Clean up any spills straight away.
- Kitchen waste should be placed in waste bins with lids (preferably foot operated). These should be emptied regularly so that they do not get too full. If the waste is left too long and allowed to build up too much, it can attract pests and bacteria can start to form.
- Protect food from bacteria and prevent bacterial growth by keeping food clean, cool and covered.
- Take great care with kitchen cloths – they are a perfect growing area for bacteria. Different cloths for different areas will help to reduce cross-contamination and it is certainly good practice to use different cloths for raw food and cooked food preparation. Using disposable kitchen towel is the most hygienic way to clean food areas.
- Also take great care with tea towels if they are used. Remember that they can easily spread bacteria, so do not use them as 'all-purpose' cloths and do not keep one on your shoulder (the cloth may touch your neck and hair and these can be sources of bacteria).
- All surfaces and equipment that come into contact with food, and items that you are likely to touch with your hands (e.g. fridge handles), should be cleaned and disinfected regularly according to your cleaning schedule.

Cleaning products

There are different cleaning products designed for different tasks.

- **Detergent** is designed to remove grease and dirt. It may be in the form of liquid, powder, gel or foam and usually needs to be added to water to use. Detergent will not kill pathogens (bacteria), although the hot water it is mixed with may help to do this. Detergent will clean and degrease surfaces so that disinfectant can work properly.

- **Disinfectant** is designed to destroy bacteria. To be effective, disinfectants must be left on a cleaned grease-free surface for the required amount of time (as per the instructions on the container).
- **Sanitiser** cleans and disinfects. It usually comes in spray form. Sanitiser is very useful for work surfaces and equipment, especially when cleaning them between tasks.

Beware! Cleaning is essential to prevent health hazards, but if it is not managed properly it can become a hazard in itself. Do not store cleaning chemicals in food preparation and cooking areas.

Avoiding contamination

The three types of food contamination listed earlier in this chapter can all be avoided by following good hygiene practices in the kitchen.

- Take care to avoid *chemical contamination* when using cleaning products.
- Make sure that items such as cloths, paper towels and fibres from mops do not get into open food, causing *physical contamination*.
- Avoid *bacterial contamination* by making sure that the same cleaning cloths and equipment are not used in raw food areas and then in high-risk food areas.

Food storage

It is important to store food at the correct temperature (see the table below).

- Check temperatures of chilled and frozen food deliveries and record them.
- Transfer chilled and frozen deliveries to fridges and freezers within 15 minutes of their arrival. Remove the outer packaging first.
- When possible, use separate fridges for storing meat, fish, dairy items etc., and make sure food is labelled and dated before it goes into the fridge.
- If you do have to use a multi-use fridge for different types of food, position the food correctly, with raw foods such as meat and poultry at the bottom.
- Temperatures between 5°C and 63°C are called the danger zone because it is possible for bacteria to multiply between these temperatures. They grow most rapidly at or around 37°C (body temperature). Keep food out of the danger zone as much as possible. Unless you are actually working on a particular food, keep it in the fridge below 5°C or hot above 63°C.

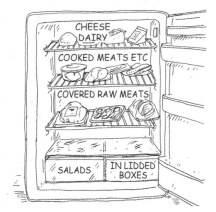

Where food should be positioned in a fridge

Defrosting

If you need to defrost frozen food:

● place it in a deep tray, cover with film and label
● put the tray at the bottom of the fridge where thawing liquid cannot drip on to anything else
● thaw food completely (no ice crystals on any part)
● cook within 12 hours.

Make sure that you allow enough time for the food to defrost properly before you cook it – it may take longer than you think!

Temperatures for storing food

Food stored in a freezer	–18°C / –23°C
Raw meat/poultry	0°C to 2°C
Raw fish and shellfish	0°C to 2°C
Cooked meats/meat products	0°C to 4°C
Cooked fish/fish products	0°C to 4°C
Dairy products/fats	0°C to 4°C
Eggs	Below 8°C
Salad items, herbs, leafy vegetables	0°C to 4°C
Cooked foods/high-risk items	0°C to 4°C
Ambient food storage, e.g. cans, dry foods Grains, general grocery items	Cool, well ventilated

Note: Although the law states that 'foods which support growth of pathogens or formation of toxins must not be stored above 8°C' it is recognised best practice to store below 5°C.

Cooking

Cooking food to a core temperature of 75°C for two minutes will kill most bacteria. This is especially important where large amounts of food are being cooked or the consumers are in a high-risk category (see page 78). However, some popular dishes on hotel and restaurant menus (e.g. steaks) are cooked to a lower temperature than this, according to individual dish and customer requirements.

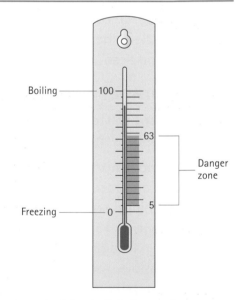

Important food safety temperatures

Cooked food being held for service must be kept above 63°C if it is going to be served hot. If food is being cooked for reheating at a later time or to serve cold, it must be protected from contamination and cooled quickly, i.e. to 8°C within 90 minutes. The best way to do this is in a blast chiller. It should then be stored below 5°C.

Any food that is to be chilled or frozen must be well wrapped or placed in a suitable container with a lid (items may also be vacuum packed). Make sure that all food is labelled and dated before chilling or freezing.

Temperatures for cooking and serving hot food
Unless told otherwise, cooked hot food should be heated to **75°C+**
Most cooked fish should be heated to **63°C** (the Environmental Health Officer may advise a higher temperature than this)
Reheated food should be heated to **75°C+**
In Scotland reheated food should be heated to **82°C+**
Food held for service should be kept at **63°C+**

Pests

When there are reports of food premises being forcibly closed down, an infestation of pests is often the reason. As pests can be a serious source of contamination and disease, having them near food cannot be allowed and is against the law.

Pests can be attracted to premises because of the food, warmth, shelter, water and possible nesting materials (e.g. cardboard boxes, packing materials). Everything possible should be done to keep them out.

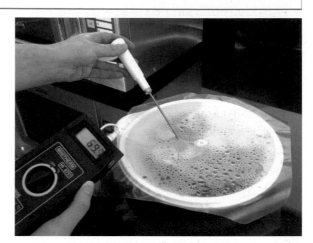

Checking the temperature of cooked food

Any suspicion of pests being present must be reported to the supervisor or manager immediately.

Signs of pest presence

Pest	Signs that they are present
Rats and mice	• Sightings of rodent • Droppings • Unpleasant smell • Gnawed wires etc. • Greasy marks on lower walls • Damaged food stock • Paw prints
Flies and wasps	• Sightings of flies and wasps • Hearing them • Sightings of dead insects • Sightings of maggots (which will grow into flies)
Cockroaches	• Sightings (dead or alive), usually at night • Unpleasant smell
Ants	• Sightings on surfaces and in food Tiny, pale-coloured Pharaoh's ants are difficult to spot but can still be the source of a variety of pathogens
Weevils	Sightings in stored products, e.g. flour/cornflour Weevils are tiny black insects that are very difficult to see but can be spotted by their movement in flour etc.
Birds	• Sighting • Droppings in outside storage areas and around refuse
Domestic pets	These must be kept out of food areas as they carry pathogens on fur, whiskers, saliva, urine etc.

How to keep pests out

How you deal with pests will depend on what they are, but here are some general guidelines and suggestions.

- Block their entry, e.g. holes around pipework and any other gaps and cavities where they could get in.
- Seal drain covers.
- Quickly repair any damage to the building or fixtures and fittings.
- Put screening or netting over windows and doors.
- Check deliveries/packaging for pests.
- Put down baits and traps to catch them (e.g. an electronic fly killer).
- Seal containers – ensure that no open food is left out.
- Do not allow waste to build up in the kitchen.
- Do not keep outside waste too close to the kitchen.
- Organise professional pest management control, surveys and reports.

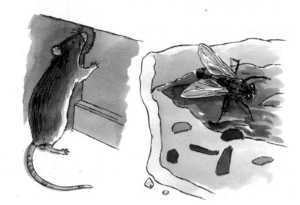

Rats and flies are common pests

Beware! Pest control measures can introduce food safety hazards. For example, the bodies of dead insects or even rodents may remain in the kitchen, potentially causing physical and bacterial contamination. Pesticides, insecticides and baits could cause chemical contamination if not managed properly. Pest control is best managed by professionals.

Food safety management systems

It is good practice for all food businesses to have a food safety management system in place. As part of the Food Standards Agency's commitment to reduce food poisoning cases by 2010 (see page 78), it became a legal requirement from January 2006 for all food businesses to operate such a system. When Environmental Health Officers inspect the premises of these businesses they will also check the food safety management system.

Hazard Analysis Critical Control Point (HACCP)

All systems must be based on the Hazard Analysis Critical Control Point (HACCP). This is an internationally recognised food safety management system that aims to identify the critical points or stages in any process. The system must provide a documented record of the stages *all* food will go through right up to the time it is eaten, and may include:

- purchase and delivery
- receipt of food
- storage
- preparation
- cooking
- cooling
- hot holding

- reheating
- chilled storage
- serving.

Once the hazards have been identified, measures are put in place to control the hazards and keep the food safe.

The HACCP system involves seven stages.

1 Identify hazards – what could go wrong.
2 Identify CCPs (critical control points), i.e. the important points where things could go wrong.
3 Set critical limits for each CCP, e.g. the temperature that fresh chicken should be at when it is delivered.
4 Monitor CCPs and put checks in place to stop problems from occurring.
5 Identify corrective action – what will be done if something goes wrong.
6 Verification – check that the HACCP plan is working.
7 Documentation – record all the above.

The system must be updated regularly, especially when new items are introduced to the menu or systems change (e.g. a new piece of cooking equipment is purchased). Specific new controls must be put in place to include any changes.

'Safer food, better business' and 'CookSafe'

The HACCP system described above may seem complicated and difficult to set up for a small business. With this in mind, the Food Standards Agency launched its 'Safer food, better business' system for England and Wales. This is based on the principles of HACCP but is in a format that is easy to understand, with pre-printed pages and charts in which to enter the relevant information, such as temperatures for individual dishes. It is divided into two parts.

1 The first part is about safe methods (e.g. avoiding cross-contamination, personal hygiene, cleaning, chilling and cooking).
2 The second part covers opening and closing checks. These are checks that procedures are in place (e.g. safe methods, recording of safe methods, training records, supervision, stock control, and the selection of suppliers and contractors) to ensure that the operation is working to the standards required to produce safe food.

A copy of 'Safer food, better business' is available from www.food.gov.uk. A similar system, called 'CookSafe', has been developed by the Food Standards Agency (Scotland) and details of this can also be found at www.food.gov.uk.

'Scores on the Doors'

'Scores on the Doors' is another strategy that has been piloted by the Food Standards Agency to raise food safety standards and reduce the incidence of food poisoning. When the strategy was piloted, various schemes were tested using a star rating of food safety. The rating was awarded based on the following criteria taken from the Food Standards Agency's statutory risk rating system:

- level of compliance of food hygiene practices and procedures
- level of compliance relating to structure and cleanliness of premises
- confidence in management of the business and food safety controls.

The star rating could then be placed in a prominent position on the door or window of premises (although this was not mandatory).

The pilot schemes were very popular, especially with customers, and in December 2008 the Food Standards Agency decided on a standard scheme to be launched throughout England and Wales. Establishments will be graded from zero stars for poor standards of food safety up to five stars for excellent standards.

It is expected that the 'Scores on the Doors' scheme will have a lasting positive impact on food safety standards. No matter how good the food is in a particular establishment, few people will want to eat there if its food safety score is low!

What the law says

New laws relevant to food handlers took effect from 1 January 2006. Almost all of the requirements in these regulations remain the same as the ones they replaced – the Food Safety (General Food Hygiene) Regulations 1995 and the Food Safety (Temperature Control) Regulations 1995.

These set out the basic food safety requirements for all aspects of a food business, from premises to the personal hygiene of staff, with specific attention to actual temperatures relating to food.

The main difference in the 2006 laws is that they provide a framework for EU legislation to be enforced in England and they require food establishments to have an approved Food Safety Management Procedure in place, with up-to-date records available.

Activity

1 What is cross-contamination?

2 Name three food poisoning bacteria.

3 Choose one recipe from this book and identify all the hygiene procedures that are needed to make sure the dish is safe to eat.

PART ②

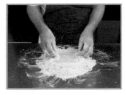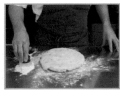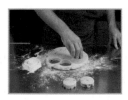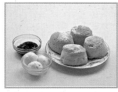

PRACTICE

Contents list:

Introduction to Part 2

In the first part of this book you have learned a lot of the theory that you will need to support you in your cooking and your work in catering. In the second part you will put much of this theory into practice by trying out different recipes and different methods of cooking.

This chapter provides you with details of the learning outcomes that will be covered in Part 2, plus some information about food preparation that you will find useful when following the recipes.

Learning outcomes covered in chapters 11–22

Listed below are the NVQ and VRQ units that will be covered in the practical chapters in the second part of this book. The icons beside the learning outcomes will also appear beside recipes in the practical chapters that relate to the objectives in these outcomes. You can refer back to these as you work through the practical chapters, to check which objectives you are covering.

VRQ Unit 107 Prepare and cook food by boiling, poaching and steaming

VRQ Unit 108 Prepare and cook food by stewing and braising

VRQ Unit 109 Prepare and cook food by baking, roasting and grilling

VRQ Unit 110 Prepare and cook food by deep frying and shallow frying

VRQ Unit 112 Cold food preparation (see Chapter 12)

NVQ 501 (1GEN1) Maintain a safe, hygienic and secure working environment

NVQ 603 (2GEN3) Maintain food safety when storing, preparing and cooking food

NVQ 515 (1FP1) Prepare vegetables

NVQ 516 (1FP2) Prepare and finish simple salad and fruit dishes

NVQ 517 (1FP3) Prepare hot and cold sandwiches

NVQ 518 (1FC1) Cook vegetables

NVQ 519 (1FPC1) Prepare and cook fish

NVQ 520 (1FPC2) Prepare and cook meat and poultry

NVQ 521 (1FPC3) Prepare and cook pasta

NVQ 522 (1FPC4) Prepare and cook rice

NVQ 523 (1FPC5) Prepare and cook eggs

NVQ 524 (1FPC6) Prepare and cook pulses

NVQ 525 (1FPC7) Prepare and cook vegetable protein

NVQ 526 (1FPC8) Prepare and cook simple bread and dough products

NVQ 527 (1FPC9) Prepare and cook grain

Learning outcomes:

- Prepare and cook food by boiling

- Prepare and cook food by poaching

- Prepare and cook food by steaming

- Prepare and cook food by stewing

- Prepare and cook food by braising

- Prepare and cook food by baking

- Prepare and cook food by roasting

- Prepare and cook food by grilling

- Prepare and cook food by deep frying

- Prepare and cook food by shallow frying

- Prepare cold food

- Present cold food

Flavouring and presenting food

Culinary herbs and spices

Herbs and spices add a huge amount of flavour, colour and aroma to foods, and allow us to cook in a great variety of styles. There are vast numbers of herbs and spices available these days from all over the world.

- Herbs are the leafy parts of plants.
- Spices are obtained from the root, stem, flower or seed of plants.

Their function is to season food. There is a huge variety of flavours. The flavour deteriorates the longer herbs and spices are stored. Freshly ground spices and fresh herbs have the best flavour.

Dried spices

Dried spices come in different forms. Some are used as dried seeds, while others come in the form of dried leaves, flowers, buds or ready-ground powder. Dried spices include:

allspice bark and roots	coriander
buds, e.g. cloves	cumin
cassia	curry leaves
cardamom	fruits or flowers, e.g. tamarind and saffron
cinnamon	ginger
cloves	kaffir lime leaves
leaves, e.g. bay leaves	mustard.
peppercorns	

There are many more than are listed here, and you will learn more about them as you do more cooking and try out different recipes. Many spices are of tropical Oriental origin. However, allspice, vanilla and chillies are originally from Central America and the West Indies.

Selecting spices

Choose whole seeds, berries, buds and bark where possible as these keep their flavour longer than powdered spices. It is better to grind spices (e.g. peppercorns, cumin seeds, cardamom pods, allspice, cloves, cinnamon sticks) as and when you need them.

Fresh roots such as ginger, galangal (a type of ginger from Thailand) and lemon grass have a very different flavour from their dried versions and should be used whenever possible.

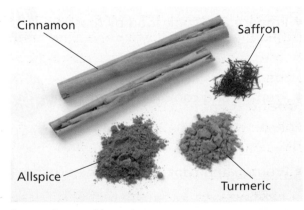

Some spices used in cookery

Preparation of spices

Dry frying

This is also known as dry roasting and is common in Indian cookery.

- Heat a suitable pan on the stove and add the spices.
- Cook for 2–3 minutes, stirring well. The spices will start to give off a rich aroma.
- Remove the pan from the heat, place the spices in a mortar and grind them with a pestle.

This increases the flavour of spices such as cumin, coriander, fennel, mustard and poppy seeds.

Grinding

Spices are normally ground with a pestle in a mortar to release their flavour and aroma. Do not grind them too early – wait until you are ready to use them. Use an electric spice grinder or coffee grinder to grind spices that are hard to grind in a pestle and mortar, e.g. cinnamon, cassia, fenugreek.

Making wet spice mixtures

Add the spices to a food processor with a little oil. Mix them in the food processor to form a smooth paste.

Grating

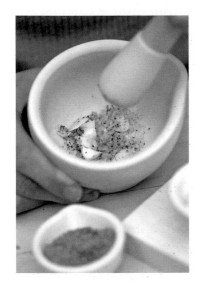

Grate fresh root spices, such as ginger and horseradish, and whole nutmegs. Peel ginger and horseradish and then grate using a fine grater.

Crushing

Some spices, such as cardamom, juniper berries and lemon grass, are often lightly crushed to release their aroma. In the case of cardamom, crushing also releases the seeds, which can then also be crushed.

Hard spices, such as juniper berries, peppercorns and cardamoms, may be placed in a polythene bag or wrapped in clingfilm and crushed with the bottom of a small saucepan or a rolling pin.

Braising

Some spices (e.g. lemon grass) are added to the recipe during cooking to give a subtle background flavour and then removed before serving. These can be bruised before they are added to the cooking pot – on a chopping board, use the back of a knife to crush the fibres.

Shredding and chopping

For some recipes, spices such as ginger, garlic and kaffir lime leaves are cut into fine slices or pieces to maximise their flavour and aroma.

Spice infusions

Some spices, or a combination of spices, are infused in a hot liquid (e.g. water, stock, milk or wine) to give it an aroma and colour. Saffron is infused to give a yellow colour. Tamarind is infused to produce a tangy juice.

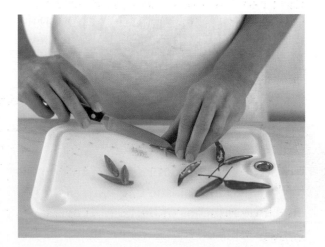

Frying in oil

Many recipes state that the spices should be fried in oil to release the flavour before the other ingredients are added.

Preparing chillies

Chillies have to be handled with care, especially if you have sensitive skin. Do not touch your eyes while handling chillies as you will suffer a nasty stinging burn. It is easier to deseed chillies before chopping them. Cut the chilli in half and scrape out the seeds using the point of a small knife.

Storing fresh spices

If possible, use fresh spices the day they are purchased, or store them in a refrigerator. Keep leaves such as curry leaves, lemon grass and kaffir lime leaves wrapped in clingfilm. Fresh ginger and chillies will keep for up to three weeks in a sealed container. Fresh spices pounded into a paste and placed in sealed containers will keep for up to six months.

Storing dried spices

Dried spices should be kept in airtight containers. Whole spices will keep for up to six months. Some spices are available in ready-mixed combinations, like those listed below.

- **Garam masala** is a mixture of hot spices used in Indian cooking. There is no standardised recipe for this mixture as there are many regional variations. The mixture is used sparingly, and generally put into foods towards the end of their cooking period. A typical mix could be cardamom, cumin, cinnamon, cloves, nutmeg, black peppercorns.
- **Chinese five spice** is a blend of fragrant spices. Again there is no standardised recipe, but a typical example would include five of the following: star anise, anise pepper, fennel or anise seed, clove, Chinese cinnamon, ginger, nutmeg, dried citrus peel.
- **Panch puran** is a combination of five aromatic seeds – cumin, mustard, fennel, fenugreek and kalonji (black onion) – fried in hot oil before being used in various meat and vegetable dishes.

Using herbs

Herbs are aromatic plants grown mainly for use in cookery. Many are also used for medicinal purposes. Some herbs grow annually and need to be sown each year. Others are perennial and grow year after year. Some common herbs used in the kitchen that are readily available are:

basil	lemon balm	rosemary
chervil	marjoram	sage
chives	mint	tarragon
coriander	oregano	thyme.
dill	parsley	

Fresh herbs add flavour to a whole range of dishes.

Storing herbs

Ideally, fresh herbs should be picked just before use. If necessary, they can be stored in a refrigerator for one to two days sealed in a plastic bag with plenty of air. Large bunches of herbs such as parsley and coriander (which may still

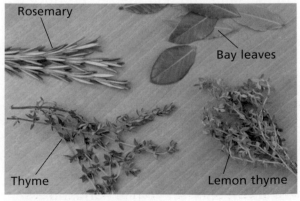

Some herbs used in cookery

have their roots attached) should be stored in water with a plastic bag over the top of them covering their leaves.

Herbs may also be dried or frozen. Dried herbs keep best in airtight jars away from the light.

Cooking with herbs

Herbs may be used whole or chopped before they are added to a dish.

- The more delicate herbs such as parsley, chervil and tarragon should normally be added towards the end of the cooking time.
- Tougher varieties, such as rosemary and thyme, are added at the beginning.

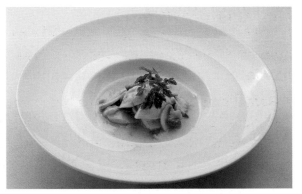

Dried herbs work well in cooked dishes such as stews and casseroles but are not suitable for salads. Dried herbs have a stronger flavour than fresh ones and should be used sparingly as a general rule. If you use dried herbs instead of fresh herbs in a recipe, use one-third of the amount of dried herbs compared with fresh herbs.

This chicken casserole is garnished with parsley

Presentation of food

The presentation of food is very important. Food may taste and smell good, but if it looks a mess on the plate it will not look appetising for the customer.

Putting the food on the plate

Food should be served on a plate or dish that is large enough:

- to allow the food to be fully appreciated
- so that any sauce or garnish can be applied to enhance the dish
- so that the food does not go over the edge of the plate or dish.

It should be placed carefully and neatly on the plate. It is important that the dish looks colourful and appetising. The food should be handled as little as possible at the presentation stage (when it is being plated up and garnished), particularly with foods that are susceptible to contamination.

Garnishing

Garnishing is also important. The aim of a garnish is to add to the visual appeal of the plate (the dish should look interesting, attractive and colourful) and also to add flavour.

- The food must look attractive and appetising.
- It must appeal to the eyes as well as the palate, so that the enjoyment of the food is not spoiled in any way.
- The colours and arrangement of food should work together.

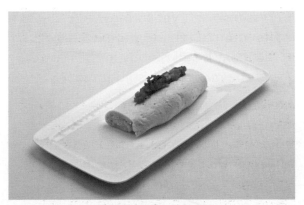

This omelette has been neatly garnished with chopped tomato

- Avoid over-garnishing.
- All garnishes should look fresh and should be handled as little as possible.
- The flavour of a garnish should be borne in mind when decorating a dish.

How do you like your meat?

Cattle (beef), sheep (lamb and mutton) and pigs (pork, gammon and bacon) are reared for fresh meat. Later in the book (Chapters 17–19) you will learn more about the different types of meat and how to cook them. Here is a brief introduction to meat in general, including the types of meat available and some cooking tips.

Amount of cooking

Images and text courtesy of Donald Russell (www.donaldrussell.com).

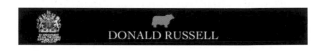

- All beef products, with the exception of minced beef and burgers, can be cooked rare, medium or well done.
- Lamb and veal can be cooked medium and well done.
- Pork, with the exception of fillets, should always be cooked well done.

You can see the differences between the differently cooked meats in their:

- internal temperature (you can use a temperature probe to test this)
- outer colour
- inner colour
- firmness (you can press the meat to test this)
- moistness (you can check the colour and amount of juices to test this)
- shape.

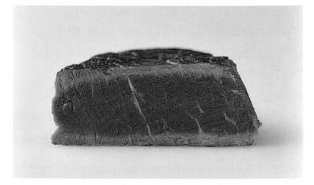

Rare meat

Rare (bleu)

- Press-test: soft.
- The internal temperature is 45–47°C.
- The meat is bloody and the juices are dark red.

Medium rare (saignant)

- Press-test: soft yet springy.
- The internal temperature is 50–52°C.
- The meat is still bloody in the centre and the meat juice is light red.

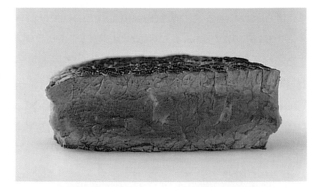

Medium rare meat

Medium (a point)

- Press-test: firm and springy.
- The internal temperature is 55–60°C.
- The centre of the meat is pink.

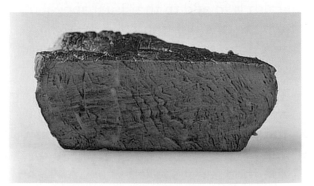

Medium meat

Well done (bien cuit)

- Press-test: firm.
- The internal temperature is 64–70°C.
- The meat is cooked throughout and the juices are clear.

Serving size guide

Suggested uncooked weights per person:

Beef, lamb, pork and veal	
Without bone	100–250 g
With bone	200–350 g
Offal	125–175 g
Sauces	50 g/100 ml

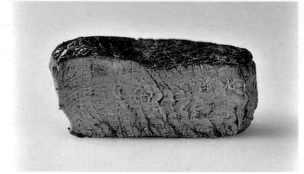

Well done meat

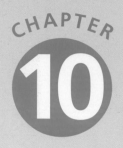

Methods of cookery

VRQ Units 107, 108, 109 and 110 (see page 92 for details)

Learning outcome: Prepare and cook food by a variety of methods

NVQ 519 (1FPC1) Prepare and cook fish; NVQ 520 (1FPC2) Prepare and cook meat and poultry; NVQ 521 (1FPC3) Prepare and cook pasta; NVQ 522 (1FPC4) Prepare and cook rice; NVQ 523 (1FPC5) Prepare and cook eggs; NVQ 524 (1FPC6) Prepare and cook pulses; NVQ 525 (1FPC7) Prepare and cook vegetable protein; NVQ 527 (1FPC9) Prepare and cook grain

Cooking methods

Different foods can be cooked in different ways. We use different cooking methods to:

- make food easy to digest and safe to eat
- make food pleasant to eat, with an agreeable flavour
- give food a good texture – tender, slightly firm, crisp, depending on the food
- give variety to our menus and our diets.

The different methods also have specific purposes and advantages.

The following ways of cooking food are described in the sections below:

- boiling
- poaching
- steaming
- stewing/casseroling
- braising
- baking
- roasting
- pot roasting
- cooking with a tandoor
- grilling (griddling)
- frying (shallow and deep)
- microwave cooking.

Stock

Stock is an important component in several cooking methods. It is the basis of all meat sauces, soups and purées. There are three main types of stock:

1 white stock is a cooking liquor made from bones, vegetables and herbs
2 brown stock is the same as white stock except you brown the bones in a pan or in the oven before you add the rest of the ingredients
3 vegetable stock is made from vegetables and herbs, without any bones.

Stocks are important foundations in professional cookery (see Chapter 11).

Boiling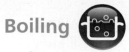

Definition

Boiling is when food is covered in water or stock, which is then heated up until the liquid starts to bubble vigorously. At this point it is boiling. Usually the heat is then turned down so that the liquid is just bubbling gently (also known as 'simmering').

Purpose

Boiling is a healthy method of cookery as it does not use any fat but when done properly will keep the flavour and nutritional value of the food.

Methods

There are two ways of boiling.

1 Place the food in boiling liquid. The liquid will stop boiling when you put the food in, so heat it up to bring it back to boiling. Then reduce the heat so that the liquid just bubbles gently (this is known as simmering) and boils the food.
2 Cover food with cold liquid. Heat it up and bring it to the boil, then reduce the heat to allow the food to simmer.

The effects of boiling

Gentle boiling helps to break down the tough fibres of certain foods. When boiling meats, some of the meat extracts dissolve in the cooking liquid.

Advantages of boiling

Older, tougher, cheaper joints of meat and poultry can be made more tasty and tender.

It is an economical way of cooking lots of food as it does not use too much fuel.

Nutritious, well-flavoured meat and vegetable stock can be produced from the cooking liquor.

It is labour saving, as boiling food does not need much attention from the cook.

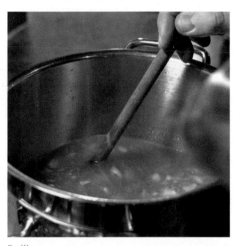

Boiling

Temperature and time control

The temperature must be controlled so that the liquid is brought to the boil and then adjusted so that it goes to a gentle boil (simmer) until the food is cooked.

Stocks, soups and sauces must only simmer.

Pasta should not be overcooked but left slightly firm (called *al dente*).

Meat and poultry should be well cooked and tender.

Vegetables should not be overcooked but left slightly crisp.

General rules

- Choose pans that are neither too small nor too large.
- When you put food into boiling liquid (e.g. when you cook green vegetables), make sure that there is enough liquid in the pot and that it is boiling before you add the food.

- When boiling meat, skim the surface of the liquid regularly during the cooking.
- You should simmer rather than boil vigorously whenever possible. This will mean that less water evaporates, so the amount of liquid will stay more or less the same and the food will not shrink too much.

⚠ Health and safety

It is important to think about health and safety when you work with large amounts of hot or boiling water. You must always be aware when there are large pots of hot water, and do everything possible to avoid any accidents.

When pots of boiling liquids are on stoves, make sure that the handles are turned in, so that sleeves and hands do not catch them.

When you place food into boiling water, you should lower them into the water gently to prevent splashing and scalding.

Ensure that the cooking pot is large enough for the water to cover the food without spilling over the edge once the water starts to boil. This will reduce the risk of being splashed by boiling water.

When removing the lid from the cooking pot, tilt it away from your face to allow the steam to escape safely. If you open it towards you the hot steam may burn your face.

RECIPE

1 Spicy parsnip soup

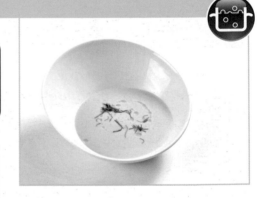

Get ready to cook
1 Wash, peel and slice the vegetables.
2 Prepare a bouquet garni.

It is important to learn the strength of garam masala. The final flavour of the spices should be gentle.

INGREDIENTS	4 portions	10 portions
Butter, margarine or oil	50 g	125 g
Onion or white leek slices	50 g	125 g
Celery	50 g	125 g
Parsnips, washed, peeled and sliced	200 g	500 g
Garam masala	¼ tsp	½ tsp
Flour	50 g	125 g
White stock or water	1 litre	2½ litres
Bouquet garni		
Salt		

Cooking
1 Melt the fat in a thick-bottomed pan.
2 Add all the vegetables and the garam masala and cover pan with a lid.

Allow them to cook gently without colouring, stirring frequently until they are soft.

3 Mix in the flour and cook slowly for 4–5 minutes, stirring frequently without allowing the flour to colour.

4 Remove from the heat and allow to cool for 3–4 minutes.

5 Gradually add the hot stock, stirring continuously over a medium heat until it boils.

6 Add the bouquet garni and season lightly with salt.

7 Simmer for 30–45 minutes, skimming when necessary.

8 Remove from the heat.

9 Taste and correct the seasoning, then taste again to check.

10 Remove the bouquet garni and carefully liquidise the soup.

11 Pass the liquid through a medium strainer (chinois).

12 Return the soup to a clean pan and reheat it.

13 Correct the consistency, which should be like single cream.

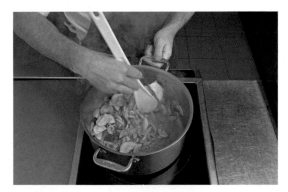
Gently cooking the vegetables

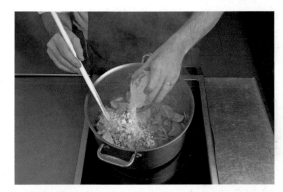
Adding the flour

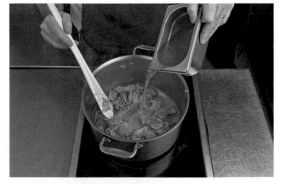
Adding the stock

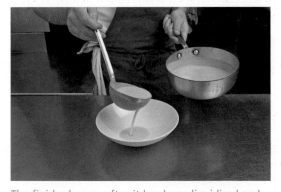
The finished soup, after it has been liquidised and strained

Poaching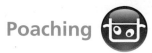

Definition

Poaching is when food in cooked in a liquid that is very hot but not boiling. It should be just below boiling point.

Poaching media

A poaching medium is the liquid in which the food is cooked. Media is the plural of medium. Several different media can be used, depending on the food.

- **Water**: eggs are usually poached in water with a little vinegar added. Fruit is poached in water with sugar.

- **Milk**: fish fillets, such as smoked haddock, may be poached in milk.
- **Stock**: some foods may be poached in stock. The stock should be suited to the food. For example, fish fillets can be poached in fish stock and chicken breast fillets in chicken stock. You can also poach poultry and fish in a rich vegetable stock.
- **Wine**: some fruit, such as pears, may be poached in wine.

Sometimes a tasty sauce can be made with the cooking liquid, e.g. a parsley or other sauce can be made from the milk in which fish is poached.

Purpose

The purpose of poaching is to cook food so that it is:

- very tender and easy to eat
- very easy to digest.

Methods

For most foods, heat the poaching liquid first. When it reaches the right temperature, lower the prepared food into the barely simmering liquid and allow it to cook in the gentle heat.

There are two ways of poaching: shallow and deep.

Shallow poaching – cook the food, such as cuts of fish and chicken, in only a small amount of liquid (water, stock, milk or wine) and cover it with greased greaseproof paper. Never allow the liquid to boil – keep it at a temperature as near to boiling as possible without actually boiling. To prevent the liquid from boiling, bring it to the boil on top of the stove, then take it off the direct heat, then place the food in the water and complete the cooking in a moderately hot oven, approximately 180°C.

Deep poaching – cook eggs in approximately 8 cm of gently simmering water. (When eggs are cooked in individual shallow metal pans over boiling water this is actually steaming rather than poaching.) You can also deep poach whole fish (e.g. salmon), slices of fish on the bone (e.g. turbot), grilled cod and salmon, and whole chicken. All of these should be covered with the poaching liquid.

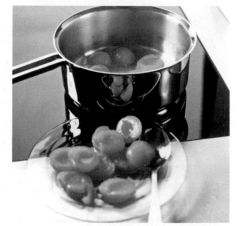

The effects of poaching

Poaching helps to tenderise the food, keep it moist and improve the texture.

Temperature and time control

The temperature must be controlled so that the cooking liquid does not become too cool or too hot. Poaching is cooking at just below simmering point.

Poaching

It is important to time the cooking correctly so that food is neither undercooked nor overcooked. If it is undercooked it will not be pleasant to eat and can sometimes be dangerous (e.g. undercooked chicken). If it is overcooked it will break up and lose some of its nutrients.

The time and temperature needed to cook the food correctly will vary slightly for different types of food.

⚠ *Health and safety*

Although poaching liquids are not quite as dangerous as boiling liquids, they are still very hot and can cause serious burns or scalds. So, as with boiling liquids, you need to be aware of pans of hot liquids.

Make sure that handles cannot be caught on sleeves or passing hands.

When you lower food into the poaching liquid, you should do so carefully to prevent splashes that can cause burns and scalds.

RECIPE

2 Poached salmon

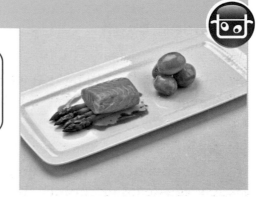

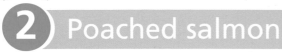

Get ready to cook

1 Wash and dry the fish fillets.
2 Grease an ovenproof dish with butter.

INGREDIENTS	4 portions	10 portions
Salmon fillets (100–150 g each)	4	10
Butter or margarine	25 g	60 g
Fish stock	Sufficient to come halfway up the fish – this will depend on the size and type of cooking vessel	
Salt		

Cooking

1 Arrange the washed and dried fish fillets in the ovenproof dish and season lightly.
2 Add sufficient fish stock to come halfway up the fish.
3 Cover with buttered greaseproof paper.
4 Cook in a moderate oven at 170°C for approximately 10 minutes. The cooking time will vary according to the thickness of the fillets. Fish should *not* be overcooked.
5 When cooked, remove the fillets, drain well, and keep warm and covered with greaseproof paper.
6 Strain off the cooking liquor into a small pan. Place on a hot stove and allow to reduce by half. Strain.

Serving suggestion

Serve with a little of the cooking liquid spooned over the fish.

Try something different

- Enrich the cooking liquid to give a light sauce. When the cooking liquid has been reduced, gradually add 25 g of softened butter, mixing well until combined. Taste and correct seasoning.
- Add chopped fresh herbs to the sauce, e.g. chives, parsley, dill or fennel.
- When the salmon is prepared for cooking, sprinkle a few finely cut slices of white

button mushrooms on the top before covering with the buttered greaseproof paper. When the fish is finally presented for serving, add a light sprinkle of freshly chopped parsley.

Activity

In groups, prepare, cook and serve five variations of poached salmon. Then taste, assess and discuss the findings.

Steaming

Definition

Steaming is another method of cooking using moist heat. Food is cooked under pressure in the steam produced by a boiling liquid (rather than placing the food itself in the boiling liquid).

Purpose

- The purpose of steaming food is to cook it so as to keep it as nutritious as possible (steaming keeps most of the nutrients in the food).
- Also, because the steaming process is gentle, it prevents the food from becoming too saturated with water.

Methods

There are four main methods of steaming.

1 **Atmospheric steaming** – steam is produced by placing water in the bottom of a saucepan and bringing it to a rapid boil. Food is placed in a container above the boiling water. The steam from the boiling water heats the container and cooks the food inside it.

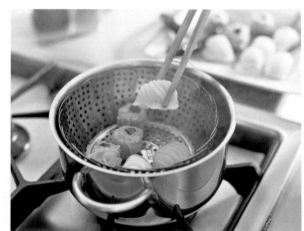

Steaming

2 **High-pressure steaming** – this is done in high-pressure steamers, such as pressure cookers. The high pressure in the steamer produces higher temperatures and forces steam through the food, which makes the food cook faster.

3 **Low-pressure steaming** – because the pressure is lower in these steamers the steam is also at a lower temperature, so the food cooks more slowly and gently.

4 **Combination steaming** – this is done in a combination ('combi') oven. This combines dry heat and steam in the oven, which helps to add a little moisture to the food as it cooks.

The effects of steaming

When food is steamed its texture is changed and it becomes edible. The texture will vary according to the type of food, type of steamer and level of heat. Sponges and puddings are lighter in texture if steamed rather than baked.

Note: Meat and sweet pudding basins must be greased. Once they have been filled they must be covered with greased greaseproof or silicone paper and foil to prevent moisture getting in and making the pudding soggy.

Advantages of steaming

The food keeps more of its nutritional value (retains its goodness).

It makes some foods lighter and easy to digest so, for example, it is a good way of cooking for people who are ill.

Low-pressure steaming reduces the risk of overcooking, which can cause food to go soft and fall apart.

High-pressure steaming enables food to be cooked or reheated quickly.

Like boiling, it is labour saving and suitable for cooking large quantities of food at one time, for example in schools and hospitals.

High-pressure steamers are also used for 'batch' cooking, where small quantities of vegetables are cooked frequently throughout the service. This means the vegetables are always freshly cooked, so they keep their colour, flavour and nutritional content.

The natural juices that result from steaming fish can be served with the fish or used to make the accompanying sauce.

Steaming uses a low heat, and a multi-tiered steamer (where several containers are placed one on top of the other in the steamer) can be used, making it economical on fuel.

Temperature and time control

When using steamers, timing and temperature is very important to make sure that the food is not undercooked. Food cooks much faster in high-pressure steamers and so there is a great danger of the food overcooking very quickly. When you are using a high-pressure steamer, wait until the pressure gauge shows that it has reached the correct pressure, then open the door very carefully to allow the steam to escape before you place the food in the steamer. This way you will be sure that the necessary cooking temperature has been reached.

⚠ Health and safety

Boiling water is used in the bottom of steamers, so the same rules of safety apply to steaming as to boiling. The steam in steamers can be very dangerous as it is extremely hot and can cause serious burns and scalds.
To avoid injuring yourself:

- make sure you know how to use steamers
- use them with great care
- check the pressure in high-pressure steamers continually
- allow the pressure to return to the correct level before opening doors or removing pressure-cooker lids

- allow time for the pressure to return to normal before opening commercial steamers; then stand well away from the door as you open it, to avoid the full impact of the escaping steam.

RECIPE

③ Plain steamed rice

INGREDIENTS	4 portions	10 portions
Basmati rice, dry weight	100 g	250 g

Cooking

1 Wash the rice and place in a saucepan.
2 Add sufficient cold water for the water level to be 2½ cm above the rice.
3 Bring to the boil over a fierce heat until most of the water has evaporated.
4 Turn down the heat as low as possible. Cover the pan with a lid and allow the rice to complete cooking in the steam.
5 Once cooked, the rice should be allowed to stand in the covered pan for 10 minutes.

Stewing/casseroling

Definition

Stewing and casseroling are slow, gentle, moist-heat methods of cooking in which the food is completely covered by a liquid. Both the food and the sauce are served together. Stews are cooked on top of the stove. Casseroles are stews cooked in the oven.

Purpose

The purpose of stewing is to:

- cook cheaper cuts of meat and poultry in a way that makes them tender and palatable
- keep many of the nutrients from the food, which go into the cooking liquid
- give a rich flavour to the food.

Methods

Stews can be cooked on a hob or in an oven.

1 When cooked on a hob, meat and vegetables are placed in a saucepan and covered with liquid (water or stock). The liquid is brought to the boil then turned down to a low simmer. A lid is placed on the pan and the food is left to cook slowly.
2 A stew may also be cooked in the oven, when it is referred to as a casserole. The term 'casserole' refers to both the baking dish and the ingredients it contains. Casserole dishes are usually deep, round, ovenproof dishes with handles and a tight-fitting lid. They can be made of glass, metal, ceramic or any other heatproof material.

Both are slow, moist methods of cooking.

The effects of stewing

In the slow process of cooking in gentle heat, the connective tissue in meat and poultry is changed into gelatine so that the fibres fall apart easily and become tender. Less liquid is used for stewing than for boiling, and the cooking temperature is slightly lower. See 'The effects of boiling' (page 101) as these also apply to stewing.

Advantages of stewing

Stewing can make cheaper, tougher cuts of meat and poultry tender and palatable, so it is an economical method of cooking. The tougher cuts of meat often have more flavour than more tender cuts of meat, which tend to dry out in stews due to the long cooking times.

If stews and casseroles are cooked correctly, very little liquid will evaporate, leaving plenty of sauce to serve up as part of the stew.

The meat and vegetable juices that escape from the food during cooking stay in the liquid. This means that any vitamins and minerals are not lost, but are served up in the tasty and nutritious sauce.

Usually, everything in a stew can be eaten, so there is very little waste. Also, because it is a gentle cooking method the food does not shrink much and keeps its flavour.

Stews reheat easily.

Stews and casseroles are labour saving because foods can be cooked in bulk and do not need to be monitored too closely.

Temperature and time control

Good stews are cooked slowly, so it is important to control the temperature properly. The liquid must barely simmer.

Use a tight-fitting lid to keep in the steam. This helps to keep the temperature correct and reduces evaporation.

General rules

All stews should have a thickened consistency. This comes from thickening agents.

Unpassed ingredients can cause thickening. For example, in stews such as Irish stew all the vegetables are left in the stew and help to make it the right consistency.

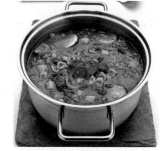

Stewing/casseroling

Flour can be added to the sauce, for brown lamb stew (navarin), for example.

Egg yolks and cream can also be used to thicken white stews, such as blanquette.

However, stews should not be over-thickened and the sauce should stay light.

Make sure you use the correct amount of thickening agents.

Adjust the consistency during cooking if necessary by adding more liquid or more thickening agent.

Do not overcook stews as this:

- causes too much liquid to evaporate
- causes the food to break up
- causes the food to lose its colour
- spoils the flavour and makes the food feel dry when it is eaten.

⚠ *Health and safety*

Stews must simmer continually as they cook, so they become very hot. You will need to stir stews regularly, so you are more likely to burn or scald yourself.

Place large stews on stovetops carefully, to avoid splashes and spills.

When you lift the lid from a pan, lift it away from you to avoid burning yourself on the steam.

When using Bratt pans, take care when stirring the large quantity of hot, semi-liquid food.

RECIPE

4 Beef goulash (Hungarian)

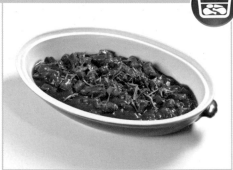

Get ready to cook
1 Trim the meat and cut it into 2 cm square pieces.
2 Peel and chop the onions.

INGREDIENTS	4 portions	10 portions
Lard or oil	35 g	100 g
Prepared stewing beef	400 g	1¼ kg
Salt		
Onions, chopped	100 g	250 g
Paprika	10–25 g	25–60 g
Flour	25 g	60 g
Tomato purée	25 g	60 g
Stock or water	750 ml	2 litres

Cooking

1 Heat the fat in a thick-bottomed pan, season the meat lightly with salt and quickly fry it until lightly coloured.
2 Add the onions, cover with a lid and cook gently for 3–4 minutes until the onions are soft.
3 Mix in the paprika and flour using a wooden or heat-proof plastic spoon.
4 Allow to cook out on top of the stove or in an oven for 2–3 minutes.
5 Mix in the tomato purée and then gradually add the stock, mixing well.
6 Bring to the boil, skim, taste, correct seasoning and cover.
7 Simmer, preferably in the oven at 110°C, for approximately 1½–2 hours, or until the meat is tender.
8 Skim, taste and correct the seasoning again.

Try something different

Add a little cream or yoghurt at the last moment.

Braising

Definition

Braising is a moist-heat method of cooking larger pieces of food. The food is only half covered with liquid, and can be cooked on the stovetop or in the oven. The food is cooked very slowly in a pan with a tightly fitted lid, using very low temperatures. A combination of steaming and stewing cooks the food. Food is usually cooked in very large pieces and carved before serving.

Purpose

The purpose of braising food is to enhance the flavour and texture.

Methods

Whole joints of meat, whole chickens and game (meat or fowl) can all be braised, as can vegetables. Tougher cuts of meat and other foods can also be braised.
There are two methods of braising: brown braising and white braising.

1 Brown braising is used, for example, for joints and portion-sized cuts of meat.
2 White braising is used, for example, for vegetables. The first thing you should do is to blanch the vegetables, then place in a braising pan with mirepoix and white stock.

For both methods, the liquid used for braising is usually a stock, but it may also be water, wine or beer.

Once you have added the liquid, place a heavy, tight-fitting lid on the cooking pan. The lid keeps the moisture in the pan and around the food, and creates steam. This prevents the food from becoming dry and tough.

The effects of braising

Braising breaks down the tissue fibre in certain foods, which softens them and makes them tender and edible. Cooking them in the braising liquid also improves the texture.

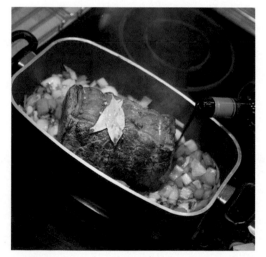

Braising

Advantages

Tougher, less expensive meats and poultry can be used.

Maximum flavour and nutritional value are retained.

Temperature and time control

It is essential to cook the food slowly. The liquid must barely simmer.

Use a tight-fitting lid to reduce evaporation and maintain the temperature.

The time needed for braising will vary according to the quality of the food.

The ideal oven temperature for braising is 160°C.

General rules

These are the same as for stewing. However, if the joint is to be served whole, you should remove the lid three-quarters of the way through cooking. Then baste the joint frequently to protect it from burning and glaze it – this makes it look attractive when it is served.

⚠ *Health and safety*

During cooking, the contents of the braising pan become extremely hot.

- Use heavy oven cloths whenever you remove the pot from the oven or lift the lid.
- When you lift the lid from the pan, lift it away from you to avoid burning yourself on the steam.
- The contents can become extremely hot, so take great care to prevent splashing when you stir them.

RECIPE

(5) Braised mushrooms 'East–West'

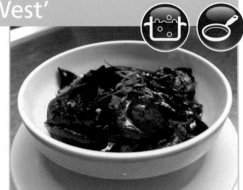

Get ready to cook

1 Place the ceps in a bowl, cover them with hot water and leave to soak for 30 minutes.
2 Squeeze the water out and cut them into wide strips. Set aside.
3 Peel and finely chop the ginger and shallots.
4 Clean and slice the button mushrooms.

Ceps are a type of wild mushroom.

Black Chinese mushrooms are a type of mushroom used in oriental cooking.

INGREDIENTS	4 portions	10 portions
Olive oil	2 tbsp	5 tbsp
Shallots, finely chopped	4	10
Fresh young ginger, finely chopped	3 cm	7 cm
Dried ceps (mushrooms)	50 g	125 g
Black Chinese mushrooms	50 g	125 g
White button mushrooms, cleaned and sliced	400 g	1 kg
Light soy sauce	2 tbsp	5 tbsp
Chives, chopped	2 tbsp	5 tbsp
Chicken or vegetable stock	120 ml	300 ml
Freshly ground black peppercorn to taste		

Cooking

1 Heat the olive oil in a medium-sized frying pan. Add the shallots and ginger, and then all the mushrooms and sauté for 3 minutes.
2 Add in the soy sauce, chives and stock. Cook over a medium heat for a further 10 minutes to completely reduce the liquid.
3 Season with pepper to taste. There is no need to add salt, because the soy sauce is salty.

Baking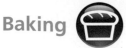

Definition

Baking is cooking food with dry heat in an oven. Although the food is cooked in a dry oven, steam plays a big part in this method of cookery.

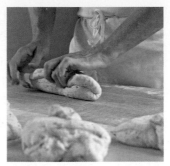
Baking

Purpose

The purpose of baking is to:

- create visual appeal through colour and texture
- produce tasty food that is enjoyable to eat.

Methods

There are three methods of baking.

1 **Dry baking** – this is done in a dry oven. The water that is already naturally in the food turns to steam when it is heated. This steam combines with the dry heat of the oven to cook the food (e.g. cakes, pastry, baked jacket potatoes).

2 **Baking with increased humidity** – certain foods, such as bread, need to be baked with increased humidity. To do this, place a bowl of water in the oven or inject steam into the oven (there will be a switch on the oven you can use to do this). The humidity of the air (the moisture in it) is increased, which in turn increases the water content of the food, keeping it moist and good to eat.

3 **Baking with modified heat** – food such as baked egg custard requires the heat in the oven to be modified (reduced). To do this, place the food in a bain-marie (tray of water). This makes the food cook more slowly and means that it does not overheat. In the case of egg custard, it also means that the egg mixture is less likely to overcook: if it overcooked it would be spoiled and could not be eaten.

Always preheat ovens prior to baking.

The effects of baking

Heating certain ingredients, such as yeast and baking powder, changes the raw structure of many foods (e.g. pastry, cakes) to an edible texture. However, there are many different ingredients, methods of mixing and types of product, so the effects of baking can also be very different.

Advantages of baking

A wide variety of sweet and savoury foods can be produced.

Bakery products make appetising goods with visual appeal and mouth-watering aromas.

Baked goods can be produced in bulk, all cooked for the same amount of time and all coming out the same colour.

Baking ovens have effective manual or automatic temperature controls.

There is straightforward access for loading and removing items from baking ovens.

Temperature and time control

Always preheat ovens to the required temperature before putting the food in. In general-purpose ovens, the top part of the oven is the hottest, so you will need to think about where you place the shelves. In convection ovens, the temperature is the same in all parts of the oven, so you can place the shelves anywhere.

Accurate timing and temperature control are essential to good baking. Make sure the oven reaches the required temperature before each additional batch of goods is placed in the oven. The time between taking out one batch of goods and putting in the next is known as 'recovery time'.

General rules

Always preheat ovens to the required cooking temperature, otherwise the product will be spoiled.

Be accurate in your weighing and measuring, and in your control of the oven temperature.

Prepare trays and moulds correctly.

Avoid opening oven doors whenever possible. Draughts may affect the quality of the product, and the oven temperature will drop. Opening the oven door too quickly may also adversely affect the presentation of products such as Yorkshire puddings and soufflés.

Utilise oven space effectively.

Avoid jarring products (particularly fruit cakes, sponges and soufflés) before and during baking, as the quality may be affected.

Keep baking trays level in the oven so that the product bakes evenly.

⚠ Health and safety

- Use thick, dry oven cloths when removing trays from the oven.
- Do not overload trays.
- Do not open oven doors too quickly as there is likely to be a lot of steam, which may burn your face.

RECIPE

6 Baked rice pudding

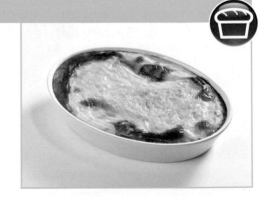

INGREDIENTS	4 portions	10 portions
Rice, short grain	50 g	125 g
Caster sugar	50 g	125 g
Milk, whole or skimmed	½ litre	1½ litres
Butter	12 g	30 g
Vanilla essence	2–3 drops	6–8 drops
Nutmeg, grated		

Cooking

1 Wash the rice and place it in a pie dish.
2 Add the sugar and milk and mix well.
3 Add the butter, vanilla essence and the nutmeg.
4 Place the dish on a baking sheet. Clean any milk from the rim of the pie dish.
5 Bake at 180–200°C until the milk starts to simmer.
6 Reduce the heat to 150°C and allow the pudding to cook slowly for 1½–2 hours.

Roasting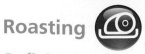

Definition

Roasting is cooking in dry heat in an oven or on a spit, with the aid of fat or oil.

Purpose

Roasting creates a distinctive taste and provides interesting variety to the menu.

Methods

Always preheat the oven before roasting.

There are two main methods of roasting food.

1 **Roasting on a spit** – this roasts meat using radiated heat. Place prepared meat or poultry on a rotating spit over or in front of fierce radiated heat.
2 **Roasting in an oven** – this roasts the food using applied dry heat, forced-air convected heat or convected heat combined with microwave energy.

During the cooking process, baste the product regularly with the cooking medium (fat or oil), and any other juices that come out of the product. This will help to keep the food moist. The basting liquid will also caramelise the surface of the product, which will enhance both the flavour and the visual appeal of the dish.

The effects of roasting

The initial heat of the oven seals the food. This prevents too many natural juices from escaping. Once the food is lightly browned, reduce the oven temperature (or the temperature of the heat source when spit roasting) to cook the inside of the food without hardening the surface.

Advantages

Good-quality meat and poultry is tender and succulent when roasted.

Meat juices from the joint can be used for gravy and to enhance flavour.

Both energy (the amount of gas or electricity used) and oven temperature can be controlled easily. You can cook different foods in the oven together, saving fuel.

Ovens with transparent doors allow you to check what is happening in the oven.

You have easy access to the food so it is straightforward to reach it, move it around and remove it from the oven.

With spit roasting, you can see exactly how the cooking is progressing and you have easy access to the food.

There is minimal fire risk because a thermostat is used to control the temperature so there is no risk of overheating.

Temperature and time control

Always preheat ovens to the required cooking temperature.

Always follow the oven temperature and shelf settings given in recipes.

The cooking time will be affected by the shape, size, type, bone proportion and quality of the food you are cooking.

Meat thermometers or probes can be inserted to determine the exact temperature in the centre of the joint.

⚠ *Health and safety*

- Use thick, dry oven cloths when removing trays from the oven.
- Do not overload trays.
- Do not open oven doors too quickly as there is likely to be a lot of steam, which may burn your face.
- Take care when removing the product from the oven as a joint, say, may have released a lot of fat that could cause burns or scalds.
- When basting the product, try to avoid splashing hot fat.

Meat carving tips

Images and text courtesy of Donald Russell, www.donaldrussell.com

Good carving comes with experience, knowledge and the right equipment. But most importantly, your joint should be allowed to rest for at least 15 minutes beforehand, as this will allow the joint to 'set', making it easier to carve.

Bone-in-joints: Hold the joint at the end of the bone, using a towel or kitchen paper for a firmer grip if necessary. Carve the meat away from the bone, into approximately 1 cm thick slices.

Boneless joints (e.g. short saddle of lamb): Hold the joint in place with a carving fork or tongs. Carve the meat across the grain into slices approximately ½ cm thick.

Racks and rib roasts: Hold the meat with the bones facing upward, using a towel or kitchen paper for a firmer grip if necessary. Carve down between the bones into even-sized cutlets. Or remove the bones completely by cutting along the bones through the meat. This will enable you to carve the roast into thin slices.

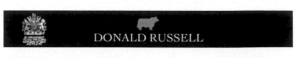

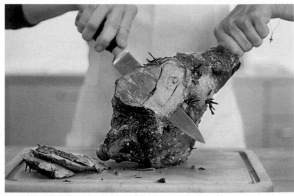

Carving a bone-in joint

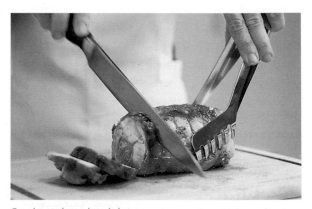

Carving a boneless joint

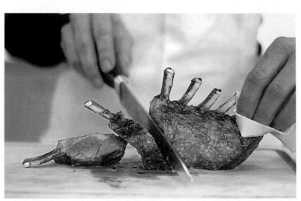

Carving a rack

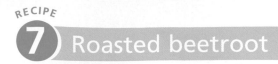 7 Roasted beetroot

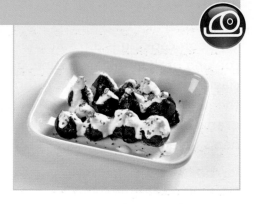

Get ready to cook

1 Trim and thoroughly wash the beetroot (but do not peel it). Dry well.
2 Preheat the oven to 200°C.

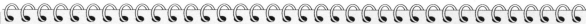

It is not necessary to peel the beetroots. If peeled they will lose colour (bleed).

INGREDIENTS	4 portions	10 portions
Small young beetroot	4	10
Olive oil	2 tbsp	5 tbsp
Grated horseradish	2 tbsp	5 tbsp
Crème fraiche	150 ml	375 ml
Chives, finely chopped	1 tbsp	2½ tbsp

Cooking

1 Place the washed beetroot in a roasting tray and sprinkle with olive oil.
2 Roast at 200°C for approximately 1½ hours until cooked.
3 Mix the horseradish in the crème fraiche.

Serving suggestion

● When the beetroot is cooked, place on a serving dish. Cut a criss-cross in the top, to halfway through.
● Spoon some crème fraîche onto each beetroot and sprinkle with chopped chives.

Try something different

You can use natural yoghurt or half-whipped cream as alternatives to crème fraiche.

Pot roasting

Definition

Pot roasting (poêlé) is cooking on a bed of root vegetables in a covered pan. This method retains the maximum flavour of all the ingredients.

Method

Place the meat on a bed of roots and herbs, coat generously with clarified butter or oil, cover with a lid and cook in an oven.

General rules

Select pans that are just the right size – neither too large nor too small.
Add the vegetables and herbs to a good stock to use as a base for the sauce.

Methods of cookery

Tandoori cooking

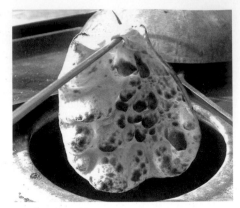

Tandoori cooking

Definition

Tandoori cooking is a traditional method of cooking used in Indian cuisine. It uses dry heat in a clay oven called a tandoor. Although the source of the heat is at the base of the oven, the heat is evenly distributed in the oven because the clay heats up and radiates heat evenly.

Purpose

Tandoori cooking giving a distinctive flavour and texture to the food.

Method

- Meat (small cuts and small joints), poultry (small cuts and whole chickens) and fish, such as prawns, are usually placed vertically in the oven.
- No fat or oil is used.
- The food is cooked quickly and the flavour is similar to that of barbecued food.
- Oven temperatures reach 375°C.
- Depending on the type, food may be marinated for 20 minutes to two hours before being cooked and, in some cases, may be brushed with the marinade during cooking.
- Depending on the spices used, the colour of the food may change. A red colour agent is used in some marinades, plus onions, garlic, herbs, spices and oil, wine or lemon juice.

Advantages

Tandoori-cooked food has a distinctive flavour that comes from both the marinade and the cooking process.

Marinating tenderises and also adds flavour to foods.

Grilling (griddling)

Definition

This is a fast method of cooking using radiant heat. It is sometimes known as broiling.

Method

Grilled foods can be cooked over heat (charcoal, barbecues, gas or electric heated grills/griddles), under heat (gas or electric salamanders, over-heated grills) or between heat (electrically heated grill bars or plates).

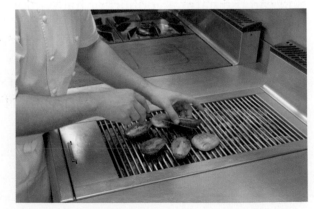

Grilling (griddling)

- **Grilling over heat** – preheat grill bars and brush with oil prior to use, otherwise food will stick to them. The bars should char the food on both sides to give the distinctive appearance and flavour of grilling. Barbecuing is a type of grilling over heat.

- **Grilling under heat/salamander** – preheat salamanders (sometimes called over-heated grills) and grease the bars. Steaks, chops and items that are likely to slip between the grill bars of an under-heated grill may be cooked under a salamander.
- **Grilling between heat** – this is grilling between electrically heated grill bars or plates, and is used for small cuts of meat.

Effects of grilling

The food keeps most of its nutrients and flavour because it is cooked so quickly. When grilling meat, the fierce heat seals the surface of the meat, helping to keep the juices in the meat. Grilled meats lose less of their juices than meat cooked any other way, as long as they are not pierced by a fork while they are cooking. Grilling is only suitable for certain cuts of best-quality meat – inferior meat cooked this way will be tough and inedible.

Advantages

The speed of grilling means that food can be cooked quickly to order.

Charring foods gives a distinctive appearance and improves the flavour.

You have good control of the cooking process because the food is visible and accessible while it is being grilled.

Grills may be situated in view of customers, which means that they can see the food cooking, which adds to the entertainment in a restaurant.

General rules

Smaller, thinner items should be cooked very quickly.

Seal and colour food on the hot part of the grill, then move to a cooler part to complete cooking.

Do not grill foods for too long. Cooking the food slowly will dry it out.

Basting of food and oiling of bars will help to prevent the food from drying out and sticking to the grill.

⚠ Health and safety

- Use tongs to turn and lift cutlets and steaks.
- Use fish slices to turn and lift tomatoes, mushrooms and whole or cut fish.
- When reaching over to, say, turn a steak at the back of the grill, be careful of the heat coming up from underneath, which may burn your forearm. (This is a good reason to wear a jacket with long sleeves.)
- If meat or fish has been marinating in an oil marinade, ensure that it is well drained before you place it on the grill. Food with too much oil on it may be a fire hazard if it is moved directly from the marinating container to the grill.

8 Grilled sardines

Get ready to cook

Prepare, clean, wash and thoroughly dry the fish.

INGREDIENTS
Sardines, three or four per portion depending on their size
Flour
Light oil

1 Pass the fish through flour, shake off surplus and place on an oiled baking sheet.

2 Brush the tops with oil and cook carefully under a hot grill, ensuring they do not burn.

3 After 2–3 minutes, remove the tray and turn the sardines with a palette knife. Return to the grill and cook for 2 minutes, until lightly browned.

Serving suggestion

Serve with quarters of lemon (pips removed).

Shallow frying

Definition

Shallow frying is cooking food in a small quantity of pre-heated fat or oil in a shallow pan (a frying pan or a sauté pan) or on a flat surface (a griddle plate).

Purpose

The purpose of shallow frying is to brown food, giving it a different colour and an interesting and attractive flavour.

Methods

There are four methods of shallow frying: shallow frying, sautéing, griddling and stir-frying.

To **shallow fry**, cook the food in a small amount of fat or oil in a frying pan or sauté pan. Fry the presentation side of the food first (the side that will be seen when it is on the plate). The side that is fried first will have the better appearance because the fat is clean. Then turn the food to cook and colour the other side.

To **sauté** tender cuts of meat and poultry, cook them in a sauté pan or frying pan in the same way as for shallow frying.

To **griddle** foods such as hamburgers, sausages and sliced onions, place them on a lightly oiled, pre-heated griddle (a solid metal plate). Turn them frequently during cooking. Pancakes can also be cooked this way but should be turned only once.

Stir-fry vegetables, strips of fish, meat and poultry in a wok or frying pan by fast frying them in a little fat or oil.

If shallow-fried food needs to be cooked in butter, you should use clarified butter. This is because clarified butter has a higher burning point than unclarified butter, so it will not burn as easily. To clarify butter, melt it and then carefully strain off the fat, leaving behind the clear liquid.

Effects of shallow frying

The high temperature used in shallow frying seals the surface of the food almost instantly and prevents the natural juices from escaping. Some of the frying medium (oil or butter) will be absorbed by the food, which will change its nutritional content (in other words, will make it more fatty).

Advantages

Shallow frying is a quick method of cooking prime cuts of meat and poultry because suitable fats or oils can be heated to a high temperature without burning.
As the food is in direct contact with the fat, it cooks rapidly.

Temperature and time control

This is particularly important, as all shallow-fried foods should have an appetising golden-brown colour on both sides. This can be achieved only by carefully controlling the temperature, which should initially be hot. The heat should then be reduced and the food turned when necessary.

General rules

When shallow-frying continuously over a busy period, prepare and cook the food in a systematic way.

Clean the pans after every use.

⚠ Health and safety

Select the correct type and size of pan. If it is too small, the food, such as fish, will not brown evenly and may break up. If it is too large the areas of the pan not covered by food will burn and spoil the flavour of the food.

Always keep your sleeves rolled down to prevent splashing fat from burning your forearms.

Add food to the pan carefully, away from you, to avoid being splashed by hot fat.

Use a thick, clean, dry cloth when handling pans.

Move pans carefully in case they jar and tip fat on to the stove.

RECIPE

9 Sautéed pork medallions

Get ready to cook
You can cut pork medallions from the pork fillet by cutting it into 2 cm slices.

INGREDIENTS
Pork loins
Oil

You can buy medallions ready prepared, or you can prepare them from a fillet as described above.

Cooking

1 Heat the oil in a suitable frying or sauté pan.
2 Sauté the medallions on both sides to a light golden brown.

Serving suggestion

These can be served with a variety of sauces and garnishes, e.g. sliced red onion lightly softened or a thickened roast gravy with thinly sliced gherkins.

Try something different

Pork chops or medallions can also be fried in a thick-bottomed pan and served with a sauce made from four parts apple purée and one part cream or natural yoghurt.

Deep frying

Definition

Deep frying is cooking small tender pieces of food, which are totally immersed in hot fat or oil, and cooked quickly. The heat of the oil penetrates the food and cooks it. Although oils and lards are 'wet', deep frying is classified as a dry method of cookery. This is because it has a drying effect on the food.

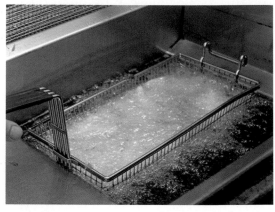

Deep frying

Methods

When we think of deep-fried foods, we tend to think first of fish and chips, which are probably the most popular kind of fried food. However, many things can be deep fried, such as morsels of lean meats, chicken fillets, whole or filleted fish, cheese and vegetables.

Most deep-fried foods need to be coated in a batter to protect them from the effects of the extremely high temperature of the fat or oil. Conventional deep-fried foods, with the exception of potatoes, are coated with either milk, flour, egg and crumbs, batter or pastry to:

- protect the surface of the food from intense heat
- prevent moisture and nutrients escaping
- modify (slow down) the penetration of the intense heat.

To deep fry:

- pre-heat the oil or fat
- once it has reached the required temperature, place the food carefully into the oil or fat
- fry it until it is cooked and golden brown
- drain the food well before serving.

Partially cooking food before deep frying is known as blanching. This method may be used with chipped potatoes. The food is partly cooked (usually by boiling) in advance of service and then finished by deep frying to order. This works particularly well with certain types of potato, where it gives the chips a floury texture inside and a crisp exterior.

Purpose

The purpose of deep frying is to produce food with an appetising golden-brown colour, which is crisp and enjoyable eat.

The effects of deep frying

Deep frying food coated with milk or egg seals the surface so that the food absorbs the minimum amount of fat.

Advantages

Blanching or partial cooking prior to deep frying enables certain foods (e.g. chips) to be prepared in advance and cooked later. This helps during a busy service and saves time.

Coating the food means that a wide variety of foods can be cooked in this way.

Foods can be cooked quickly and handled easily for service.

Coated foods are sealed quickly, preventing the enclosed food from becoming greasy.

Temperature and time control

When deep fat frying it is essential to maintain the fat at the right temperature.

When batches of food are being fried one after another, the temperature of the fat must be allowed to recover after one batch has been removed before the next batch is cooked. If the fat is not allowed to reheat sufficiently, the food will look pale and unappetising and will be soggy to eat. This is especially important if you are cooking food from frozen.

Timing is important too. If you are cooking thicker pieces of food, you should lower the temperature. This allows the food to cook thoroughly on the inside without burning on the outside.

The reverse is also true – the smaller the pieces of food, the hotter the frying temperature needs to be and the shorter the cooking time.

Types of oil used

A variety of oils and fats can be used for deep fat frying. Beef dripping was traditionally used for deep frying as it gives a good flavour. However, in recent years this has been replaced with vegetable oil, which is healthier. There are several varieties of vegetable oil:

- sunflower
- corn
- maize
- rapeseed
- olive.

Often a mix of vegetable oils is used.

Some establishments deep fry in goose fat. This has become popular because of the flavour it adds to the fried food, in particular chips.

General rules

Never over-fill fryers with fat or oil, or with the food to be cooked.

The normal frying temperature is between 175°C and 195°C. A slight heat haze will rise from the fat when it reaches this temperature.

Do not attempt to fry too much food at one time.

After removing a batch of food, allow the fat to heat up again before adding the next batch.

Ensure that you are using the right amount of fat for the amount of food you are cooking. If you cook too much food in too little fat, the amount of food will reduce the temperature drastically and spoil the food.

Reduce frying temperatures during slack periods to conserve fuel.

Do not fry the food too far in advance of serving it – fried foods soon lose their crispness.

Strain oil and fat after use to remove any food particles. If these are left in the fat they will burn when the fat is next heated, spoiling the appearance and flavour of the food.

Always cover oil or fat when not in use to prevent exposure to the air making it rancid.

⚠ Health and safety

Deep frying can be a very dangerous method of cooking, especially if those doing it are not correctly trained. Hot fat can cause serious burns, either through spills or accidents.

Commercial deep fryers have built-in safety features, such as thermostatic controls and fat-level indicators. These safety features make commercial fryers preferable to pots on stoves.

Always keep a close eye on a deep fryer and never leave it unattended.

Monitor the temperature – if it is too high, the fat may easily ignite and cause a fire.

Never allow fat to heat up so much that it starts to smoke. Smoke means that the oil is too hot. It will also give the food a bad taste.

Do not move a deep fryer that is either on or still hot.

Avoid sudden movements around deep fryers, as they may be bumped or items may be dropped into the hot fat.

Stand back when placing food into the fryer to avoid steam and splash burns.

Avoid putting your face, arms or hands over the deep fryer.

Before using a deep fryer, know how to put out a fat fire.

- Remember: oil and water do not mix, so do not try to put out a fat fire with water.
- To put out a fat fire, cover the pot or fryer with a lid or fire blanket.
- Then use the correct fire extinguisher and use it correctly. Fire-extinguishing equipment should be kept nearby and staff should be trained in how to use it.

RECIPE
10 Deep-fried chicken

Get ready to cook
1 Prepare the batter (page 199).
2 Mix together the flour and dried spices.
3 Heat the fat to 175°C.

INGREDIENTS
Chicken pieces of your choice, e.g. boneless cuts, suprêmes
Flour
Dried spices, e.g. paprika, Chinese five spice
Light batter (page 199)
Fat in deep fryer

Cooking

1 Coat the chicken pieces in (pass them through) the mixture of flour and spices.
2 Pass them through the batter.
3 Deep fry them at a temperature of 175°C.
4 Drain well and serve.

Microwave cooking

Definition

This is a method of cooking and reheating food using electromagnetic waves in a microwave oven powered by electricity.

Purpose

The purpose of microwaving is to:

- cook raw, prepared or pre-cooked foods quickly
- reheat food safely – all the food is heated at the same time
- defrost frozen food.

Advantages

Microwave ovens cook certain foods between 50 and 70 per cent faster than conventional ovens.

It is a quick way to reheat foods.

It is a fast method of defrosting foods.

It is economical in terms of electricity as less energy is required.

It is labour saving because there is less washing-up as food can be cooked in serving dishes.

Hot meals can be available 24 hours a day and offered on a completely self-service basis. This can increase consumer satisfaction and reduce costs.

Food is cooked in its own juices, so flavour and goodness are retained.

It minimises food shrinkage and drying out.

It can be used flexibly with conventional cooking methods.

Disadvantages

It is not suitable for all foods.

Limited oven space restricts its use to cooking small quantities of food.

Many microwave ovens do not brown food, although browning elements are available in certain models.

Microwaves can penetrate only 5 cm into food (from all sides), so the food will not cook evenly and parts of the food may not be cooked.

Points for special attention

It is essential to follow the manufacturer's instructions regarding cooking time.

You must remove certain foods from the microwave before the cooking is finished. The cooking finishes after they are removed, so standing time is important. For example, during this time fish turns from opaque to flaky and scrambled eggs turn creamy. Tender, crisp vegetables do not need to stand.

You must pierce the skin of baked potatoes and whole unpeeled apples in order to release pressure and prevent them from bursting.

Do not cook eggs in their shells or they will burst.

Cover foods when possible to reduce condensation inside the oven and prevent splashing. Microwave clingfilm is available for this purpose.

Factors that affect efficient cooking

Use suitable containers made of glass, china or plastic. Only use metal or foil if the instructions specify that the cooker can take metal without causing damage. For best results use straight-sided, round, shallow containers.

Even-shaped items cook uniformly; arrange uneven-shaped items with the thickest part to the outside of the dish.

Keep food as level as possible; do not pile it into mounds.

Allow sufficient space to stir or mix the food if necessary.

Turn dense foods such as corn on the cob during cooking, as they take longer to cook if they are not turned.

Foods with a higher water content cook faster than those that are drier.

⚠ *Safety*

Do not operate the oven when it is empty.

Remember to cover foods and pierce foods that are likely to burst.

Be sure always to follow the manufacturer's instructions.

Activity

1 What are the differences between poaching, boiling and steaming?

2 List three types of food, other than vegetables, that can be boiled

3 Name three liquids, other than water, that may be used for poaching.

4 What is high-pressure steaming? What safety measures are needed with this method?

5 What is the difference between baking and roasting?

6 Describe a salamander.

7 What is the difference between stewing and braising?

8 Name two meat dishes that would be stewed, and two that would be braised.

9 Why should food be coated before deep frying?

10 Name five types of oils or fats that can be used for deep frying.

CHAPTER 11

Stocks, soups and sauces

The skills covered in this chapter provide the foundation of all practical work for NVQ and VRQ.

Stock

Introduction

Stock is the base of soups, sauces, gravies, and many meat, poultry and fish dishes. Meat stock is made from the juices of meats, vegetables and herbs, extracted by long, gentle simmering with water. Chicken, fish and vegetable stocks do not have to be cooked for so long.

Key points to remember when making stocks

- Use only fresh bones and vegetables.
- Continually remove scum and fat from the surface of the stock as it cooks.
- Always simmer gently.
- Never add salt.
- If the stock is going to be kept, strain and cool it quickly then store it in a refrigerator.

Convenience stocks are available in chilled, frozen, powder and condensed forms. It is important to taste these to check that you are satisfied with their quality before using them.

RECIPE

1 Stock (white and brown)

Get ready to cook

1 Chop the bones into small pieces and remove any fat or marrow.
2 Wash and peel the vegetables. Leave them whole for white stock and chop them for brown stock.
3 Prepare a bunch of herbs (bouquet garni).

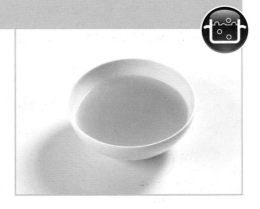

INGREDIENTS	To make 4½ litres	To make 10 litres
Raw, meaty bones, chopped into small pieces	1 kg	2½ kg
Water	5 litres	10½ litres
Onion, carrot, celery, leek (whole for white stock and chopped for brown stock)	400 g	1½ kg
Faggot of herbs (bouquet garni)		

127

Cooking white stock

1 Place the bones in a large pot, cover with cold water and bring to the boil.
2 As soon as the water comes to the boil, take pot to the sink and drain away the water.
3 Wash the bones and clean the pot.
4 Return the bones to the pot, cover them with water and bring them back to the boil again.
5 Reduce the heat so that the water is simmering gently.
6 Skim the surface to remove any scum as and when required. Also wipe round the top and inside of the pot.
7 After 2–3 hours add the vegetables and the faggot of herbs.
8 Simmer for 3–4 hours, skimming regularly.
9 When the cooking is finished, skim the stock again and strain it.

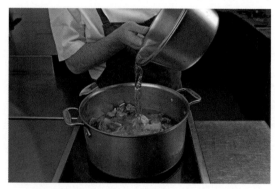

Covering the bones with water

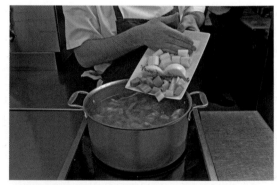

Adding vegetables and herbs

You can add the following to the brown stock:

● squashed tomatoes and washed mushroom trimmings

● a calf's foot and/or a knuckle of bacon.

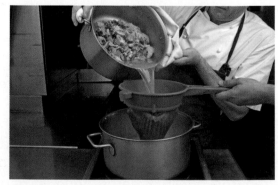

Straining the stock

Cooking brown stock

1 Brown the chopped bones well on all sides. You can do this by frying them in a little fat or oil in a frying pan, or by roasting them in a hot oven.
2 Strain off any fat and place the bones in a large pot.
3 If there is any sediment in the bottom of the frying pan or roasting tray, brown this and then deglaze (swill out) the pan with ½ litre of boiling water.

4 Simmer for a few minutes and then add this liquid to the bones.

5 Cover the bones with cold water and bring it to the boil.

6 Reduce the heat so that the water is simmering gently.

7 Simmer for 2–3 hours, skimming the surface to remove any scum as and when required.

8 Fry the vegetables in a little fat or oil until brown. Drain off any fat and add them to the bones with the bunch of herbs.

9 Simmer for 3–4 hours, skimming regularly.

10 When the cooking is finished, skim the stock again and strain it.

Storage suggestion

If you are going to keep the stock, cool it quickly, pour it into a suitable container and put it in the fridge.

RECIPE

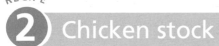 **Chicken stock**

Ingredients

These are the same as for white stock, but replace meat bones with chicken.

Chicken stock can be made from either:

- an old boiling fowl

- raw chicken carcasses or chicken winglets, or a combination of both.

Cooking

The cooking instructions are the same as for white stock. However, depending on what sort of chicken you use:

1 Allow the boiling fowl to three-quarters cook before adding the vegetables. The time will vary according to the age of the bird.

2 Simmer the carcasses and/or winglets for 1 hour, then add the vegetables and simmer for a further hour.

Storage suggestion

If you are going to keep the stock, cool it quickly, pour it into a suitable container and put it in the fridge.

3 Fish stock

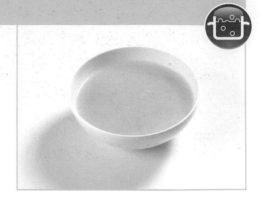

Get ready to cook

1 Slice the onions.
2 Wash the fish bones thoroughly.

INGREDIENTS	To make 4½ litres	To make 12 litres
Oil, butter, margarine	50 g	125 g
Onions (sliced)	200 g	500 g
Fresh white fish bones	2 kg	4 kg
Lemon juice	1	2
Bay leaf	1	2
Parsley stalks	4–6	12–15
Water	4½ litres	12 litres

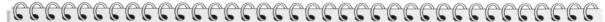

Cooking the stock for longer than 20 minutes will spoil the flavour.

Cooking

1 Place the oil, butter or margarine in a thick-bottomed pan.
2 Add the onions, fish bones, lemon juice, bay leaf and parsley stalks.
3 Cover the ingredients with oiled greaseproof paper and a tight-fitting lid, and sweat them gently without colouring for 5 minutes.
4 Add the water and bring it to the boil.
5 Reduce the heat so that the water is simmering gently.
6 Simmer for 20 minutes, then skim and strain.

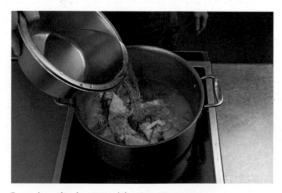

Covering the bones with water

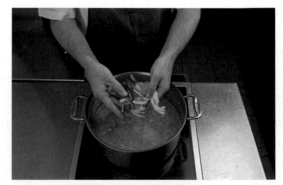

Adding onions and herbs

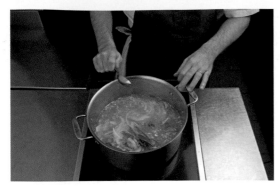

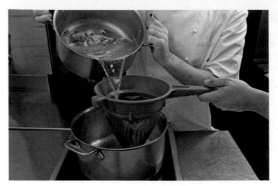

Simmering the stock   Straining the stock

Storage suggestion

If you are going to keep the stock, cool it quickly, pour it into a suitable container and put it in the fridge.

Soups

Introduction

Different flavoured stocks can be used as a base to make a large variety of soups. Almost any of the vast range of fresh vegetables and dried pulses (peas and beans) can be added to soups. Grains, pasta and many herbs and spices can also be used.

Croutons

Croutons are cubes of toasted or fried bread often served with soup and sometimes served with salad.

Make croutons by cutting stale bread into ½ cm cubes and shallow frying in fat. Alternatively, the croutons can be lightly toasted under a grill.

RECIPE

4 Mutton broth

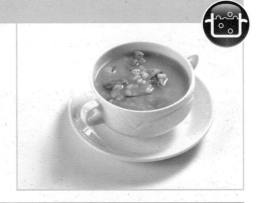

Get ready to cook

1 Trim off any fat from the meat.
2 Wash the barley.
3 Wash and peel the vegetables, and cut into small neat squares (brunoise).
4 Prepare a bunch of herbs (bouquet garni).

INGREDIENTS	4 portions	10 portions
Scrag end of mutton	200 g	500 g
Mutton or lamb stock or water	1 litre	2½ litres
Barley	25 g	60 g
Carrot, turnip, leek, celery, onion	200 g	500 g
Bunch of herbs, chopped parsley		

Instead of chopped parsley, you could use basil and oregano if you prefer.

131

Cooking

1 Place the meat in a saucepan and add cold water.
2 Heat this to a fast boil.
3 As soon as the water starts to boil, remove the pan from the heat, drain the meat and wash it under cold running water.
4 Clean the pan.
5 Replace the meat and cover with cold water or stock.
6 Bring the water or stock to the boil and skim.
7 Add the barley to the pan and then reduce the heat and simmer for 1 hour.
8 Add the vegetables, the bunch of herbs and seasoning.
9 Continue simmering for 30 minutes or until meat is tender. Skim off any fat or scum as necessary.
10 Once cooked, remove the meat from the pan and allow it to cool.
11 Remove the meat from the bone and cut it into neat cubes the same size as the vegetables. Return the meat to the broth.
12 Skim off any fat, taste and correct the seasoning.

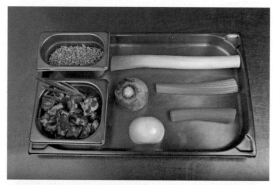

All the ingredients, ready to cook

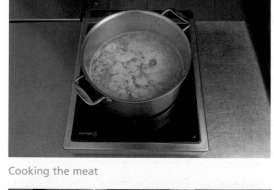

Cooking the meat

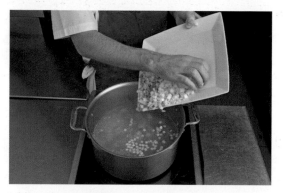

Adding the vegetables

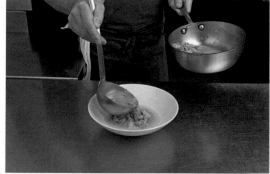

The finished broth

Serving suggestion

Add fresh chopped parsley and serve.

Try something different

● Scotch broth – use lean beef and beef stock in place of mutton. Use barley and vegetables as for mutton broth.
● Chicken broth – use chicken and well-flavoured chicken stock. Add washed rice 12–15 minutes before the broth is cooked. Use vegetables as for mutton broth.

Activity

Suggest a different broth of your own choice.

RECIPE

5 Split pea soup

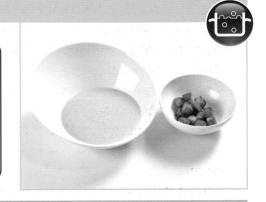

Get ready to cook

1 Check and wash the peas. If pre-soaked, change the water.
2 Wash, peel and chop the onions and carrots.
3 Prepare a bunch of herbs (bouquet garni).
4 Prepare the croutons.

INGREDIENTS	4 portions	10 portions
Split peas	200 g	500 g
White stock or water	1½ litres	3¾ litres
Onions, chopped	50 g	125 g
Carrots, chopped	50 g	125 g
Bunch of herbs		
Knuckle of ham or bacon (optional)		
Salt		
Stale bread sliced (to make croutons)	1 slice	2½ slices
Butter, margarine or oil (to fry croutons)	50 g	125 g

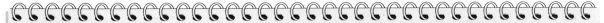

Any type of pulse can be made into soup, e.g. split pea (yellow or green), haricot beans, lentils.

Some pulses may need to be soaked overnight in cold water.

Cooking

1 Place the peas in a thick-bottomed pan.
2 Add the stock or water. Bring to the boil and skim.
3 Add the remainder of the ingredients and a little salt.
4 Simmer until tender, skimming when necessary.
5 Remove the bunch of herbs and ham.
6 Liquidise the soup and pass it through a conical strainer.
7 Return the soup to a clean pan and bring it back to the boil.
8 Taste and correct the seasoning and consistency. If too thick, dilute with stock.

Serving suggestion

Serve with fried or toasted croutons.

Try something different

Add either of the following:

- a chopped fresh herb from parsley, chervil, tarragon, coriander, chives
- a spice or a combination, e.g. garam masala.

Activity

Name as many types of pulse as you can. There are at least 21.

RECIPE

6 Vegetable soup

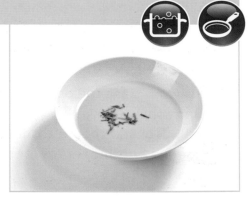

Get ready to cook

1 Peel, wash and slice the vegetables.
2 Prepare a bunch of herbs (bouquet garni).
3 Prepare the croutons.

INGREDIENTS	4 portions	10 portions
Butter, margarine or oil	50 g	125 g
Mixed vegetables (onion or leek, carrot, celery, turnip), peeled, washed and sliced	300 g	1 kg
White stock	1 litre	2½ litres
Potatoes, peeled and sliced	100 g	300 g
Bunch of herbs		
Salt		
Stale bread sliced (to make croutons)	1 slice	3 slices
Butter, margarine or oil (to fry croutons)	50 g	125 g

Cooking

1 Place the fat into a thick-bottomed pan. Allow it to melt over moderate heat.
2 Add all the vegetables apart from the potatoes. Put a lid on the pan.
3 Sweat the vegetables (in other words, allow them to soften without colouring), stirring frequently with a wooden spoon.
4 Remove from the heat and allow to cool.
5 Mix in the hot stock and return to the heat. Stir it until it comes back to the boil.
6 Add the potatoes, the bunch of herbs and a little salt.
7 Simmer for 30–45 minutes, skimming when necessary.
8 Remove the herbs.
9 Liquidise or pass through a sieve and then through a medium-mesh strainer.
10 Return to a clean pan, re-boil, taste and correct seasoning and consistency.

Serving suggestion

Serve with croutons.

Try something different

This is a basic soup from which many variations may be made.

- Do not use turnips if you find the flavour too strong.
- Add other vegetables, e.g. broccoli, spinach, parsnips, tomatoes or tomato purée.
- Add cooked pulses.
- Add small pasta.
- Vary the herbs in the faggot (bouquet garni).
- Add a little spice or a mixture of spices at the beginning when sweating the vegetables.
- Add some chopped pimentos – red, yellow and green peppers can all be added to the soup.

Activity

1 Write and prepare your own idea for a tasty, substantial vegetable soup.

2 In a group, prepare three or four of your ideas.

3 Taste, discuss and assess them.

RECIPE

 7 Tomato soup

Getting ready to cook

1 Peel, wash and roughly chop the vegetables.
2 Prepare a bouquet garni.
3 Prepare the croutons.

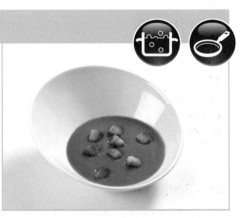

INGREDIENTS	4 portions	10 portions
Butter, margarine or oil	50 g	125 g
Bacon trimmings (optional)	25 g	60 g
Onion and carrot, washed peeled and roughly chopped	100 g of each	250 g of each
Flour	50 g	125 g
Tomato purée	100 g	250 g
Stock	1½ litres	3½ litres
Bouquet garni		
Salt		
Stale bread sliced (to make croutons)	1 slice	3 slices
Butter, margarine or oil (to fry croutons)		

- A slightly sweet/sharp flavour can be added to the soup by preparing what is known as a gastric (gastrique). In a thick-bottomed pan, reduce 100 ml of malt vinegar and 35 g caster sugar until it is a light caramel colour. Mix this into the completed soup.

- Some tomato purée can be stronger than others, so you may have to add a little more or less when making this soup.

Cooking

1 Melt the fat in a thick-bottomed pan.
2 Add the bacon, carrots and onions, and lightly brown them.
3 Mix in the flour and cook to a sandy texture.
4 Mix in the tomato purée, then remove the pan from the heat and allow the mixture to cool.
5 Return the pan to the heat and gradually mix in the hot stock. Stir it until it is boiling.
6 Add the bouquet garni and a little salt and simmer for 1 hour.
7 Skim the soup and remove the bouquet garni.
8 Liquidise or pass the soup firmly through a sieve, then through a medium-mesh conical strainer.
9 Return the soup to a clean pan and reheat it.
10 Taste the soup to check seasoning and consistency.

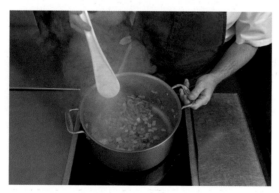

Sweating the vegetables

Mixing in the flour

Serving suggestion

Serve with fried or toasted croutons.

Try something different

Try adding:

- the juice and lightly grated peel of 1–2 oranges
- cooked rice
- a chopped fresh herb, e.g. chives.

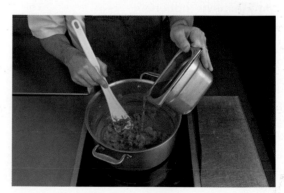

Adding the stock

Leave out the flour and the tomato purée to make a modern tomato soup. Use 250 g of chopped fresh, ripe plum tomatoes, or 250 g of tinned plum tomatoes to make four portions.

Activity

1 Prepare, cook and taste the recipe for tomato soup with and without a gastric. Discuss and assess the two versions.

2 Name and prepare a variation of your own.

There are a number and variety of ready-prepared soups on the market and also soups in powdered and condensed form. If you have to make use of a convenience product, always taste and appraise it first.

In some situations, you can combine a freshly prepared soup with a suitable convenience product, e.g. large-scale cookery, an outdoor festival for 1000.

RECIPE

 Leek and potato soup

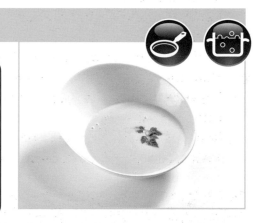

Get ready to cook

1 Wash and trim the leeks and cut the white and light green part into ½ cm squares (paysanne).
2 Wash and peel the potatoes and cut into ½ cm squares 2 mm thick.
3 Prepare a bouquet garni.

INGREDIENTS	4 portions	10 portions
Butter, margarine or oil	25 g	60 g
Leeks, trimmed and washed	400 g	1½ kg
White stock	750 ml	2 litres
Potatoes, peeled and washed	200 g	½ kg
Bouquet garni		
Salt		

Cooking

1 Melt the fat in a saucepan. Add the leeks, cover with a lid and cook slowly without colouring until soft (sweat).
2 Add the stock, potatoes, bouquet garni and a little salt.
3 Simmer for approximately 15 minutes.
4 Remove the bouquet garni, then taste and correct the seasoning before serving.

RECIPE

9 Dhal and spinach soup

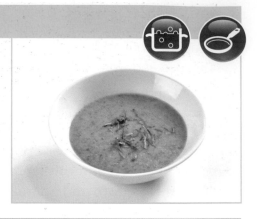

Get ready to cook

1 Finely chop the onions.
2 Wash, peel and slice the potatoes.
3 Crush and chop the garlic, chop the chilli and grate the ginger.

INGREDIENTS	4 portions	10 portions
Cumin seeds	2 tsp	5 tsp
Coriander seeds	2 tsp	5 tsp
Ghee or vegetable oil	1 tbsp	2½ tsp
Onions, finely chopped	300 g	750 g
Garlic cloves, crushed and chopped	2	5
Red chillies, chopped	2	5
Curry leaves	8	20
Black mustard seeds	2 tsp	5 tsp
Fenugreek seeds	½ tsp	1¼ tsp
Ground turmeric	1 tsp	2½ tsp
Red lentils (dhal)	200 g	500 g
Potatoes, peeled and cut into slices	400 g	1 kg
Chicken stock	1¼ litres	3 litres
Spinach	1 kg	2½ kg
Tamarind paste	2 tbsp	5 tbsp
Coconut milk	150 ml	375 ml
Grated fresh ginger	1 tbsp	2½ tsp

Cooking

1 Place the cumin and coriander seeds in a frying pan. Cook until fragrant.
2 When fragrant, crush the seeds in a blender or a pestle and mortar.
3 Place the ghee or vegetable oil in a large saucepan. Add the onions, garlic, chillies, curry leaves, mustard and fenugreek. Cook until the onions are lightly brown.
4 Add the turmeric and crushed cumin and coriander and cook for another minute.
5 Add the lentils, potatoes and chicken stock.
6 Bring to the boil and simmer until the potatoes are tender.
7 Add the spinach and cook for two minutes.
8 Using a liquidiser or hand blender, purée the soup.
9 Add the tamarind paste and the coconut milk and stir in.
10 Correct the consistency with stock or water. You may also add more coconut milk if required.

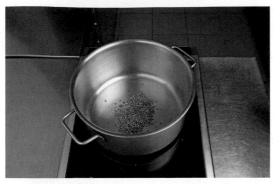

Cooking the cumin and coriander

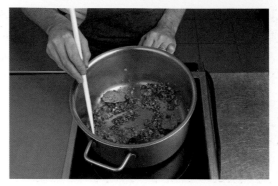

Cooking the onions, garlic and herbs in ghee

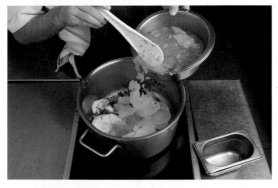

Adding the stock

RECIPE

(10) Butternut squash soup

Get ready to cook

1 Peel and finely dice the butternut squash.
2 Wash the leeks and shred them finely.
3 Wash and chop the chives.

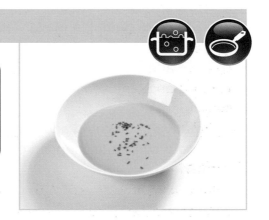

INGREDIENTS	4 portions	10 portions
Butternut squash, peeled and finely diced	2	5
Leeks, finely shredded	2	5
Garlic cloves, peeled and chopped	2	5
Vegetable stock	1 litre	2.5 litres
Vegetable oil	60 ml	150 ml
Double cream or natural yoghurt	250 ml	625 ml
Chopped chives	1 tsp	2½ tsp
Ground black pepper		

Cooking

1 Place the vegetable oil in a suitable pan and sauté the squash lightly for 5 minutes.
2 Add the leeks and garlic, and sauté for a further 3 minutes, stirring occasionally.
3 Season with black pepper.
4 Add the vegetable stock. Bring to the boil. Simmer for 10–12 minutes until the squash is cooked.

5 Liquidise the soup and strain.
6 Put the soup into a clean saucepan and bring to the boil.
7 Remove from the heat and add the cream or yoghurt.
8 Correct the consistency and check the flavour. Add a little salt if required.

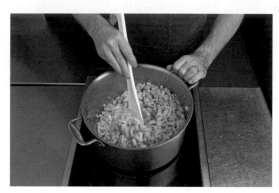

Frying the vegetables

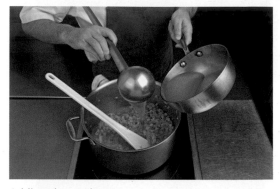

Adding the stock

Serving suggestion

Serve sprinkled with chopped chives or with a little chopped fresh coriander, basil or oregano.

Try something different

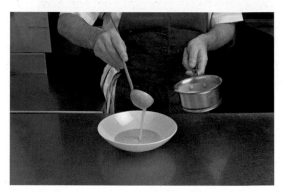

The finished soup, with a good consistency

- You could use pumpkin in place of butternut squash.
- You can add a bouquet garni during cooking and remove it before liquidising.
- Alternatively you could add a little ground mixed spice or ground cinnamon.
- You could add some chopped coriander, basil or oregano when the soup is simmering.

RECIPE

 11 Spicy tomato soup

Get ready to cook

1 Peel and roughly chop the tomatoes.
2 Peel and dice the onion and garlic.
3 Slice the chilli.

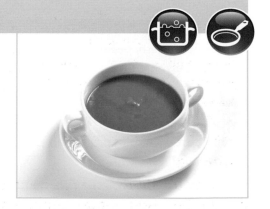

INGREDIENTS	4 portions	10 portions
Onions, peeled and diced	2	5
Cloves of garlic, peeled and diced	2	5
Olive oil	90 ml	225 ml
Tomatoes, peeled and roughly chopped	2 kg	5 kg
Bay leaves	1	3
Black pepper	1 tsp	2 tsp
Red chilli, sliced	½	1
Chicken stock or vegetable stock	1 litre	2½ litres
Cornflour	1 tbsp	2½ tbsp

Cooking

1 Sweat the onion and garlic in a large pan with the oil until soft and translucent.
2 Add the tomatoes, bay leaf, pepper and chilli.
3 Add the stock and bring to the boil.
4 Lower the heat and simmer for approximately 30–40 minutes.
5 Pass the soup through a sieve and return it to the pan.
6 Mix the cornflour with a little water to make a smooth paste.
7 Stir in the cornflour and heat gently to thicken.
8 Taste and adjust the seasoning before serving.

RECIPE

12 Sweet potato soup

Get ready to cook

1 Remove the seeds from the peppers and dice into even-sized pieces.
2 Peel and dice the sweet potato.
3 Peel and dice the onions and chop the garlic.

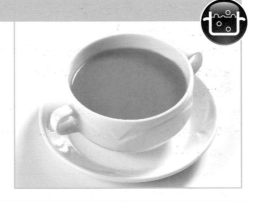

INGREDIENTS	4 portions	10 portions
Onions, peeled and diced	1	3
Sweet potatoes, peeled and diced	1 kg	2½ kg
Red peppers, deseeded and diced	2	5
Garlic cloves, chopped	2	5
Vegetable or chicken stock	1 litre	2½ litres
Salt and pepper to season		

Cooking

1 Sweat the onions until soft and translucent.
2 Add the sweet potato, peppers and garlic, and cook gently for 10–15 minutes on a low heat.
3 Add the stock and simmer for approximately 40 minutes.
4 Purée the vegetables either in the pan with a stick blender or in a liquidiser.
5 Pass through a sieve.
6 Return to pan and season to taste.

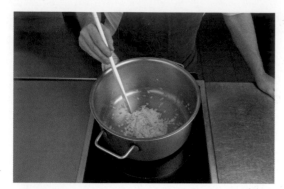

Sweating the onions

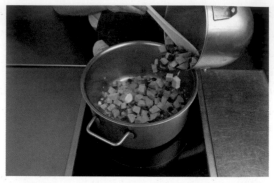

Adding the vegetables

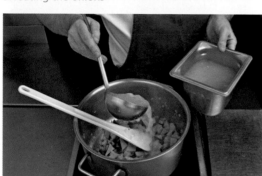

Adding the stock

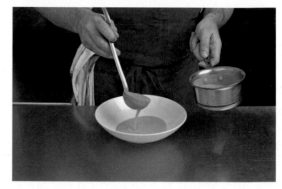

The finished soup, after it has been liquidised and passed

RECIPE

13 Split pea and butternut squash soup

Get ready to cook

1 Soak the peas overnight in enough water to cover them.
2 Peel and roughly dice the tomatoes, onion and butternut squash.

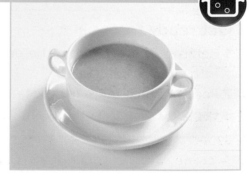

INGREDIENTS	4 portions	10 portions
Split peas (soaked)	250 g	625 g
Water	1 litre	2½ litres
Onions, peeled and roughly diced	1	2
Vegetable oil	90 ml	225 ml
Butternut squash, peeled and roughly diced	1	2
Tomatoes (large), peeled and roughly diced	6	15
Tarragon, chopped	1 tsp	2½ tsp
Coriander, chopped	1 tbsp	2½ tbsp
Cumin	½ tsp	1 tsp
Chilli powder	½ tsp	1 tsp

Cooking

1 Drain the peas and cook in water for approximately 30–40 minutes.
2 In a separate pan, sweat the onion in oil until soft and translucent.

3 Add the diced squash, diced tomato, tarragon, coriander, cumin, chilli powder.
4 Add the water and bring to the boil.
5 Add the vegetable mixture to the pan of peas and cook for approximately 40 minutes.
6 Purée the vegetables either in the pan with a stick blender or in a liquidiser.
7 If it is too thick, adjust the consistency by adding more water.

Try something different
You could use pumpkin in place of butternut squash.

RECIPE
 14 Garden marrow soup

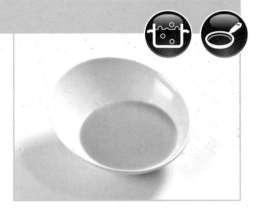

Get ready to cook
1 Peel and roughly dice the onion.
2 Peel and cube the marrow.

INGREDIENTS	4 portions	10 portions
Onions, peeled and roughly diced	1	2
Vegetable oil	90 ml	225 ml
Marrow (large), cut into cubes	1	2½
Mild curry powder	½ tbsp	2½ tbsp
Chicken or vegetable stock	1 litre	2½ litres
Salt and pepper		

Cooking
1 Sweat the onion in the oil until translucent.
2 Add the cubed marrow and fry gently.
3 Stir in the curry powder.
4 Add the stock and simmer for approximately 40 minutes.
5 Purée the vegetables either in the pan with a stick blender or in a liquidiser.
6 Season with salt and pepper.
7 Adjust the consistency if necessary by adding a little water.

Sauces

Introduction
A sauce is a liquid that has been thickened in some way, maybe by a roux or cornflour or arrowroot. (A roux is a combination of fat and flour gently cooked over a low heat for a short time.) Some types of accompaniment that are called sauces are not really sauces (e.g. apple sauce, mint sauce, horseradish sauce). Recipes for several of these types of 'sauce' that can be served with meat or poultry are given in the meat and poultry chapters.

Sauces that will be used for coating foods (e.g. jus-lié – thickened gravy) should be as thin as possible and should coat the food only lightly.

15 Béchamel (basic white sauce)

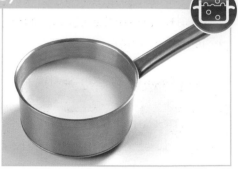

Get ready to cook

Push a clove into an onion, with the sharp end going into the onion, leaving the round end studding the outside of the onion.

INGREDIENTS	1 litre	2½ litres
Margarine, butter or oil	100 g	400 g
Flour	100 g	400 g
Milk, warmed	1 litre	4½ litres
Onion studded with cloves	1	2–3

Cooking

1 Melt the fat in a thick-bottomed pan.
2 Mix in the flour with a wooden or heat-proof plastic spoon.
3 Cook for a few minutes, stirring frequently. As you are making white roux you should not allow the mixture to colour.
4 Remove the pan from the heat to allow the roux to cool.
5 Return the pan to the stove and, over a low heat, gradually mix the milk into the roux.
6 Add the studded onion.
7 Allow the mixture to simmer gently for 30 minutes, stirring frequently to make sure the sauce does not burn on the bottom.
8 Remove the onion and pass the sauce through a conical strainer.

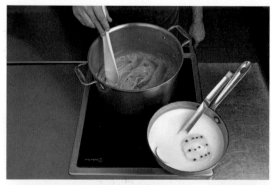

Mixing in the flour to make a roux

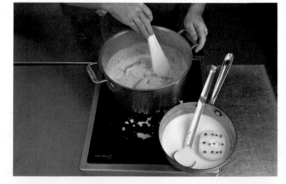

Mixing in the milk

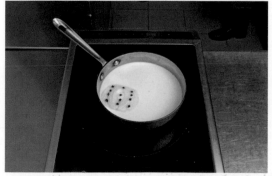

Cooking the sauce with the studded onion

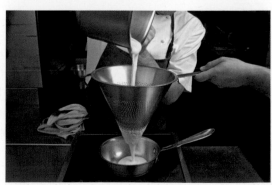

Passing the sauce through a strainer

Storage suggestions

To prevent a skin from forming, brush the surface with melted butter. When ready to use, stir this into the sauce. Alternatively, cover the sauce with clingfilm or greaseproof paper.

Try something different

Béchamel is a basic white sauce that can be used as the basis for many other sauces. The suggestions below are for half a litre of béchamel, which is enough for 8 to 12 portions of sauce.

Sauce	Served with	Additions per ½ litre
Egg	Poached or steamed fish	2 diced hard-boiled eggs
Cheese	Poached fish or vegetables	50 g grated Cheddar cheese
Onion	Roast lamb or mutton	100 g chopped onions cooked without colouring, either by boiling or sweating in fat
Parsley	Poached fish or boiled ham	1 teaspoon chopped parsley
Cream	Poached fish or vegetables	Add cream or natural yoghurt to give the consistency of double cream
Mustard	Grilled herrings	Add diluted English or continental mustard to give a spicy sauce

Activity

1 As a group, make all six of these sauces. Taste, discuss and assess them.

2 Suggest a variation of your own, using béchamel and a dish with which it might be served.

RECIPE

16 Velouté

This is a basic white sauce made from white stock and a blond roux.

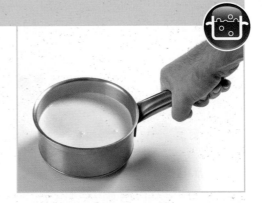

INGREDIENTS	4 portions	10 portions
Margarine, butter or oil	100 g	400 g
Flour	100 g	400 g
Stock (chicken, fish)	1 litre	4½ litres

Cooking

1 Melt the fat in a thick-bottomed pan.

2 Mix in the flour.

3 Cook out to a sandy texture over a gentle heat, allowing the lightest shade of colour (blond roux).

4 Remove the pan from the heat to allow the roux to cool.

5 Return the pan to the stove and, over a low heat, gradually add the hot stock.

6 Mix until smooth and simmering.

7 Cook for 1 hour on a low heat, making sure the sauce does not burn on the bottom, and pass through a fine conical strainer.

Storage suggestions

To prevent a skin from forming, brush the surface with melted butter. When ready to use, stir this into the sauce. Alternatively, cover the sauce with clingfilm or greaseproof paper.

Try something different

A velouté-based sauce can be used for egg, fish, chicken and mutton, with the following additions.

Sauce	Served with	Additions per ½ litre
Caper	Boiled leg of mutton or lamb	2 tbsp capers
Aurora	Poached eggs, chicken	1 tsp tomato purée 60 ml cream or natural yogurt or crème fraiche 2–3 drops of lemon juice
Mushroom	Poached chicken	100 g sliced button mushrooms lightly cooked in a little fat or oil

Activity

1 Suggest an alternative of your choice.

2 Prepare, taste, discuss and assess it.

RECIPE

17 Fish velouté

This is a basic white sauce made from white fish stock and a blond roux.

INGREDIENTS	
Blond roux:	
● margarine, butter or oil	100 g
● flour	100 g
Fish stock	1 litre

Cooking

1 Prepare a blond roux and allow to cool.

2 Gradually add the hot stock and mix to the boil.

3 Simmer for 1 hour.

4 Pass through a fine conical strainer.

Storage suggestions

To prevent a skin from forming, brush the surface with melted butter. When ready to use, stir this into the sauce. Alternatively, cover the sauce with clingfilm or greaseproof paper.

18 Roast gravy

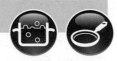

Roast gravy is traditionally made from the residue that roast joints leave in their roasting pans (see Chapter 18, page 232), but it can also be made with raw bones if you need a larger quantity, as in this recipe.

INGREDIENTS	4 portions	10 portions
Raw meat bones, chopped small	200 g	500 g
Brown stock or water	500 ml	1½ litres
Onions, roughly chopped	50 g	125 g
Carrots, roughly chopped	50 g	125 g
Celery, roughly chopped	25 g	60 g

Get ready to cook
Wash, peel and roughly chop the vegetables.

Cooking

1 Brown the bones in a little fat in a roasting tray in the oven or in a heavy frying pan on the stove at 180°C.
2 Drain off the fat and place bones in a saucepan.
3 Deglaze the tray or pan with stock or water to ensure that the tasty brown residue is not wasted.
4 Pour the deglaze liquid into the saucepan with the bones and cover the bones with stock or water.
5 Bring to the boil, skim and allow to simmer.
6 Lightly fry the vegetables in a little fat in a frying pan or add them to the bones when these are partly browned.
7 Simmer for 1½–2 hours, strain and skin any excess fat off the surface.

Try something different

If your roast gravy does not have enough flavour when tasted, add little of a suitable convenience product to help. Many convenience gravy products are available, but you should taste and assess these before using them.

19 Thickened gravy

> You can make a light brown sauce by lightly thickening a well-flavoured roast brown stock with arrowroot or cornflour diluted in a little water.

INGREDIENTS	Amount per ½ litre of gravy
Brown stock	½ litre
Tomato puree	1 tsp
Mushroom trimmings	1 heaped tsp
Thyme	a small pinch
Arrowroot or cornflour	1 heaped tsp

Cooking

1 Simmer the required amount of stock in a thick-bottomed pan.

2 Add the tomato purée, mushroom trimmings and thyme.

3 Dilute the arrowroot or cornflour in a basin with a little cold water and gradually add this to the simmering gravy, stirring continuously until it re-boils.

4 Simmer for 5–10 minutes and pass through a fine-mesh conical strainer.

Try something different

This basic sauce can be used for a number of variations.

Rosemary or lavender can be used in place of thyme.

Small, finely sliced gherkins can be added to make a sharp sauce to serve with burgers, sausages, etc.

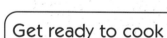

20 Tomato, mushroom and tarragon sauce

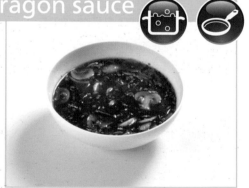

Get ready to cook

1 Remove the eyes (where the stem was attached) from the tomatoes using the tip of a small knife.

2 Plunge the tomatoes into rapidly boiling water for 8–10 seconds.

3 Remove them from the boiling water and immediately plunge them into cold water. Leave them in the water until they are cold.

4 Once cold, peel and cut the tomatoes into quarters, remove the seeds and cut them into ½ cm dice.

5 Finely chop the onions and garlic, and slice the mushrooms.

INGREDIENTS	4 portions	10 portions
Butter, margarine or oil	25 g	60 g
Shallots or onion, finely chopped	10 g	25 g
Garlic clove, finely chopped (optional)	½	1
Button mushrooms, sliced	50 g	125 g
Tomatoes, skinned, deseeded and diced	100 g	250 g
Thickened gravy	250 ml	625 ml
Tarragon, chopped	1 sprig	2 sprigs

Cooking

1 Melt the fat in a small thick-bottomed pan.
2 Add the shallots/onions and cook gently for 2–3 minutes, without colouring, until soft.
3 Add the garlic and mushrooms. Cover with a lid and cook gently for 2–3 minutes.
4 Strain off any fat.
5 Add the tomatoes and gravy, and simmer gently for 5–10 minutes.
6 Taste and season as required.

Try something different

If a gentler flavour of garlic is required, do not add the chopped garlic but instead add a whole peeled garlic clove at point 5 and remove it before point 6.

Serving suggestion

This sauce can be served with fried chicken breasts, steaks or chops.

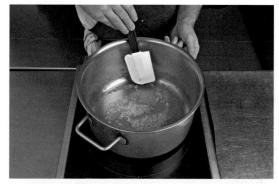

Gently cooking the shallots

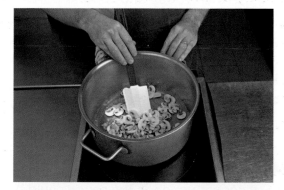

Adding the garlic and mushrooms

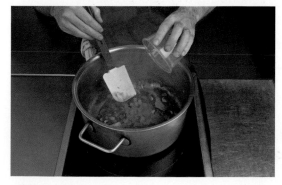

Adding the tomatoes and gravy

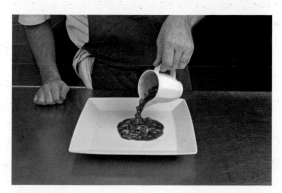

The finished sauce

21) Tomato sauce

Gastric is made by reducing 100 ml sherry vinegar and 35 g caster sugar to a light caramel.

INGREDIENTS	
Carrots	90 g
Celery	30 g
Garlic, clove	½
Vegetable oil	25 g
Butter	25 g
Thyme	1 g
Bay leaf	½
Tomato purée	12 g
Plum tomatoes	200 g
Chicken stock	750 g
Juniper berries	2
Cream	75 g
Gastric	5 g
Salt	

Cooking

1 Sweat the carrots, celery and garlic in the oil and butter.
2 Add the thyme, bay and tomato purée. Cook for 5 minutes.
3 Add the tomatoes. Cook for 5 minutes.
4 Add the stock and juniper berries. Reduce by a third.
5 Add the cream. Bring the sauce to the boil.
6 Liquidise the sauce.
7 Season with gastric and salt.

Activity

1 Suggest other foods the sauce could be served with.

2 Suggest ways of making other sauces from a thickened gravy base, together with the foods you would serve them with.

3 Prepare, cook, taste and assess some of your ideas.

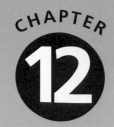

Cold food preparation

Introduction

Cold foods are probably the most popular and versatile dishes that we prepare and serve.

- In many countries, cold meats and cheeses of all types are eaten with breakfast.
- Where food is served all day, cold items, including self-serve salad counters, will often feature.
- In establishments where lunch and dinner is offered, menus will often include cold hors d'oeuvre, which may be a single item, e.g. melon, prawns or smoked salmon, or a selection of assorted items and a variety of salads.
- Cold main courses include:
  - meats, e.g. ham, beef, pork, salami, chicken, turkey and pâtés, terrines and pies
  - dairy products (e.g. a cheese board with celery) and eggs (e.g. cold hard-boiled, Scotch eggs and a selection of egg-based quiches)
  - fish, e.g. salmon, crab, prawns
  - a good selection of breads or/and rolls (e.g. white, brown, wholemeal), which are often served with cold meals.
- Sandwiches are a quick, timesaving snack that are available from many food outlets. There is a huge variety of both breads (rolls, slices, crusty, seeded, bagels, etc.) and fillings on offer (see page 153). In hotels, dainty, finger-sized sandwiches sprinkled with cress are offered for afternoon teas.

Quality points

- **Freshness** – Foods should be bought frequently, stored correctly (usually in refrigerators below 5°C) and checked carefully to ensure that they are in good condition (with no blemishes) and within the use by date.
- **Smell** – The smell should always be fresh and appetising.
- **Preparation** – Dishes should be prepared according to recipes and specifications, cut into even-sized portions and trimmed if necessary, with minimum waste.
- **Appearance** – Dishes should be neatly dressed and simply garnished.

Advantages of serving cold food

Cold food is popular in every kind of food service operation for the following reasons.

- **Visual appeal** – Food can be attractively displayed, carefully arranged and neatly garnished.
- **Efficiency** – It can be prepared in advance, allowing a large number of people to be served in a short space of time.
- **Adaptability** – If cold foods are served from a buffet, the range of foods can be simple or complex and wide-ranging.

Preparation

Well-planned organisation is essential to ensure adequate pre-preparation (known as mise-en-place), so that foods are assembled with a good workflow and are ready on time. Before, during and after being assembled, the foods must be kept in a cool place or refrigerator to minimise the risk of food contamination and growth of bacteria. High standards of personal, food and equipment hygiene must be maintained with all cold work.

Activity

1 Make a poster or checklist for new kitchen staff, highlighting ten ways they can avoid cross-contamination in a kitchen. Include some illustrations.

2 Suggest six kitchen areas or items that should be both *cleaned* and *disinfected*.

3 You have been asked to put a food delivery in a multi-use fridge. Draw a fridge with four shelves and show where you would put the different foods delivered:

raw chicken, cooked ham, cream, salmon fillets, cooked vegetable quiche, eggs, cheese, cooked pasties, pâté, fresh pasta, rump steak, milk, sausages, butter, frozen chicken drumsticks that need to be defrosted for use tomorrow

4 There is already some cream cheese in the fridge with a 'use by' date of today, and some yoghurt with a 'use by' date of yesterday. What should be done with these items?

5 If you found the temperature display on the fridge reading 10°C, what would you do?

(Refer back to Chapter 8 if you need some help in answering these questions.)

Cold foods can either be pre-plated or served from large dishes and bowls. In both cases presentation is important. The food should appear fresh, neatly arranged and simply, not overly, garnished. Keep the cold service area tidy, removing empty dishes and bringing new items.

Types of hors d'oeuvre

A wide variety of foods, different combinations of foods and recipes can be served as hors d'oeuvre and salads. Hors d'oeuvre can be divided into three categories:

1 single cold food items (smoked salmon, pâté, melon, etc.)
2 a selection of well-seasoned cold dishes
3 well-seasoned hot dishes.

Hors d'oeuvre may be served for luncheon, dinner or supper, and the wide choice of dishes, their colour appeal and versatility, make many items and combinations of items suitable for snacks and salads at any time of day.

Preparing salad items

Lettuce – Cut off a slice from the root stem, remove any wilted outer leaves and discard these, then remove the rest of the leaves. Wash these carefully and dry them in a salad spinner.

Cucumber – Peel with a vegetable peeler or leave unpeeled, according to the chef's requirements, and cut into thin slices on a mandolin or with a sharp knife.

Tomato – Remove the stems and cut out the stem bases with the point of a sharp, small knife. Leave the skins on, or peel by plunging them into boiling water for ten seconds, then removing them and cooling them under cold running water. Cut into slices or segments.

Cress – Wash carefully, dry in a salad spinner or in a clean, dry tea towel or between sheets of absorbent kitchen paper, and remove any black pieces or stems.

Radish – Trim the green foliage to leave approximately ½cm, then wash and dry.

Peppers – The colour of peppers changes according to their ripeness, from green (the least ripe), to orange and red (the ripest and the best to use for salads). Cut into quarters, remove the seeds and pith, and cut into fine strips.

Other cold options

Dairy – A sensible selection of cheese should be available. It is better to have a small selection, which can be kept fresh, rather than a large number, which can soon turn dry looking and unappetising. These can be replaced as they are used. Cheese biscuits or fresh bread and/or rolls should be offered, together with sticks of celery.

Eggs – Hard-boiled, pickled or Scotch eggs and a variety of quiches can, with a self-service salad, provide an appetising and healthy meal.

Vegetarian dishes – Some people prefer not to eat fish, meat or poultry. There is a large variety of foods (e.g. pulses, seeds, herbs and spices) from which many interesting and appetising dishes can be made.

Sandwiches

The traditional sandwich is made by spreading butter or a butter substitute on two slices of bread, placing a filling on one slice and covering it with the other. The crusts may or may not be removed and the sandwich then cut into two or four pieces.

Types of bread

There is a wide variety of breads available (e.g. white, brown, wholemeal, granary, seeded) and many bakers will bake bread according to your specification (e.g. tomato, basil, rosemary, walnut and olive) and will slice it ready for use.

Fillings

There is an almost endless variety of sandwich fillings that can be used – single food items such as ham, cheese, corned or roast beef, and mixed foods such as ham and tomato, egg and cress, and chicken and lettuce.

The fillings may also include flavourings and sauces such as mustard (English or continental), horseradish sauce, various pickles and chutneys, and mayonnaise.

Types of sandwich

Toasted sandwiches can be made in two ways.

1 Add the filling between two slices of hot, freshly buttered toast.
2 Use an item of equipment called a sandwich toaster. Put the filling in between two slices of bread and toast the whole sandwich in the sandwich toaster. Some toasters will seal the sandwich, remove the crusts and cut the sandwich in half.

A **club sandwich** is made from three slices of hot buttered toast.

- On the first slice, place slices of grilled, crispy streaky bacon, slices of tomato and lettuce.
- Put the second slice of toast on top of this and layer it with slices of hard-boiled egg, mayonnaise and slices of cooked chicken breast.
- Finally, put the third slice of toast on top. Then press down carefully on the sandwich, make it as compact as possible, cut it in halves or quarters, and serve with potato crisps.

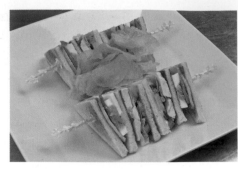

A club sandwich

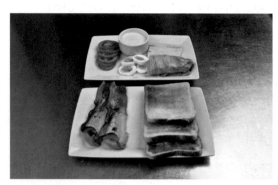

The ingredients for a club sandwich

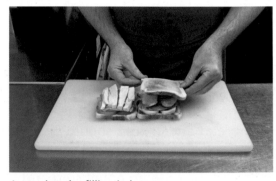

Arranging the filling in layers

To make a **bookmaker sandwich**, place an underdone thin sirloin steak (known as a minute steak because it only needs a minute over a fierce heat to cook) between two slices of toast from a bloomer loaf.

Use three or four slices of bread, toasted or untoasted, to make **double-decker** and **triple-decker sandwiches**.

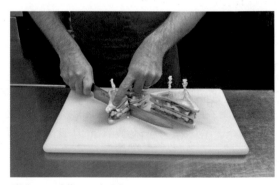

Slicing a club sandwich

To prepare **open sandwiches**, butter a slice of any type of bread and top this with a variety of foods, such as:

- smoked salmon, lettuce, potted shrimps, slice of lemon
- cold roast beef, sliced tomato, gherkin fan
- shredded lettuce, slices of hard-boiled egg, cucumber slices and mayonnaise
- pickled herring, slices of hard-boiled egg, sprinkled with chopped gherkins, capers and parsley.

Fish

Fish is available fresh, frozen, pickled and tinned.

- **Precooked fresh salmon** – A portion can be served neatly dressed and garnished with lettuce leaves, cucumber slices and quarters of tomato, accompanied by mayonnaise.
- **Frozen crab meat and prawns** must be defrosted, preferably in a refrigerator, before use.

Prawns precooked from fresh or frozen can be served:

- accompanied by mayonnaise and brown bread and butter
- removed from the shells, combined with various ingredients (e.g. shredded lettuce, thin slices of cucumber or/and tomato) and mixed with a thinned mayonnaise or vinaigrette.

Crab pre-prepared from fresh or frozen should be checked carefully for any pieces of shell. It can then be served either:

- in neat portions on a lettuce leaf, accompanied by mayonnaise or vinaigrette
- mixed with a little seasoning and/or mayonnaise or vinaigrette and served in neat portions on a lettuce leaf.

- **Canned fish** – Canned salmon, sardines and tuna are particularly useful in cold dishes. Simply remove them from their cans, dress them neatly and serve with lettuce leaves.

RECIPE

1 Soused (pickled) herring or mackerel

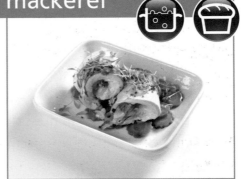

Get ready to cook

1 Clean, scale and fillet the fish.
2 Peel and wash the onion and carrots, and cut into neat, thin rings.

INGREDIENTS	4 portions	10 portions
Herrings or mackerel	2	5
Salt and pepper		
Button onions	25 g	60 g
Carrots, peeled and fluted	25 g	60 g
Bay leaf	½	1½
Peppercorns	6	12
Thyme	1 sprig	2 sprigs
Vinegar	60 ml	150 ml

Cooking

1 Wash the fish fillets well and season with salt and pepper.
2 Roll up with the skin outside.
3 Place in an earthenware dish.
4 Blanch the onion and carrots for 2–3 minutes.
5 Add to the fish with the remainder of the ingredients.
6 Cover with greaseproof paper or aluminium foil and cook in a moderate oven for 15–20 minutes.
7 Allow to cool.
8 Place in a dish with the onion and carrot.

Serving suggestion

Garnish with picked parsley, dill or chives.

Salads and salad dressings

Introduction

Salads may be made from a wide variety of foods – raw or cooked. They may be served as an accompaniment to hot and cold foods and as dishes in their own right. They can be served for lunch, tea, high tea, dinner, supper and snack meals. Salads can be divided in two types:

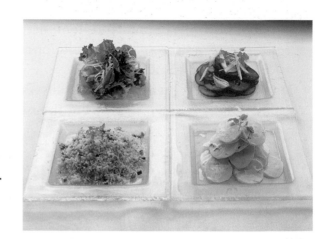

1 simple, using one ingredient
2 mixed, or composite, using more than one ingredient.

Some salads may form part of a composite hors d'oeuvre.

Accompaniments include dressings and cold sauces. There are two basic sauces used with cold food, both of which have many variations. These are:

1 vinaigrette
2 mayonnaise.

Commercial mayonnaises and vinaigrettes are available in many brands. If you decide to use one of these, always taste it to check that you like it before using it.

RECIPE

2 Vinaigrette

INGREDIENTS	4–6 portions
Olive oil	3–6 tbsp
Vinegar	1–2 tbsp
French mustard	1 tsp
Salt	1 tsp

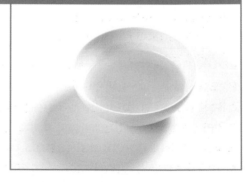

Preparing the dish

Combine all the ingredients thoroughly, either whisking with a fork or shaking well in a container such as a jar.

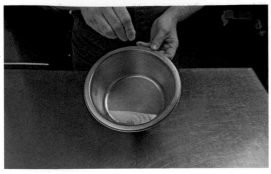

Adding seasoning to the vinegar

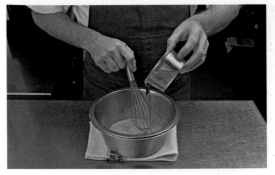

Slowly whisking the vinaigrette

Try something different

You could use:

- English in place of French mustard
- chopped fresh herbs, chives, parsley, tarragon, etc
- different oils, e.g. sesame oil
- different vinegars, or lemon juice instead of vinegar.

Activity

Suggest two more variations to a basic vinaigrette.

RECIPE

3 Mayonnaise

Because of the risk of salmonella food poisoning, it is strongly recommended that pasteurised egg yolks are used.

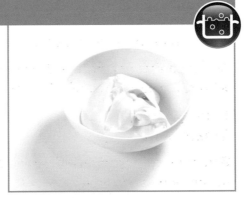

INGREDIENTS	8 portions
Egg yolks, very fresh or pasteurised (see note above)	2
Vinegar or lemon juice	2 tsp
Small pinch of salt	
English or continental mustard	½ tsp
A mild-flavoured oil such as corn oil or the lightest olive oil	250 ml
Boiling water	1 tsp

Preparing the dish

1 Place yolks, vinegar, salt and mustard in a bowl and whisk until thoroughly mixed.
2 Whisk continuously and vigorously while slowly adding the oil.
3 Whisk in the boiling water.
4 Taste and correct seasoning if necessary.

Try something different

Add:

- fresh chopped herbs
- garlic juice – peel a clove garlic and press it using a garlic press,
- thick tomato juice.

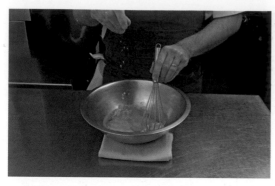

Beating the egg yolks and mixing in the vinegar and seasoning

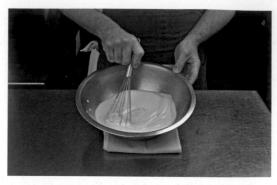

Starting to whisk in the oil

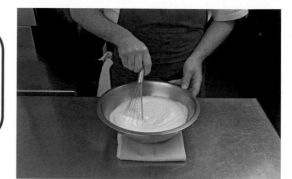

Gradually adding more oil

Activity

1 Suggest three further variations.

2 Deliberately curdle some mayonnaise and reconstitute it.

If the mayonnaise becomes too thick while you are making it, whisk in a little water or vinegar.

Mayonnaise may separate, turn or curdle for several reasons:

- you have added the oil too quickly
- the oil is too cold
- you have not whisked it enough
- the egg yolks were stale and weak.

To reconstitute (bring it back together) either:

- take a clean basin, pour in 1 teaspoon of boiling water and gradually but vigorously whisk in the curdled sauce a little at a time
- in a clean basin, whisk a fresh egg yolk with 1/2 a teaspoon of cold water then gradually whisk in the curdled sauce.

RECIPE 4 Potato salad

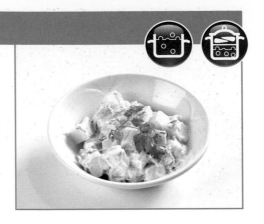

Get ready to cook

1 Wash and peel potatoes (or cook in skins and then peel).
2 Cook potatoes by boiling or steaming.
3 Cut potatoes into ½–1 cm dice or slices.
4 If desired, blanch the onion by placing in boiling water for 2–3 minutes, cooling and draining. This will reduce its harshness.
5 Prepare the vinaigrette (see recipe 2).

INGREDIENTS	4 portions	10 portions
Potatoes, cooked and cut into dice	200 g	500 g
Vinaigrette	1 tbsp	2½ tbsp
Mayonnaise or natural yoghurt	125 ml	300 ml
Onion or chive, chopped (optional)	10 g	25 g
Parsley or mixed chopped fresh herbs	½ tsp	1½ tsp
Salt		

Preparing the dish

1 Put the potatoes into a bowl and sprinkle on the vinaigrette.
2 Mix in the mayonnaise, onion and chive.
3 Finally, chop and mix in the parsley or other herbs and season to taste.

Try something different

At the end, add chopped mint or chopped hard-boiled egg.

Activity

Suggest two or three more additions.

RECIPE 5 Vegetable salad

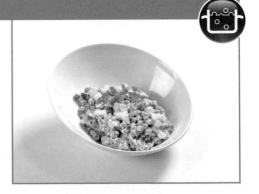

Get ready to cook

1 Peel and wash the carrots and turnips, and cut into neat dice.
2 Top and tail the beans and cut into ½ cm pieces.
3 Prepare the vinaigrette (see recipe 2).

INGREDIENTS	4 portions	10 portions
Carrots	100 g	250 g
French beans	50 g	125 g
Turnip	50 g	125 g
Peas	50 g	125 g
Vinaigrette	1 tbsp	2–3 tbsp
Mayonnaise or natural yoghurt	125 ml	300 ml
Salt		

Preparing the dish

1 Cook the carrots, beans and turnips separately in lightly salted water, then refresh and drain well.
2 Cook, drain and refresh the peas. Drain well.
3 Mix all the vegetables in a basin with the vinaigrette and then add and mix in the mayonnaise or yoghurt.
4 Taste and correct the seasoning if necessary.

Try something different

Potato can be used in place of turnip.

A little of any or a mixture of the following can be chopped and added: chives, parsley, chervil, tarragon.

Activity

Suggest two or three more ingredients that could be added.

RECIPE

6 Beetroot salad

Get ready to cook
1 Wash the beetroot.
2 Prepare the vinaigrette (see recipe 2).

INGREDIENTS
Beetroot (quantity as required)
Vinaigrette, if desired

Preparing the dish

1 Cook the beetroot in their skins in a steamer or gently simmering water until tender.
2 Cool and test by rubbing the skin between your fingers and thumb. When cooked, the skin should peel (rub) off easily.
3 Cut into ½ cm dice and either serve plain or lightly sprinkled with vinaigrette.

Try something different

Sprinkle with chopped onion, or chive and parsley, or other fresh herbs.

7 Tomato salad

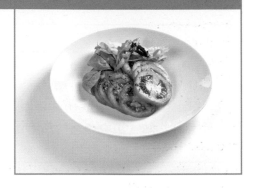

Get ready to cook

1 Wash and dry the tomatoes.
2 Remove the stem eyes.
3 Leave the skins on, or peel by plunging them into boiling water for ten seconds, then removing them and cooling them under cold running water.
4 Slice the onion and, if desired, blanch it.

INGREDIENTS	4 portions	10 portions
Tomatoes	200 g	500 g
Lettuce leaves		
Vinaigrette	10 g	25 g
Onions (sliced) or chives (optional)		
Finely chopped parsley and/or fresh mixed herbs		

The amount of lettuce required will depend on type and size.

Preparing the dish

1 Slice the tomatoes.
2 Arrange them neatly on washed, well-drained lettuce leaves.
3 Sprinkle on the vinaigrette and the onion.
4 Chop the parsley or other herbs and sprinkle these on.

8 Green salad

There are a large number of salad leaves available, including different varieties of lettuce. You can use whichever you choose, or a mixture of several.

1 Green salad is a mixture of salad leaves, well washed and dried, served on a plate or in a bowl with vinaigrette served separately.
2 Tossed green salad is the same as green salad but with the vinaigrette added. It is tossed in a salad bowl using two salad servers, to coat the leaves in the dressing.
3 Tossed green salad with herbs is a tossed salad with chopped fresh herbs mixed in.

Cold food preparation

RECIPE

9 Coleslaw

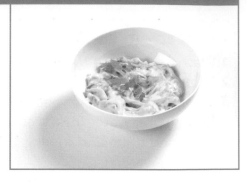

Get ready to cook

1 Trim off the outer cabbage leaves.
2 Wash and peel the carrot.
3 Finely shred the onion, and blanch and refresh it to remove the harsh taste (optional).

INGREDIENTS	4 portions	10 portions
Cabbage, white or Chinese	200 g	500 g
Carrot	50 g	125 g
Onion (optional)	25 g	60 g
Mayonnaise or natural yoghurt	125 ml	300 ml
Salt		

Preparing the dish

1 Cut the cabbage into quarters and cut out the hard centre stalk.
2 Wash the cabbage, finely shred it and drain it well.
3 Cut the carrot into fine strips (known as julienne – for large quantities this can be done in a food processor).
4 Mix all ingredients.
5 Taste and season *very* lightly with salt, only if necessary.

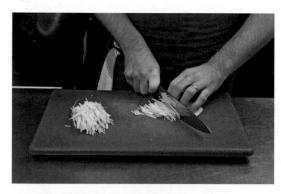

Finely shredding the cabbage

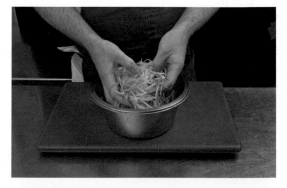

Mixing the shredded vegetables

Activity

Prepare batches of coleslaw:

1 without the onion

2 with the onion

3 with the onion blanched.

In a group, taste and assess the different coleslaws and note down your findings.

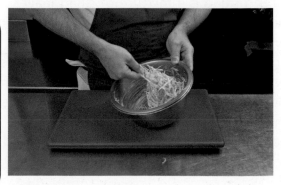

Stirring in the mayonnaise

10 Rice salad

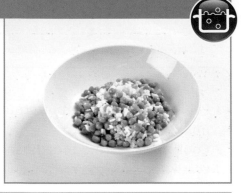

Get ready to cook

1 Cook the rice (see page 192).
2 Cook the peas.
3 Skin the tomatoes (see page 153).
4 Prepare the vinaigrette (see recipe 2).

INGREDIENTS	4 portions	10 portions
Tomatoes	100 g	250 g
Long grain rice, cooked	100 g	250 g
Peas, cooked	50 g	125 g
Vinaigrette	1 tbsp	2½ tbsp
Salt		

Preparing the dish

1 Cut the tomatoes into quarters, remove the seeds and cut into ½ cm dice.
2 Mix the tomatoes with the rice, peas and vinaigrette.
3 Taste and correct the seasoning.

11 Green bean salad

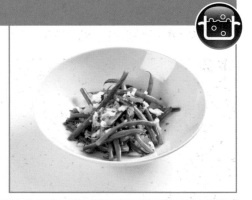

Get ready to cook

1 Cook the green beans.
2 Chop and blanch the onions.
3 Prepare the vinaigrette (see recipe 2).

INGREDIENTS	4 portions	10 portions
Green beans, cooked	200 g	500 g
Vinaigrette	1 tbsp	2½ tbsp
Onion, chopped and blanched if required	15 g	40 g
Chives		
Salt		

Preparing the dish

1 Combine all ingredients.
2 Taste and season as necessary.

Activity

Prepare six salads and present them in three or four different ways.

Try something different

This recipe can also be made using any type of dried bean. Many dried beans are available ready cooked in cans.

Make a three-bean salad using three different types of dried bean, e.g. red kidney, black-eyed, flageolet.

Cold food preparation

Warm Asian bean salad with satay dressing

Get ready to cook

1 Peel and deseed the butternut squash and cut into 2 cm dice.
2 Cook and shell the broad beans
3 Wash and slice the radishes.
4 Roughly chop the spring onions.
5 Roast and chop the cashew nuts.

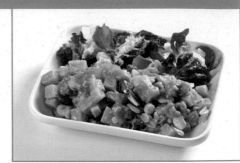

INGREDIENTS	4 portions	10 portions
Butternut squash, peeled, deseeded and cut into 2 cm dice	250 g	625 g
Broad beans, cooked and skinned	240 g	600 g
Clear honey	1 tbsp	2 tbsp
Lime, grated zest and juice	½	2
Peanut satay	80 g	200 g
Coriander, chopped	½ tbsp	1½ tbsp
Spring onions, chopped	6	15
Radishes, thinly sliced	4	10
Roasted cashew nuts, roughly chopped	50 g	125 g

Satay is peanut sauce. You can buy this ready made or you can make it yourself. To make it, add the following ingredients to a food processor and blend until smooth:

4 tbsp peanut butter

2 tbsp sesame oil

1 tbsp soy sauce

1 tbsp honey

1 tbsp milk or water

1 garlic clove, peeled and crushed/chopped

¹/₂ lime, juice only

Preparing the dish

1 Blanch the butternut squash in boiling water for 3–4 minutes and drain.
2 Place the butternut squash in a large bowl with the cooked broad beans.
3 Prepare the dressing by mixing together the honey, lime juice and peanut satay.
4 Roughly chop the coriander and add this, along with the chopped spring onions, sliced radish and cashew nuts, to the squash and broad beans.
5 Mix in half the dressing.

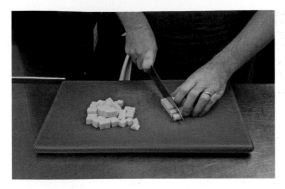

Dicing the squash

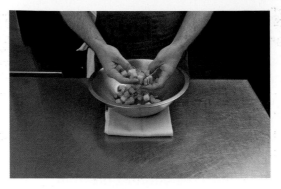

Mixing the squash and beans

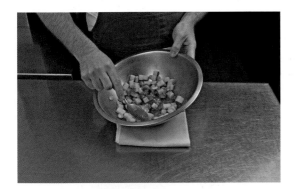

Mixing in the dressing

Serving suggestion

Serve on plates, on a bed of mixed salad leaves. Drizzle over the remainder of the dressing and serve.

13 Spicy squash salad

Get ready to cook

1 Preheat the oven to 200°C.
2 Peel and deseed the butternut squash and cut into small chunks.
3 Deseed the peppers and cut into rough slices.

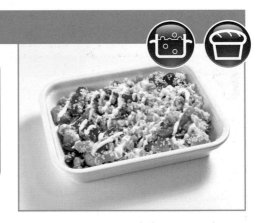

INGREDIENTS	4 portions	10 portions
Oil	¾ tbsp	2 tbsp
Harissa paste	1½ tbsp	4 tbsp
Butternut squash, peeled, deseeded and cut into chunks	400 g	2 (approx. 1½ kg)
Red peppers	1	3
French beans or sliced runner beans	125 g	300 g
Couscous	125 g	280 g
Vegetable stock	400 ml	1.2 l
Lemon juice	1 tbsp	3 tbsp
Yoghurt	125 g	300 g
Garlic, crushed	½ clove	2 cloves
Chickpeas	300 g	800 g

Preparing the dish

1 Mix the oil and the Harissa paste together, and use to coat the squash and pepper.
2 Spread the vegetables on a baking tray and bake until just tender.
3 Cook the green beans in boiling water until just tender.
4 Put the couscous in a bowl and cover with boiling vegetable stock. Leave for 5 minutes to allow the couscous to absorb the stock and fluff up.
5 In a separate bowl, mix together the lemon juice, yoghurt and garlic.
6 Combine the couscous, squash, peppers, green beans and chickpeas in a bowl and drizzle with the yoghurt dressing.

RECIPE

 Asian rice salad

Get ready to cook

1 Lightly cook the peas.
2 Cook the rice lightly in salted water. Drain and cool.
3 Very finely dice the courgette and finely slice the spring onion, cutting on the slant – for this salad the pieces must be small.
4 Peel and finely chop the garlic and ginger.
5 Roughly chop the herbs.

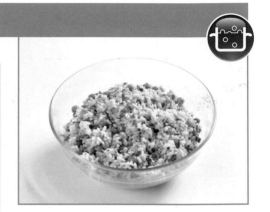

INGREDIENTS	4 portions	10 portions
Flat-leaf parsley, chopped	2 tbsp	5 tbsp
Coriander, chopped	2 tbsp	5 tbsp
Mint, chopped	1 tbsp	2½ tbsp
Garlic, finely chopped	1 clove	4 cloves
Ginger, finely chopped	2 cm	5 cm
Reduced salt soy sauce	2½ tbsp	6 tbsp
Lime juice	1 tbsp	2½ tbsp
Honey	1 tbsp	2½ tbsp
Sunflower oil	4 tbsp	10 tbsp
Basmati rice, cooked	400 g	1 kg
Courgettes	1	3
Peas, lightly cooked	125 g	300 g
Spring onions	2	5

Preparing the dish

1 Blitz the herbs, garlic, ginger, soy sauce, lime juice and honey in a food processor.
2 Slowly add the oil to create a glossy mixture.
3 To the rice add the courgettes, peas and spring onions and combine.
4 Stir through the dressing.

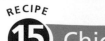

15 Chicken and honey salad

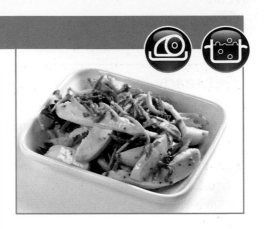

Get ready to cook

1 Lightly cook the potatoes in boiling water until just tender. Cut lengthways into quarters.
2 Lightly cook the green beans in boiling water until just tender. Drain and cool under cold running water.
3 Roast or boil and then skin and slice the chicken.
4 Cook and chop the bacon.

INGREDIENTS	4 portions	10 portions
Lettuce leaves or other salad leaves (baby spinach, or red and green loose leaf)	100 g	250 g
Potatoes (Mayan Gold, Charlottes or another waxy variety)	400 g	900 g
Fine green beans	125 g	300 g
Cooked chicken breasts, skinned, sliced into strips	1½	4
Honey and mustard dressing – can be bought ready made		
Crispy precooked bacon to garnish	5 pieces	12 pieces

Preparing the dish

1 Divide the lettuce into four portions and place in salad bowls.
2 Scatter the potatoes and beans over the salad leaves.
3 Toss the cooked chicken in the honey and mustard dressing and spoon over the other salad items.

Serving suggestion

Garnish with chopped bacon.

Honey and mustard dressing can be bought ready made or you can make it in the right quantity by combining

- honey (1 tsp/2½ tbsp)
- mustard herb (1 tsp/2½ tsp)
- a little oil or vinaigrette, as required.

16 Spicy nasi goreng

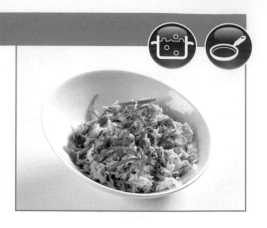

Get ready to cook

1 Cook the rice in lightly salted boiling water until just tender. Drain and cool.
2 Blitz the garlic, 1 chilli and 1 onion (or ½ of each for four portions) in a food processor to make a paste.
3 Slice the remaining onion, spring onions and chilli.

INGREDIENTS	4 portions	10 portions
Small eggs	2	4
Sunflower oil	2 tbsp	5 tbsp
Onion	1	3
Red chilli, sliced	1	3
Yellow pepper, seeded and sliced	½–1	2
Carrots, sliced julienne	1½	4
Long grain rice, cooked	250 g	600 g
Reduced-salt soy sauce	1½ tbsp	4 tbsp
Garlic	1 clove	4 cloves
Spring onions, sliced	1½	4
Coriander, chopped	1½ tbsp	4 tbsp

This can be served hot, or cold as a salad.

Preparing the dish

1 Heat a wok or large frying pan and lightly scramble the eggs. Remove and set aside.
2 Heat the oil in the wok and stir-fry the onion, chilli, peppers and carrots for 2 minutes.
3 Add the rice and cook for a further 3 minutes.
4 Stir in the soy sauce, the garlic, onion and chilli paste, spring onions and eggs.
5 Garnish with the chopped coriander.

17 Pesto pasta salad

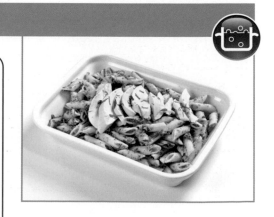

Get ready to cook

1 Cook the pasta al dente in boiling, lightly salted water. Drain and mix with oil.
2 Cook the chicken breasts by poaching, steaming, shallow frying or roasting. Remove the skin.
3 Slice the remaining onion, spring onions and chilli.

INGREDIENTS	4 portions	10 portions
Green pesto	70 g	200 g
Lemon juice	1 tbsp	3 tbsp
Reduced-fat mayonnaise	2½ tbsp	6 tbsp
Penne pasta	400 g	800 g
Extra virgin olive oil	1 tbsp	2 tbsp
Cooked chicken breasts	1–1½	3
Parsley, chopped	1 tbsp	5 tbsp

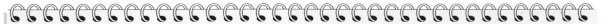

Ready-made pesto and reduced-fat mayonnaise can be purchased.

Preparing the dish

1 Mix pesto, lemon juice and mayonnaise together and stir into the pasta.

2 Cut the chicken into thin slices and combine with the pasta.

3 Chop the parsley and stir through the pasta.

Try something different

If you leave out the chicken and mayonnaise this can be served as a simple pasta salad with pesto.

RECIPE

18 Greek salad

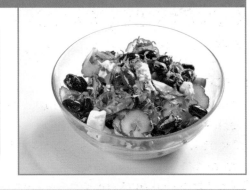

Get ready to cook

1 Wash the tomatoes and cut them in half lengthwise. Cut out the core, and cut each half into four wedges.

2 Wash and slice the cucumber.

3 Dice the feta cheese.

INGREDIENTS	4 portions	10 portions
Large tomatoes – preferably vine tomatoes	2	6
Cucumber, sliced	½	1
Feta cheese, diced	150 g	400 g
Olive oil	60 ml	150 ml
Lemon juice	2 tbsp	6 tbsp
Salt and black pepper		
Oregano, to garnish	1 level tbsp	3 level tbsp
Pitted black olives, to garnish	6	15

If you are not keen on the idea of eating olives, just try them and see what you think. They go particularly well with the other flavour and textures in this salad.

Preparing the dish

1 Put the tomatoes into a large salad bowl and add the cucumber and feta cheese.
2 Spoon over the olive oil and lemon juice.
3 Season lightly with salt and black pepper. Go easy on the salt, as feta cheese is already salty!
4 Toss gently to mix.

Serving suggestion

Sprinkle the salad with fresh oregano and decorate with olives.

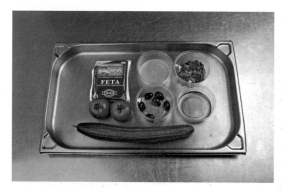

All the ingredients ready to use

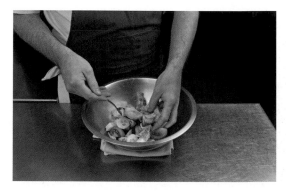

Mixing together the ingredients

RECIPE

19 Garden salad

Get ready to cook

Bring the peas to the boil and cook until just tender. Drain and refresh.

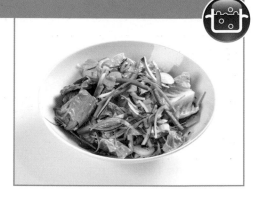

INGREDIENTS	4 portions	10 portions
Medium lettuce, crispy variety like iceberg or cos, torn into pieces	½	1
Carrot, cut into fine julienne	1	2
Red cabbage, chopped finely	125 g	350 g
Radish, thinly sliced	2	8
Onions, thinly sliced	1	3
Red pepper, thinly sliced	1	2
Green pepper, thinly sliced	1	2
Celery, thinly sliced	1 stick	3 sticks
Frozen peas, cooked	250 g	500 g

Preparing the dish

1 Wash and dry the lettuce and then tear into pieces.
2 Cut the carrots into julienne and finely slice the rest of the vegetables.
3 Combine the ingredients in large bowl with the peas.

Serving suggestion

Drizzle with a salad dressing of your own choice, e.g. vinaigrette, or serve plain.

Try something different

This works well with bean sprouts for added crunch.

Add flakes of canned tuna to make an interesting tuna salad.

Add beans such as chickpeas or butter beans for a different texture.

It also works well with 300 g (125 g) of feta cheese.

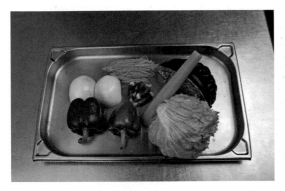

All the ingredients, ready to use

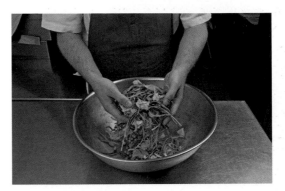

Combining the ingredients

RECIPE

20 Rice and bean salad

Get ready to cook

1 Rinse the kidney beans.
2 Deseed and dice the green pepper into small pieces.
3 Chop the onions and garlic.

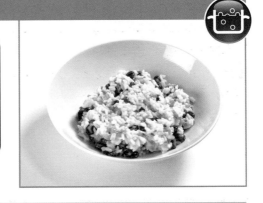

INGREDIENTS	4 portions	10 portions
Canned kidney beans, rinsed	125 g	300 g
Thyme	4 sprigs	6 sprigs
Creamed coconut	40 g	100 g
Bay leaves	1	3
Onions, chopped	1 small	2 medium
Garlic, chopped	1 clove	3 cloves
Ground allspice	⅓ level tsp	1 level tsp
Water	250 ml	600 ml
Long grain rice	375 g	900 g
Green pepper, deseeded and diced into small pieces	1 small	2 medium

Preparing the dish

1 Put the kidney beans, thyme, creamed coconut, bay leaves, onion, garlic and allspice in a large pan and stir in the water.
2 Bring to the boil and stir in the rice.

3 Reduce the heat, cover and simmer for approximately 30 minutes, until all the liquid is absorbed.

4 Remove from heat and stir in the diced pepper.

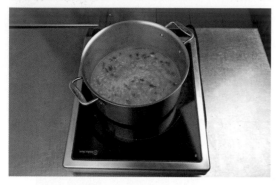
Cooking the ingredients

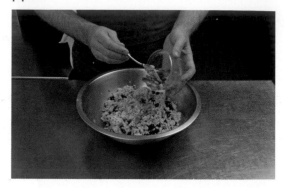
Adding the green pepper

RECIPE

(21) Spicy potato salad

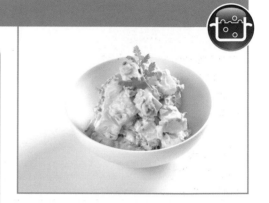

Get ready to cook

1 Cook the potatoes until just tender. If using main crop, cut into even-sized pieces.

2 Deseed the peppers and dice into small pieces.

3 Finely chop the celery, parsley, shallots, spring onions and garlic.

4 Thinly slice the chilli.

INGREDIENTS	4 portions	10 portions
Potatoes (new is best, but you can use a firm main crop potato), cooked	2 kg	1½ kg
Red pepper, deseeded and diced	1 small	2 large
Celery, finely chopped	3 sticks	5 sticks
Spring onions, finely chopped	1	4
Shallot or onion, finely diced	1 small	2 medium
Green chilli, thinly sliced	1 small	2 medium
Garlic, chopped	½ clove	2 cloves
Chives or the green of the spring onion, chopped	1 tsp	3 tsp
Parsley, chopped	1–2 tbsp	2 tbsp
Mayonnaise	2 tbsp	6 tbsp
Low-fat crème fraiche or sour cream	¾ tbsp	2 tbsp
Mild mustard	⅓ tsp	1 tsp
Sugar	⅓ tsp	1 tsp

Preparing the dish

1 Add the vegetables and herbs to the potatoes.

2 Mix the mayonnaise, crème fraiche, mustard and sugar in a bowl.

3 Add the dressing to the potatoes and gently combine.

Serving suggestion

Garnish with chopped chives or chopped spring onion.

22 Spicy vegetable chow mein salad

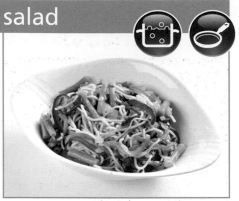

Get ready to cook

1 Cook the noodles in boiling, lightly salted water until tender. Allow to cool.
2 Finely chop the onion and celery.
3 Deseed and dice the peppers into even-sized pieces.
4 Cook the green beans in boiling, lightly salted water until just tender. Allow to cool.

INGREDIENTS	4 portions	10 portions
Sunflower oil	1 tbsp	4–6 tbsp
Garlic, crushed	1 clove	3 cloves
Onion, finely sliced	1 small	2 medium
Celery, thinly sliced	½ stick	2 sticks
Red pepper, thinly sliced	½	1
Green pepper, thinly sliced	½	1
Fine green beans	125 g	300 g
Chinese five spice powder	¼ level tsp	1 level tsp
Vegetable stock cube	½	2
Black pepper	⅛–½ tsp	½ tsp
Egg noodles	200 g	500 g
Reduced-salt soy sauce	½ tbsp	2 tbsp

Preparing the dish

1 Heat the oil in a wok or large frying pan and stir-fry the garlic, onion, celery and peppers for 3 minutes.
2 Add the green beans, five spice powder, crumbled stock cube and black pepper.
3 Combine well and cook gently for 5 minutes to allow stock cube to dissolve.
4 Add the noodles and soy sauce.
5 Carefully combine all ingredients.

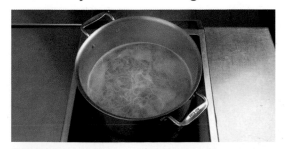

Cooking the noodles

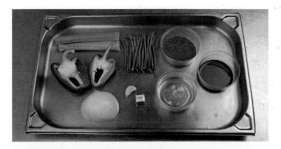

All the other ingredients, ready to cook

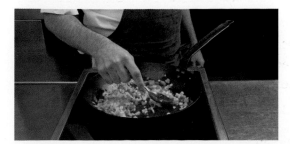

Stir-frying

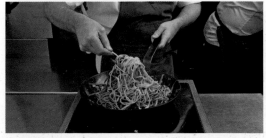

Combining the salad

Cold food preparation

Egg dishes

Introduction

Sizes

Hens' eggs, which are mainly used in cookery, are graded in four sizes: small, medium, large, very large.

Quality points

- Egg shells should be clean, strong, well shaped and slightly rough.
- When broken, there should be a high proportion of thick white to thin white. As an egg ages, the thick white gradually changes into thin white and water passes from the white into the yolk.
- The yolks should be firm, round (not flattened) and of a good, even, fresh-looking colour. As an egg ages, the yolk loses strength and begins to flatten. Water evaporates from the egg and is replaced by air.

Nutritional information

Eggs provide the energy, fat, minerals and vitamins needed for the body to grow and repair itself.

Hens can pass salmonella bacteria into their eggs, which could cause food poisoning. To reduce this risk, pasteurised eggs may be used where appropriate, e.g. in omelettes and scrambled eggs.

Egg recipes

RECIPE

1 Scrambled eggs

The reason for removing the eggs from the heat when they are only lightly cooked is because after the pan is removed from the stove it will still be hot and the eggs will continue cooking. Cooking scrambled eggs is a delicate task, and they can easily be overcooked and spoiled.

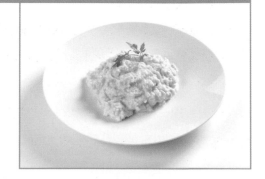

INGREDIENTS	4 portions	10 portions
Eggs (medium or large)	6–8	15–20
Salt – use sparingly		
Milk (optional)	2 tbsp	5 tbsp
Butter, margarine or oil	50 g	125 g

Cooking

1 Break the eggs into a basin, lightly season with salt and thoroughly mix using a whisk, adding the milk if using.

2 In a thick-bottomed pan, melt half of the fat.

3 Add the eggs and cook over a gently heat, stirring continuously with a heat-proof spatula or wooden spoon until the eggs are lightly cooked.

4 Remove from the heat, taste and correct the seasoning.

5 Mix in the remaining fat.

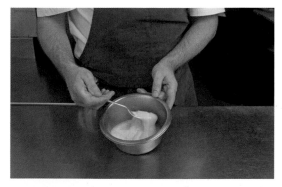

Beating the eggs

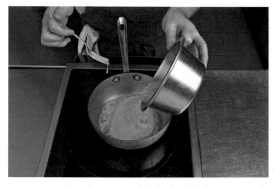

Adding the eggs to the hot pan

Serving suggestion

Serve on slices of hot buttered toast or in individual egg dishes.

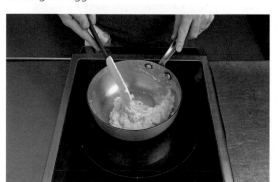

Stirring the eggs

Activity

As a group, try the following.

1 Cook two scrambled eggs following the recipe.

2 Cook two scrambled eggs as quickly as possible.

3 Cook two scrambled eggs using butter.

4 Cook two scrambled eggs using margarine or oil.

Taste, compare and discuss the four versions.

RECIPE

2 Fried eggs

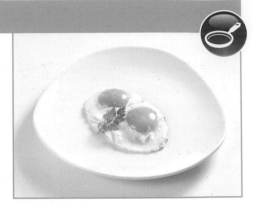

INGREDIENTS

Butter, margarine or oil – 25 g per egg
Eggs – allow one or two eggs per portion

- Only fresh, top-quality eggs should be used for frying.
- For the best flavour use butter or sunflower oil.

Cooking

1 Melt the butter, margarine or oil in a small non-stick frying pan.

2 Remove the eggs from their shells and add them carefully and gently to the pan, without breaking the yolks.

3 Cook slowly over a moderate heat and serve on a warmed plate.

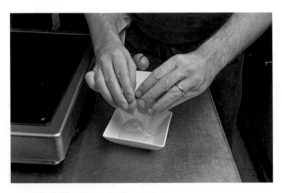

Breaking the eggs into a bowl, ready to use

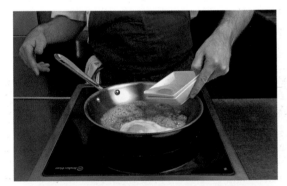

Frying the eggs

Activity

As a group, try the following.

1 Fry one egg following the recipe.

2 Fry one egg using butter.

3 Fry one egg using oil.

4 Fry one egg using margarine.

Taste, compare and discuss the four versions.

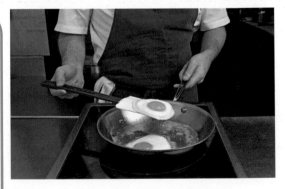

Trimming the fried eggs to a neat shape

3 Boiled eggs (in their shells)

INGREDIENT

Allow one or two eggs per portion

Cooking

For soft-boiled eggs:

1 Place the eggs in a saucepan. Cover with cold water and bring to the boil.
2 Simmer for 2–2½ minutes.
3 Remove from the water and serve in egg cups.

For medium-soft eggs:

1 Place the eggs carefully into a pan of boiling water.
2 Re-boil, simmer for 4–5 minutes and remove.

For hard-boiled eggs:

1 Place the eggs carefully into a pan of boiling water.
2 Re-boil and simmer for 8–10 minutes.
3 Refresh until cold under running water.

4 Poached eggs

INGREDIENTS

Allow one or two eggs per portion

Malt vinegar – three tablespoons per litre of water

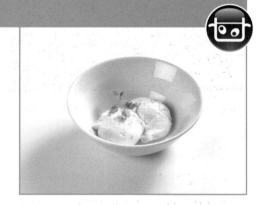

- Only use top-quality fresh eggs for poaching because of the large amount of thick white, which helps them to stick together in the simmering water.

- Using vinegar (an acid) helps to set the egg white and also makes it more tender.

Cooking

1 Heat a shallow pan of water at least 8 cm deep.
2 Add one tablespoon of malt vinegar per litre of water.
3 Carefully break the eggs into the gently simmering water.
4 Cook for approximately 3–3½ minutes, until lightly set.
5 Remove carefully using a perforated spoon. Place on a clean, dry cloth to drain off any water.
6 To keep the eggs and serve them later, gently place them in a bowl of very cold water. When they are needed, remove them with a slotted spoon and place them into gently simmering water for 1–1½ minutes. Drain and serve.

Serving suggestion

Serve on hot, buttered toast.

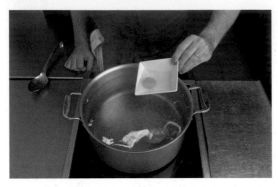

Placing the eggs into water that contains vinegar

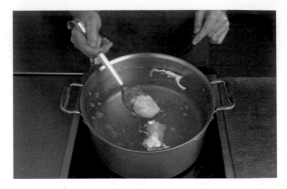

Removing the eggs from the water

Activity

Poach two eggs: one as fresh as possible, the other stale and out of its 'sell by' date. Assess the results.

RECIPE

(5) Omelette

INGREDIENTS

2–3 eggs per portion
Small pinch of salt
Butter, margarine or oil

There are many variations that can be made by adding other ingredients to the eggs when mixed, such as:

- chopped soft herbs – parsley, chives, chervil
- mushrooms – sliced and cooked in butter
- cheese – grated and added to the omelette before it is folded.

Cooking

1. Break the eggs into a basin and season lightly with salt.
2. Mix thoroughly with a fork or whisk until whites and yolks are thoroughly combined and no streaks of white can be seen.
3. Heat a non-stick omelette pan and wipe thoroughly clean with a dry cloth.
4. Add the butter, then turn up the heat to maximum until the butter is foaming but not brown.
5. Add the eggs and cook quickly, stirring continuously with a fork or heat-proof spatula until lightly set. Remove from the heat.
6. Using the fork, carefully fold the mixture in half at a right angle to the handle of the pan.

7 Pointing the pan slightly downwards, sharply tap the pan handle with the other hand to bring the edge of the omelette up to the bottom of the pan.

8 Carefully using the fork, bring up the opposite edge of the omelette as near to the first edge as possible.

9 Take a warm plate in one hand and, holding the pan under the handle, carefully tip the folded omelette onto the plate.

10 Neaten the shape if necessary, using a clean teacloth, and serve immediately.

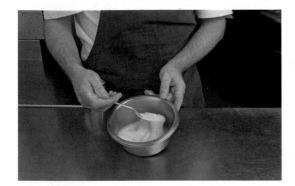
Mixing the eggs

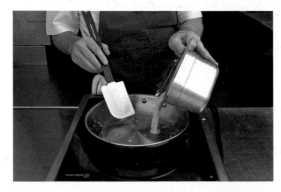
Adding the eggs to the hot pan

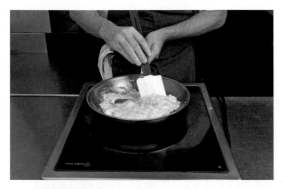
Stirring the eggs

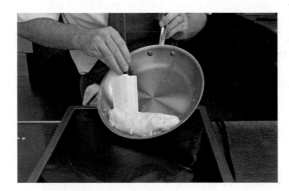
Folding the omelette

Activity

Practice is the only way to achieve a satisfactory omelette.

Suggest three variations. Prepare all three, and taste, discuss and assess them.

RECIPE

6 Red onion and sweetcorn frittata

Get ready to cook

1 Finely chop the onion and carrot.
2 Peel the tomatoes (see page 153), then de-seed and finely dice them.
3 Peel the potatoes and cut into 1 cm cubes.
4 Cook the diced potatoes in boiling water. Drain well.

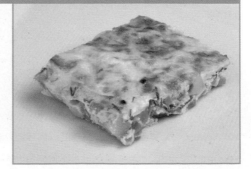

INGREDIENTS	4 portions	10 portions
Red onions, finely chopped	½ (or 1 if small)	1
Carrots, finely chopped	50 g	125 g
Oil for frying	5 ml	15 ml
Ground paprika	⅛ tsp	¼ tsp
Fresh, ripe tomatoes, peeled, deseeded, finely diced	2	5
Sweetcorn	20 g	50 g
Potatoes, diced	100 g	250 g
Parsley, chopped	1 tsp	1½ tsp
Eggs	3	5
Milk	250 ml	625 ml
Cheddar cheese, grated	100 g	250 g

Cooking

1 Shallow fry the onions and carrots in the oil without colouring.

2 Sprinkle with paprika and drain off any excess oil.

3 Add the diced tomatoes, sweetcorn, potatoes and chopped parsley to the pan and combine all the ingredients.

4 Place the mixture into a suitable ovenproof dish.

5 Whisk the eggs and milk together and season with black pepper.

6 Pour the eggs and milk over the vegetables in the ovenproof dish.

7 Sprinkle with cheddar cheese.

8 Bake in the oven at 180°C for approximately 15 minutes or until the mixture has set.

9 Allow to rest slightly before cutting into portions and serving.

Serving suggestion

Frittata may be served hot or cold with salad.

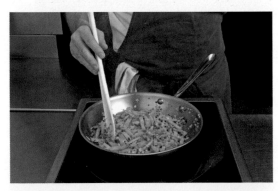

Shallow frying the onions and carrots

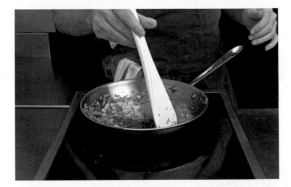

Adding the other vegetables

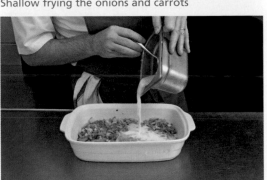

Pouring the eggs and milk over the vegetables

7 Steamed eggs with chicken and spring onions

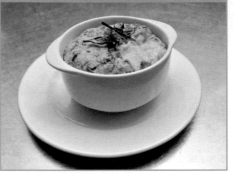

Get ready to cook

1 Cook and shred the chicken.
2 Lightly beat the eggs.
3 Peel the shallots, slice them thinly and fry until crispy.
4 Chop the garlic and spring onion.

INGREDIENTS	4 portions	10 portions
Whole eggs, lightly beaten	400 ml	1 litre
Chicken or fish stock	400 ml	1 litre
Salt and pepper to taste		
Chicken breast, cooked and shredded	100 g	250 g
Shallots, thinly sliced and fried until crispy	4	10
Garlic, chopped	2 cloves	5 cloves
Light soy sauce	10 ml	25 ml
Sesame oil	1 tsp	2 tsp
Spring onions, chopped	2	5

Cooking

1 Combine the eggs, salt, ground pepper and chicken/fish stock.
2 Using a fork, gently stir the mixture, slowly breaking the yolks. Mix well without creating too many air bubbles.
3 Pass the mixture through a fine strainer.
4 Stir in the cooked chicken.
5 Pour the mixture into small ramekins and steam on a medium heat for 20 minutes or until set.

Serving suggestion

Remove the contents from the ramekins (or serve them in the ramekins) and drizzle with light soy sauce and sesame oil, then sprinkle with fried shallots, garlic and chopped spring onions.

Egg dishes

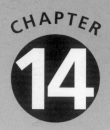

Pasta

Introduction

Pasta is made from a strong wheat flour called durum wheat flour. Water, olive oil and egg are added to the flour to make a dough.

There are two types of pasta available:

1 dried, which is made into over 50 different shapes (traditionally cooked 'al dente', which means firm to the bite)
2 fresh, also available in a variety of shapes and flavours.

Both dried and fresh pasta can be bought, as can a wide variety of sauces.

Traditionally, freshly grated Parmesan cheese is served with pasta, and freshly milled pepper is also offered.

Pasta recipes

RECIPE

 Spaghetti with a vegetable and meat sauce

> **Get ready to cook**
> Clean, peel and chop the vegetables.

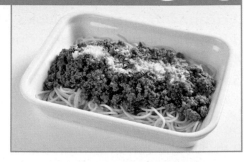

INGREDIENTS	4 portions	10 portions
Light olive oil	1 tbsp	2½ tbsp
Beef or pork mince	200 g	500 g
Onion, cut into neat pieces	100 g	250 g
Carrot, cut into neat pieces	1000 g	250 g
Celery, cut into neat pieces	50 g	125 g
Tomato purée	1 tbsp	2½ tbsp
Beef stock or thickened gravy	100 ml	250 ml
Salt and freshly ground pepper		
Spaghetti, dried	100 g	250 g
Parsley, freshly chopped	½ tbsp	1½ tbsp

There are many variations to this recipe, such as:

- adding chopped mushrooms to the vegetables
- adding a small pinch of oregano or rosemary, or a small pinch of chopped chives, etc.
- using half beef and half pork.

Cooking

1 Heat the olive oil in a thick-bottomed pan to a medium heat.
2 Add the minced meat and cook, stirring well, for 10 minutes.
3 Add the chopped vegetables and continue cooking, stirring well, until they are softened.
4 Mix in the tomato purée and add the stock.
5 Simmer until the meat is tender, then season lightly with salt and pepper and taste. Adjust seasoning if necessary.
6 Cook the spaghetti in plenty of slightly salted boiling water until al dente, then drain in a colander.
7 Mix the chopped parsley into the meat sauce.

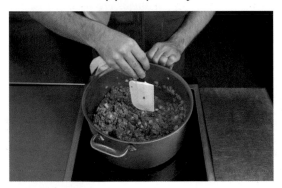

Cooking the meat

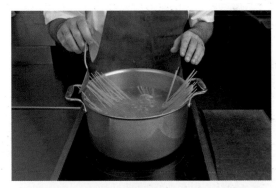

Cooking the spaghetti

Serving suggestion

1 Serve the spaghetti in a serving dish or individual dishes and pour the sauce into the centre.
2 Serve immediately, offering freshly ground Parmesan cheese and freshly ground pepper.

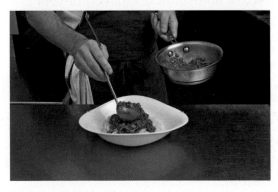

Serving the spaghetti and sauce

Activity

1 As a group, make your own version of a meat and vegetable spaghetti.
2 Taste it and discuss what you think of it.

RECIPE

2 Penne with tomato sauce

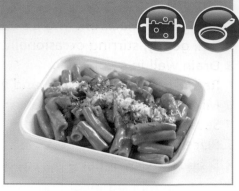

Get ready to cook

Prepare the tomato sauce, as described on page 150.

INGREDIENTS (MAIN COURSE PORTIONS)	4 portions	10 portions
Dried penne	400 g	1 kg
Tomato sauce (see page 150)	250 ml	625 ml
Olive oil	1 tbsp	2 tbsp

Cooking

1 Boil the penne in plenty of slightly salted water until 'al dente'.

2 Boil the tomato sauce.

3 Drain the penne in a colander.

4 Return the pasta to the pan.

5 Add the tomato sauce and olive oil, and mix well with the pasta.

Serving suggestion

Serve with freshly ground Parmesan cheese and offer freshly ground pepper.

Try something different

Add a *little* finely chopped red chilli to the tomato sauce.

Activity

Prepare and serve a variation of your choice to your group. The group should taste it and give their opinions.

RECIPE

3 Macaroni pasta bake

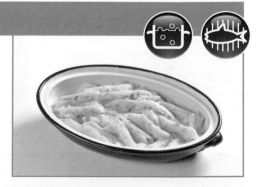

Get ready to cook

Prepare the béchamel sauce, as described on page 144.

INGREDIENTS (FIRST COURSE PORTIONS)	4 portions	10 portions
Macaroni	100 g	250 g
Oil or butter (optional)	25 g	60 g
Grated cheese	100 g	250 g
Diluted English or continental mustard	¼ tsp	1 tsp
Thin béchamel sauce (see page 144)	500 ml	1¼ litres
Salt, milled pepper		

Cooking

1 Plunge the macaroni into a saucepan of lightly salted boiling water.

2 Boil gently, stirring occasionally, for approximately 10–15 minutes (until al dente).

3 Drain well in a colander.

4 Return to a clean dry pan and add the oil or butter.

5 Mix with half the cheese, the mustard and the béchamel.

6 Season lightly and taste to check.

7 Place in an earthenware dish and sprinkle with the remainder of the cheese.

8 Brown lightly under a grill or in a hot oven.

Try something different

Add a layer of sliced tomatoes or lightly cooked sliced mushrooms to the top of the finished macaroni before adding the final grated cheese and browning.

Activity

Prepare and serve a dish of macaroni bake to your own idea. The group should taste it and give their opinions.

RECIPE

 4 Farfalle with chives and bacon

Get ready to cook

1 Grill the bacon until crisp then cut into small pieces.

2 Chop the chives.

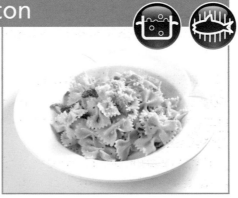

INGREDIENTS (MAIN COURSE PORTIONS)	4 portions	10 portions
Farfalle	400 g	1 kg
Streaky bacon rashers, grilled	10	25
Butter or oil	50 g	125 g
Fresh chives, chopped	2 tbsp	5 tbsp
Parmesan, freshly grated	50 g	125 g

Cooking

1 Cook the pasta in lightly salted boiling water.

2 Drain the pasta and place in a warm bowl.

3 Mix in the butter, chives and Parmesan.

4 Taste and correct the seasoning. Sprinkle with chives and crisp bacon and serve.

Activity

Make a list of as many pre-prepared types of pasta or pasta products as you can think of. (Refer back to Chapter 7 if you need help with this.)

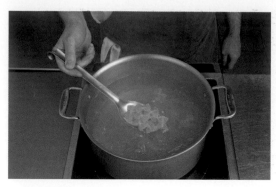
Cooking the pasta

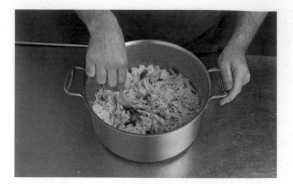
Mixing in the other ingredients

5 Green tagliatelle with sausage and cream

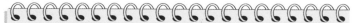

A thin béchamel sauce can be used in place of cream.

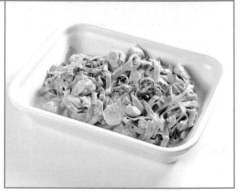

INGREDIENTS (MAIN COURSE PORTIONS)	4 portions	10 portions
Plump sausages with skins removed	4	10
Butter or oil	25 g	60 g
Single cream or crème fraiche	250 ml	625 ml
Green tagliatelle	400 g	1 kg
Parmesan	50 g	100 g
Chives, chopped	½ tsp	1 tsp

Cooking

1 Fry the sausages in a pan in the butter or oil. As they cook, break them up with a fork until they are slightly crisp.

2 Mix in the cream, allow it to thicken and then remove from the heat.

3 Boil the tagliatelle.

4 Drain well and transfer it to a bowl.

5 Pour over the sausages and cream and mix in the butter and Parmesan.

6 Taste, correct seasoning and serve sprinkled with chopped chives.

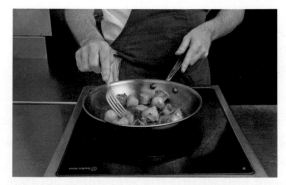
Frying the sausages and breaking them up

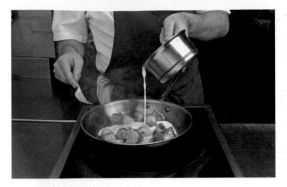

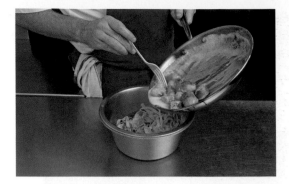

Mixing in the cream

Combining the ingredients, ready to serve

RECIPE

6 Pasta spirals with stir-fried asparagus and peanut sauce

Get ready to cook

1 Trim the asparagus and cut into 2½ cm lengths.
2 Cut the beans into 2½ cm lengths.
3 Deseed and finely chop the chilli.
4 Peel and crush the garlic.
5 Peel the ginger and chop this and the spring onions.

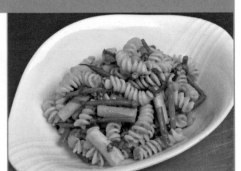

INGREDIENTS	4 portions	10 portions
Pasta spirals	375 g	1 kg
Asparagus, trimmed and cut into 2½ cm lengths	225 g	675 g
French beans, cut into 2½ cm lengths	225 g	675 g
Vegetable oil	1 tbsp	2½ tbsp
Red chilli, deseeded and finely chopped	1	2½
Clove of garlic, crushed and chopped	1	2¼
Ginger, fresh and chopped	½ tsp	1¼ tsp
Spring onions, chopped	1 tsp	2½ tsp
Water	2 tbsp	5 tbsp
Light soy sauce	2 tbsp	5 tbsp
Peanut butter	2 tbsp	5 tbsp
Fresh basil, chopped	1 tsp	2½ tsp
Toasted sesame seed oil	1 tbsp	2½ tbsp

Cooking

1 Cook the pasta spirals in boiling water until al dente. Drain and keep warm.
2 Blanch the asparagus and French beans in boiling water and drain.
3 Heat the oil in a wok. Quickly fry the chilli, garlic, ginger and spring onions for 1 minute.
4 Add the asparagus and French beans. Cook for another minute.
5 Mix the water, light soy sauce and peanut butter together. Stir into the vegetables.

6 Add the basil and sesame seed oil.

7 Stir in the pasta and toss all the ingredients together.

Serving suggestion

Serve on suitable plates and garnish with chopped fresh basil.

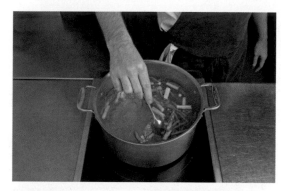

Blanching the asparagus and beans

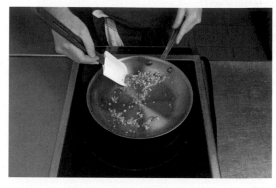

Frying the spring onions and spices

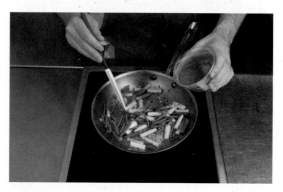

Adding the soy sauce mixture

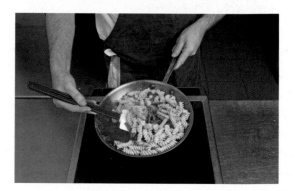

Adding the pasta

RECIPE

7) Penne with peas and cream

Get ready to cook

Cook the peas in a little water.

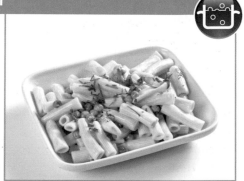

A non-dairy cream or olive oil (2 tbsp/5 tbsp) may be used as an alternative to cream.

INGREDIENTS (MAIN COURSE PORTIONS)	4 portions	10 portions
Penne	400 g	1 kg
Butter	50 g	125 g
Single cream	150 ml	375 ml
Freshly grated Parmesan cheese	100 g	250 g
Peas, shelled or frozen, cooked	200 g	500 g

Cooking

1 Cook the penne al dente in plenty of boiling salted water. Drain in a colander and place in a warm bowl.
2 Mix in the butter, cream, half the cheese and the peas.

Serving suggestion

Serve in an appropriate dish or dishes and sprinkle the remaining cheese on top.

8 Tuna pasta bake

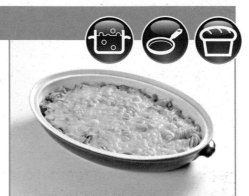

Get ready to cook

1 Peel and finely chop the onion.
2 Deseed the peppers and cut them into ¼ cm dice.
3 Slice the mushrooms.
4 Chop the tinned tomatoes.

INGREDIENTS	4 portions	10 portions
Pasta spirals	120 g	300 g
Onion, finely chopped	80 g	200 g
Oil for frying	1 tbsp	2 tbsp
Red pepper, deseeded and finely diced into ¼ cm	½	1
Green pepper, deseeded and finely diced into ¼ cm	½	1
Canned plum tomatoes, chopped	80 g	200 g
Tomato juice	250 ml	625 ml
Fresh oregano, chopped	1 tsp	2 tsp
Sugar	pinch	pinch
Flaked cooked tuna, or drained canned tuna	160 g	400 g
Cheddar cheese, grated	160 g	400 g
Button mushrooms, sliced	40 g	100 g
Tomato purée	40 g	100 g

Cooking

1 Cook the pasta in boiling water. Refresh in cold water and drain.
2 Fry the onions in the oil without colouring.
3 Add the peppers and chopped tomatoes and cook for another 3 minutes.
4 Add the juice from the tomatoes or use tomato juice.
5 Chop the fresh oregano and add this and the sugar.
6 Add the tuna and season with pepper.
7 Stir three-quarters of the cheese into the sauce and mix well.
8 Reheat the pasta by plunging it into boiling water. Drain well and place in an ovenproof serving dish.
9 Pour over the tomato mixture and sprinkle with the remainder of the cheese.
10 Finish in an oven at 200 °C until the cheese is golden brown.

Rice and grains

Introduction

Rice is a type of grain. There are many others.

- Grains are cereal crops, mostly grasses cultivated for their edible seeds or grains.
- Grains are rich in nutrients and can make a good contribution to a healthy diet.
- Store grains in airtight containers in a cool, dry and dark place.

Types of grain

Barley is available as whole or pot barley. Pot barley is polished pearl barley. Barley flakes and kernels are also produced. Barley can be cooked in water (one part grain to three parts water) for 45–60 minutes as an alternative to rice, pasta or potatoes, and is also used in broths and stews.

Buckwheat is gluten free and can be cooked and served like rice, or it can be added to stews or casseroles. Buckwheat flour can be added to cakes, muffins and pancakes.

Corn/maize is available as fresh sweetcorn or corn on the cob, when it is eaten as a vegetable. Dried corn is made into cornflakes or popcorn. Flour made from corn is used to make the Italian dish polenta, which can be used in place of pasta or potatoes.

Millet comes in several varieties and is a species of small-seeded cereal crop or grain. It is useful for replacing certain cereal grains in the diet for those with an intolerance to wheat and wheat products. Millet flakes can be made into porridge and millet flour is sometimes made into pasta.

Oats are produced in various forms – oatmeal, rolled oats, jumbo oat flakes. All forms can be used in the same way. The main uses of oatmeal are:

- as a main ingredient in baking
- in making oat cakes or bannocks
- to make a nut roast, with groundnuts
- in stuffing or dressing for poultry
- in black/blood puddings or haggis
- as porridge.

Wheat flour (crushed wheat grains) is used for bread, cakes, biscuits, pastry, cereals and pasta. Wheat is also available in other forms.

- Bulgar wheat is parboiled then cracked by cutting the whole grains with steel blades. It then only needs to be soaked in boiling water or stock before use.
- Semolina is a grainy yellow flour ground from hard or durum wheat and is the main ingredient of dried pasta.
- Couscous is made from semolina grains that have been rolled, dampened and coated with fine wheat flour. It is soaked in two parts of water or stock to one part couscous, then steamed. It is popular in Middle Eastern and North African cookery.

Quinoa (pronounced keen-wa) has small round grains similar to millet, with a mild taste and a firm and slightly chewy texture. It is cooked in three parts water to one part grain for 15 minutes. It can be used in place of other cereals, risotto rice or pasta, and in vegetable stuffings and salads.

Some recipes using grains other than rice can be found in Chapter 22. Further information can be obtained from The Vegetarian Society at www.vegsoc.org.

Rice

Rice is the main food crop for about half of the world's population. There are around 250 varieties of rice, but initially we need only deal with two types.

1 Short grain – a short, rounded grain with a soft texture, suitable for sweet dishes and risotto (an Italian speciality). Arborio is a type of short grain rice.
2 Long grain – a narrow long grain with a distinctive flavour, such as basmati. It has a firm structure, which helps to keep the grains separate when cooked. It is used for plain boiled or steamed rice served with savoury curry-type dishes.

A third variety used in cooking is whole grain, used for savoury dishes, but the recipes in this chapter all use either short or long grain rice. You may also have heard of wild rice. In fact this is not a rice, but an aquatic grass used for special dishes or salads. Rice flour can be used for thickening soups.

Rice can be cooked by steaming (see Chapter 10). This can be done in a rice cooker, following the manufacturer's instructions.

Nutritional information

Rice is a very useful and versatile carbohydrate. When added to dishes it helps to proportionally reduce the fat content (i.e. because you are eating more carbohydrate you are likely to eat less fat).

Warning

Once rice is cooked, you should keep it hot at a temperature above 65°C, but for no longer than two hours. If it is kept at a lower temperature than this, or for longer than two hours, the spores of a bacterium found in the soil may change back to bacteria and could result in food poisoning.

Avoid storing and reheating cooked rice unless it has it has been done in strict hygiene and temperature-controlled conditions.

Activity

1 Food should be kept out of 'danger zone' temperatures as much as possible. What temperature range is called the 'danger zone'?

2 Suggest three good working practices that will prevent food from being in this zone for too long.

(Refer back to Chapter 8 if you need help answering these questions.)

Rice recipes

1 Plain boiled rice

INGREDIENTS	4 portions	10 portions
Basmati rice, dry weight	100 g	250 g

Cooking

1 Pick and wash the rice and place in a saucepan. (Picking the rice means checking that there is nothing in it that should not be there!)
2 Add to plenty of lightly salted boiling water.
3 Stir to the boil then simmer gently until tender (approximately 12–15 minutes).
4 Pour into a sieve and rinse well, first under cold running water then very hot water.
5 Drain off all water and leave the rice in a sieve placed over a bowl and covered with a clean tea cloth.

2 Braised rice (pilau)

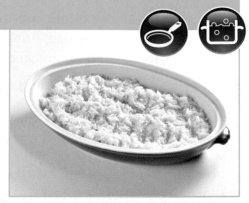

> **Get ready to cook**
> Peel the onion and chop finely.

INGREDIENTS	4 portions	10 portions
Oil, butter or margarine	50 g	125 g
Onion, finely chopped	25 g	60 g
Rice, long grain	100 g	250 g
White stock, preferably chicken	200 ml	500 ml
Salt		

Cooking

1 Place half the fat into a thick-bottomed pan.
2 Add the onion and cook gently without colouring until the onion is soft (2–3 minutes).
3 Add the rice and stir to mix. Cook over a gentle heat without colouring for 2–3 minutes.
4 Add *exactly* twice the amount of stock to rice.
5 Season lightly with salt, cover with greased paper and bring to the boil.
6 Place in a hot oven (230–250°C) until cooked (approximately 15 minutes).
7 When cooked, remove immediately to a cool container or pan. If the rice is left in the pan in which it was cooked, the heat will be sufficient for the rice to continue cooking, which will result in it overcooking and being spoilt.
8 Carefully mix in the remaining half of the fat using a two-pronged fork.
9 Taste, correct the seasoning and serve.

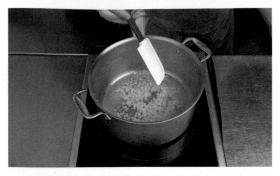

Gently cooking the onion

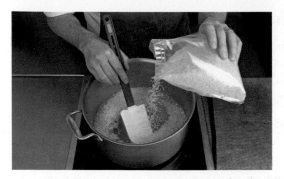

Stirring in the rice

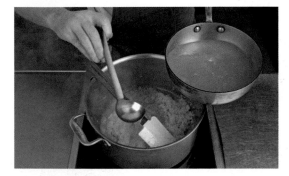

Adding the stock

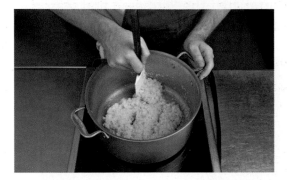

Finishing the dish

Try something different

A pilau can be varied by adding, for example:

- sliced mushrooms, which would be added at the same time as the onions
- freshly grated cheese (10–100 g) which would be added with the fat at the end.

Activity

1 Cook and compare a dish of plain boiled rice and a dish of steamed rice (page 108).

2 Cook two dishes of pilau, one with a good, richly flavoured chicken stock and the other with water. Taste and compare them.

RECIPE

3 Risotto (a traditional Italian dish)

Get ready to cook
Peel the onion and chop finely.

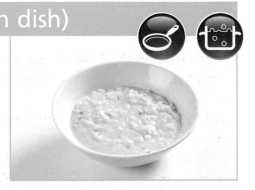

INGREDIENTS	4 portions	10 portions
Onion, finely chopped	½	2
Butter	75 g	150 g
Short grain rice, e.g. Arborio	200 g	500 g
Chicken stock	1 litre	2½ litres
Parmesan, freshly grated	50 g	125 g
Salt		

Cooking

1 In a thick-bottomed pan, lightly sweat the onion in half the butter, without colouring.
2 Add the rice and stir with a heat-resistant spatula until it is thoroughly coated with butter.
3 Pour in a large ladle of boiling stock and stir until completely absorbed.
4 Repeat this procedure, adding more stock until the rice has swollen and is almost cooked. Check by tasting it. It will usually take about 20 minutes.
5 When cooked, remove the pan from the heat and stir in the other half of the butter, half the Parmesan and season lightly.
6 Leave to rest for 2–3 minutes to allow the rice to swell.

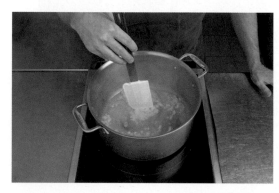

Sweating the onion

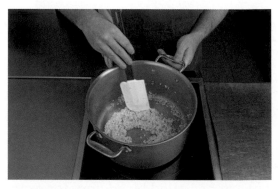

Stirring in the rice

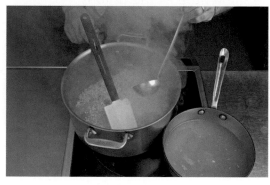

Adding some of the stock

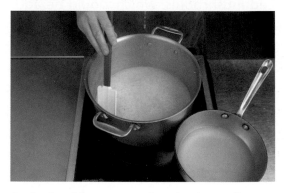

Gradually adding more stock as the rice swells

Serving suggestion

Serve with more Parmesan.

Try something different

This is a basic dish that lends itself to many additions, e.g. sliced mushrooms, prawns.

4 Risotto with lemon grass, capers and green olives

Get ready to cook

1 Peel the onion and chop finely.
2 Crush and chop the garlic and lemon grass.

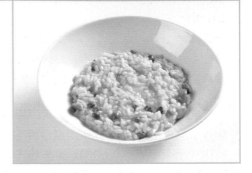

INGREDIENTS	4 portions	10 portions
Onion, finely chopped	50 g	125 g
Vegetable oil		
Garlic, crushed/chopped	1 clove	2 cloves
Lemon grass, crushed and chopped	3 stalks	6 stalks
Arborio rice	450 g	1125 g
White stock	650 ml	1625 ml
Ground black pepper		
Capers	2 tbsps	5 tsps
Stoned green olives	100 g	250 g

Cooking

1 Sweat the onions in the vegetable oil with the garlic until soft.
2 Add the lemon grass to the onions.
3 Add the rice and stir for 2 minutes until the rice is translucent.
4 Add a little stock and cook the rice until the stock has been absorbed.
5 Repeat with more stock until it has all been used and/or the rice is soft. Season with ground black pepper.
6 Add the capers and olives to the rice and serve.

Fish

Introduction

There are two types, or varieties, of fish:

- oily – round in shape, e.g. herring, mackerel, sardine, salmon
- white – of which some are flat (e.g. plaice, lemon sole) and some round (e.g. cod, haddock, hake).

It is important for fish to be as fresh as possible and kept in a refrigerator below 5°C. If freshness is lost, the quality and flavour can be affected by ammonia, which if eaten could result in food poisoning.

Quality points

Whole fish should:

- have clear, bright eyes that are not sunken
- have bright red gills
- have scales firmly attached to the skin, none missing
- smell fresh – no trace of ammonia smell.

Fillets of fish should:

- be neat and trim with firm flesh (not soft and spongy)
- be white and translucent (if it is white fish), with no discolouration such as brown marks.

Frozen fish should:

- be hard, with no signs of thawing
- be packaged properly, with no signs of damage
- not show any signs of freezer burn, i.e. dull white dry patches.

Cooking fish

Poaching

Poaching is very gentle, which is very suitable for fish, because it is delicate. Poaching is suitable for:

- whole fish, e.g. salmon, trout
- certain cuts on the bone, e.g. salmon, cod
- certain fillets, whole or cut into portions, e.g. haddock or lemon sole.

There is a recipe for poached salmon in the 'methods of cookery' chapter (Chapter 10).

Steaming

Small whole fish or fillets can be steamed with aromats, e.g. steamed fish with garlic, or spring onions and garlic (recipe 1). See also recipe 10, steamed gingered snapper.

RECIPE

1 Steamed fish with garlic and spring onion

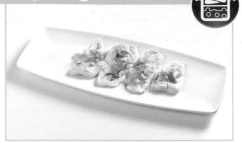

Get ready to cook

1 Peel and chop the ginger.
2 Peel and thinly slice the garlic.
3 Chop the spring onions.
4 Wash and dry the fish well.

INGREDIENTS	4 portions	10 portions
White fish fillets, e.g. plaice, lemon sole	400 g	1½ kg
Salt		
Ginger, peeled and freshly chopped	1 tbsp	2½ tbsp
Spring onions, finely chopped	2 tbsp	5 tbsp
Light soy sauce	1 tbsp	2½ tbsp
Garlic, peeled and thinly sliced (optional)	1 clove	2 cloves
Light oil	1 tbsp	2½ tbsp

Cooking

1 Rub the fish lightly with salt on both sides.
2 Put the fish in foil on plates or dishes.
3 Sprinkle the ginger evenly on top.
4 Put the plates into a steamer, cover tightly and steam gently until just cooked (5–15 minutes, according to the thickness of the fish). Do not overcook.
5 Remove the plates and foil and sprinkle on the spring onions and soy sauce.
6 Brown the garlic slices in hot oil in a small frying pan and pour over the dish (optional).

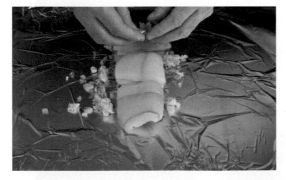

Placing the fish and other ingredients on foil ready to cook

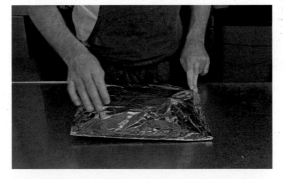

Forming a parcel of foil to protect the fish as it steams

Activity

Suggest two or three variations, then prepare, cook, serve, taste, assess and discuss them.

Shallow frying

This can be used for small whole fish or fillets, e.g. whole trout, plaice fillets.

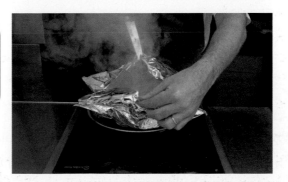

As the fish cooks, steam builds up in the parcel. When it is ready, breaking the foil releases the steam

197

2 Shallow frying fish

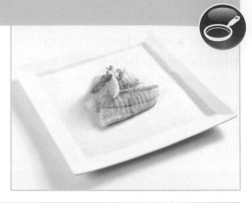

Get ready to cook

Prepare, clean, wash and thoroughly dry the fish.

INGREDIENTS	4 portions	10 portions
White fish fillets or small whole fish	400 g	1½ kg
Flour		
Light oil	1 tbsp	2½ tbsp

Cooking

1 Completely cover the fish with flour and shake off all surplus. If using non-stick pans it is not essential to flour the fish.
2 Heat the frying medium (usually a light oil) in the frying pan.
3 Shallow fry on both sides (presentation side first) and serve.

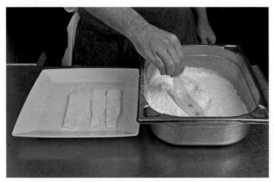

Passing the fish through the flour

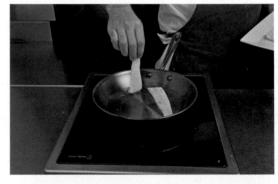

Placing the fish into the frying pan

Do not overcrowd the pan because this will cause the temperature of the oil to drop, which will affect the way the fish cooks. The fish should not be overcooked but should have an appetising light golden-brown colour.

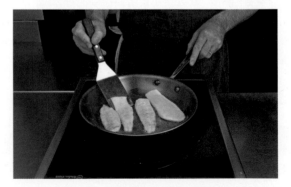

Turning the fish to cook the other side

Serving suggestion

When cooked and placed on the serving plates or dishes, add:

- a slice of lemon (remove the yellow and white pith and any pips first)
- a sprinkling of lemon juice.

Try something different

Once the fish is cooked, carefully heat 10–25 g butter per portion in a frying pan until it turns a nutty brown colour. You could add a squeeze of lemon juice. Pour this over the plated-up fish, sprinkle with chopped parsley and serve.

Deep frying

This is suitable for cuts and fillets of white fish, e.g. cod, haddock. The fish must be coated with something that prevents the cooking fat or oil from penetrating into the fish. You can coat the fish with:

- batter
- milk and flour
- flour, beaten egg and fresh white breadcrumbs.

RECIPE

3 Batter for frying

INGREDIENTS	4 portions	10 portions
Flour	200 g	500 g
Salt, a pinch	5 g	12 g
Egg	1	2–3
Water or milk	250 ml	625 ml
Oil	2 tbsps	5 tbsps

Preparing the batter

1 Sift the flour and salt into a basin.
2 Make a well (a small hollow) in the dried ingredients and pour in the egg and the milk or water.
3 Gradually mix in the flour, using a wooden spoon or whisk.
4 Beat the mixture until it is smooth.
5 Mix in the oil and allow the mixture to rest for ½–1 hour before using.

Try something different

Add yeast (5 g for four portions) or stiffly beaten egg whites to the batter, along with chopped fresh herbs, grated ginger or garam masala.

If a yeast batter is used, you must allow time for the yeast to ferment (bubble) and raise (lighten) the batter.

RECIPE

4 Frying fish in batter

Get ready to cook

1 Prepare your batter as above.
2 Prepare, clean, wash and thoroughly dry the fish.
3 Cut into 100 g portions.

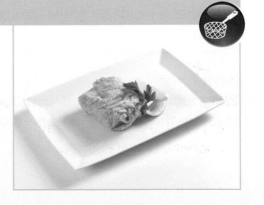

INGREDIENTS	4 portions	10 portions
White fish fillets	400 g	1½ kg
Flour		
Batter		
Light oil in deep fryer		

Cooking

1 Pass the prepared fish through flour (cover it in flour).
2 Shake off any surplus and then pass it through the batter.
3 Taking great care, gently lower the fish, away from you, into deep oil at a controlled temperature of 175°C.
4 Allow to cook until the fish turns a golden brown.
5 Remove carefully on to kitchen paper and allow to drain well.

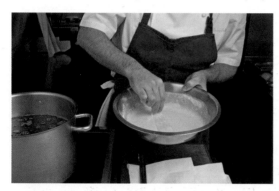

Dipping floured fish into batter

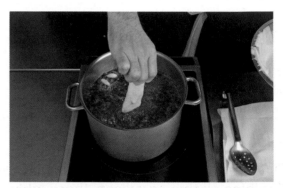

Lowering the fish into hot, deep oil (for greater safety, use a temperature controlled fryer at this point)

Serving suggestion

Serve with either quarters of lemon (pips removed) or tartar sauce. Make the tartar sauce by chopping 25 g capers, 50 g gherkins and a sprig of parsley, and adding these to 250 ml of mayonnaise (see page 157).

Grilling

Grilling fish is cooking it under radiant heat. It is a fast method suitable for small whole fish or fillets, whole or cut in portions.

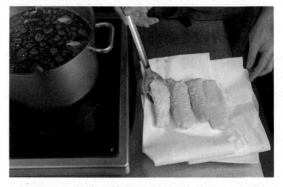

Carefully removing the fish and draining it on kitchen paper

Activity

There is a recipe for grilled sardines in the 'methods of cookery' chapter (Chapter 10). Name six other fish that could be grilled whole or in fillets.

Baking fish

Many fish (whole, filleted, portioned) can be oven baked. To retain their natural moisture the fish should be protected from direct heat.

5 Baked cod with a cheese and herb crust

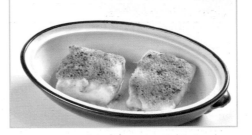

Get ready to cook

1 Prepare, clean, wash and thoroughly dry the fish.
2 Grate the cheese and chop the parsley.

INGREDIENTS	4 portions	10 portions
Cod fillet portions, 100 g each	4	10
Fresh white breadcrumbs	100 g	250 g
Butter, margarine or oil	100 g	250 g
Cheddar cheese, grated	100 g	250 g
Parsley, chopped	1 tbsp	1 tbsp
Salt		
Herb mustard	1 heaped tsp	2 heaped tsp

Cooking

1 Place the fillets on a greased tray or ovenproof dish.
2 Combine all the ingredients thoroughly. Season lightly with salt and press an even layer onto the fish.
3 Bake in an oven at 180°C for approximately 15–20 minutes until cooked and the crust is a light golden brown.

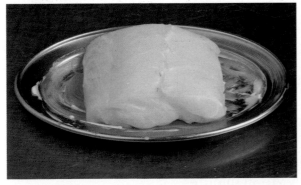

Placing the fish on a greased dish

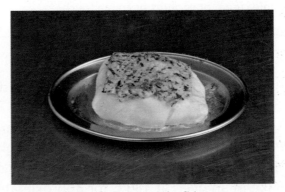

Pressing a layer of crust on to the fish

Serving suggestion

Serve with quarters of de-pipped lemon, or a suitable sauce such as tomato (page 150) or egg (page 145).

Try something different

- Add a good squeeze of lemon juice before cooking.
- Add 2 tbsp/5 tbsp milk before cooking.
- Brush with beaten egg before adding the topping.
- Cover with slices of peeled tomato before cooking.
- Use mustard powder in place of herb mustard.

Fish

- Add chopped fresh herbs, e.g. chives, dill, fennel.
- Add a touch of spice, e.g. garam masala.

Activity

In groups, prepare, cook, taste and assess four variations of your choice.

RECIPE

6 Baked fish pie

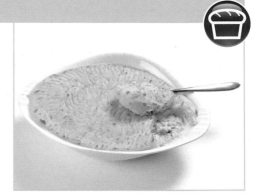

Get ready to cook

1 Prepare, clean, wash and thoroughly dry the fish. Cut it into small even pieces.
2 Prepare the mashed potato (page 276).
3 Cook and slice the hard-boiled egg (page 177).
4 Slice the mushrooms and chop the parsley.

INGREDIENTS	4 portions	10 portions
Cod or fresh haddock fillet	200 g	500 g
Butter or margarine	50 g	125 g
Salt		
White button mushrooms, thinly sliced	50 g	125 g
Egg, hard-boiled (page 177)	1	2–3
Parsley, chopped		
Single cream or yoghurt or crème fraiche	125 ml	320 ml
Potato, mashed (page 276)	200 g	500 g

Cooking

1 Place the fish into greased ovenproof dish(es).
2 Lightly season with salt.
3 Sprinkle on the mushrooms, chopped hard-boiled egg and parsley.
4 Pour on the cream, créme fraiche or yoghurt.
5 Neatly cover or pipe the mashed potato on top of the fish.
6 Bake in an oven at 180°C for approximately 20–30 minutes.

To achieve a golden colour, brush the potato with beaten egg or milk before baking.

Try something different

- Use any type of white fish or salmon, or a combination of two or three types of fish.
- Add chopped fresh herbs, e.g. dill, fennel, chives.
- Add prawns or shrimps.

Activity

In groups, prepare, cook, taste and assess four of your own variations on a pie.

RECIPE

7 Fish cakes

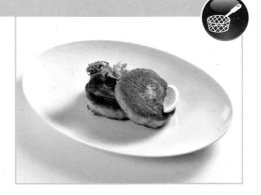

Get ready to cook

1 Prepare, clean, wash and thoroughly dry the fish, then poach it.
2 Prepare the mashed potato (page 276).
3 Beat the eggs.

INGREDIENTS	4 portions	10 portions
Cooked white fish and or salmon	200 g	500 g
Potato, mashed (page 276)	200 g	500 g
Flour	25 g	60 g
Eggs, beaten	1	2
Fresh white breadcrumbs	50 g	125 g

Cooking

1 Combine the fish and potatoes. Taste and correct the seasoning.
2 Using a little flour, form the mixture into a long roll on a clean work surface.
3 Divide the mixture into 4 or 8/10 or 12 pieces and mould into balls.
4 Pass the balls through flour, beaten egg and breadcrumbs.
5 Using a palette knife, flatten each shape firmly. Neaten the shapes and shake off surplus crumbs.
6 Deep fry in hot oil at 185°C for 2–3 minutes until golden brown.

Serving suggestion

Serve the fish cakes with a suitable sauce, e.g. tomato (page 150) or tartar (page 200).

Try something different

Bake the fish cakes in a hot oven at 250°C for 10–15 minutes. If oven baked, it is not necessary to pass them through the flour, egg and breadcrumbs. They should be shaped and placed on lightly greased baking trays.

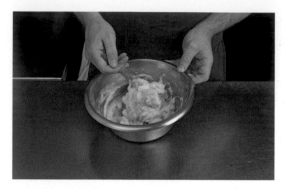

Combining the fish and potatoes

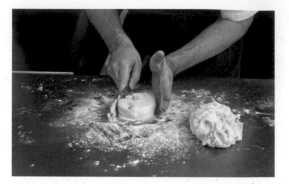

Forming the fish cakes

Activity

In groups, prepare, cook, taste, serve and assess four variations of your choice.

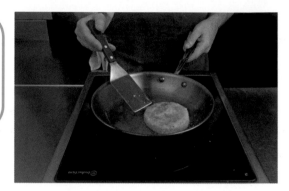

Shallow frying the fish cakes (this is an alternative to deep frying)

RECIPE

8 Coley on mustard mash served with a poached egg

Get ready to cook

1 Wash and peel the potatoes and cut into even pieces.

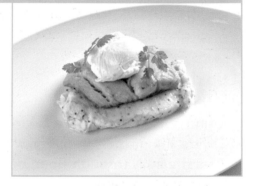

INGREDIENTS	4 portions	10 portions
Potatoes, peeled and cut into even pieces	1 kg	2½ kg
Low-fat fromage frais	100 g	250 g
Wholegrain mustard	1 tbsp	2½ tbsp
Flour	2 tbsp	5 tbsp
Ground black pepper		
Coley, 100 g portions	4	10
Vegetable oil	15 ml	40 ml
Eggs, poached	4	10
Vinegar	1 tbsp	2½ tbsp

Cooking

1 Cook the potatoes in lightly salted water and then mash them. Add the fromage frais and the mustard and mix well.
2 Season the flour with black pepper and pass the coley through it.
3 Cook the fish in the hot vegetable oil for approximately 3–4 minutes on each side.
4 Poach the eggs (page 177).
5 Divide the mash between four plates. Place it in the centre of each plate.
6 Place the coley on top of the mash.
7 Place a poached egg on top of the fish.

Serving suggestion

Garnish the fish or serve it with French beans, glazed carrots, baby sweetcorn, etc.

Try something different

Use other fish, such as salmon, cod, plaice, lemon sole, haddock or monkfish.

Add a little chilli powder or chopped fresh herbs to the flour before passing the fish through it.

RECIPE

9 Salmon, spinach and potato bake

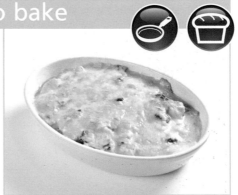

Get ready to cook

1 Fast cook the potatoes by steaming or boiling with their skins on. Cool, peel and then slice.
2 Cook the salmon and flake it.
3 Finely chop the onions.
4 Wash and top the spinach.
5 Grate the cheese.

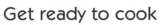

INGREDIENTS	4 portions	10 portions
Vegetable oil for frying	5 ml	15 ml
Onions, finely chopped	30 g	75 g
Spinach, fresh	30 g	75 g
Flour	25 g	50 g
Margarine or butter	25 g	50 g
Milk	250 ml	500 ml
Potatoes, peeled, cooked and thinly sliced	280 g	700 g
Salmon, cooked and flaked	280 g	700 g
Cheddar cheese, grated	80 g	200 g

Cooking

1 Heat the oil in a suitable pan and cook the onions until tender.
2 Add the spinach to the onions and cook until melted.
3 Drain off excess oil.
4 With the flour, margarine and milk, make a white sauce (page 146).

5 Place a layer of potato over the base of a suitable greased ovenproof serving dish.
6 Add the flaked salmon to the cooked onion and spinach.
7 Sprinkle half the fish mixture over the sliced potatoes and cover with the white sauce (béchamel).
8 Repeat the layer and finish with a layer of white sauce.
9 Sprinkle with grated cheese and bake in an oven at 180°C for 20–30 minutes.
10 Serve immediately.

RECIPE

⑩ Steamed gingered snapper

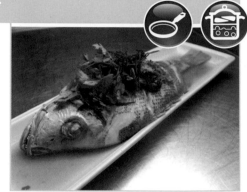

Get ready to cook
1 Clean the fish.
2 Peel the garlic and ginger. Cut the ginger into julienne and thinly slice the garlic.
3 Slice the spring onions thinly.

INGREDIENTS	4 portions	10 portions
Garlic, peeled and thinly sliced	40 g	100 g
Vegetable oil	1 tbsp	3 tbsp
Red snapper, whole, cleaned and scored	1	3
Ginger root, peeled and sliced into julienne	4 cloves	10 cloves
Fish stock	60 ml	150 ml
Spring onions, thinly sliced	4	10
Coriander, fresh and roughly chopped	100 g	250 g
Light soy sauce	80 ml	200 ml
Sesame oil	2 tsp	1 tbsp

Cooking

1 Fry the sliced garlic in the vegetable oil until fragrant and light brown.
2 Score the fish through the thickest part of the flesh on both sides and place it on a large sheet of oiled aluminium foil.
3 Sprinkle the fish with half of the julienne ginger and fried garlic. Drizzle with half the fish stock and garlic oil. Fold the foil loosely to enclose the fish completely.
4 Place the wrapped fish in a large steamer and steam it, covered, for 25 minutes or until the flesh turns opaque.

Serving suggestion

Unfold the foil and transfer the fish onto a serving platter. Chop the coriander leaves and sprinkle the fish with these and the remaining ginger, spring onion, remaining stock and sesame oil.

Try something different

Use sea bass, cod or haddock instead of snapper.

Lamb

A butcher's guide to lamb cuts and joints

Lamb is meat from a sheep under one year old. Over the age of one the animal is called a hogget and the meat is known as mutton.

Images and text courtesy of Donald Russell (www.donaldrussell.com).

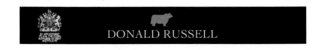

Leg
A traditional leg of lamb is cut from the hind part (the rear) of the animal.

Liver and kidney
The butcher can supply them prepared and fully kitchen-ready.

Loin
This tender cut is the equivalent of sirloin in beef. Lean and full of flavour, there are several loin cuts available. These include valentine steaks, noisettes and lamb mini-steaks, or simply lamb loin on its own.

Fillet
Very tender and mild in flavour, lamb fillets are tiny finger-shaped pieces that are ideal for pan-frying.

Saddle
The saddle is cut from the back part of the animal. Trim and remove all the bones, trim the meat, hand roll it and tie it so it keeps its shape during cooking, as shown on the next page.

Noisettes
These are a delicious lamb cut, tied with string for a neat-looking presentation that holds its shape during cooking.

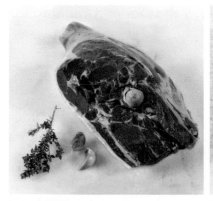

Leg of lamb

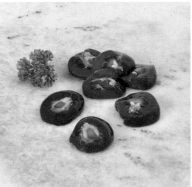

Lamb kidneys

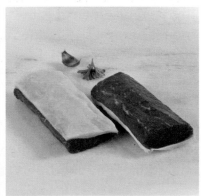

Loin of lamb

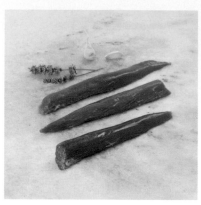

Fillet of lamb

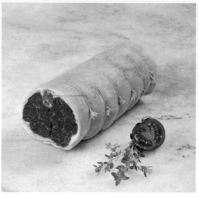

A trimmed and rolled saddle of lamb

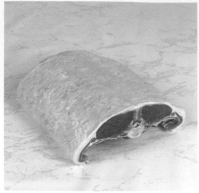

A saddle of lamb with the bone still in (source: Meat and Livestock Commission)

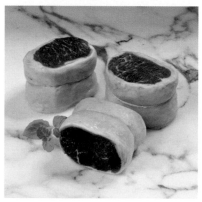

Noisettes of lamb

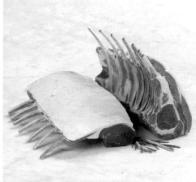

French-trimmed rack of lamb

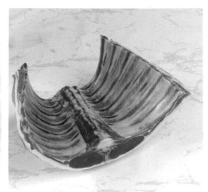

A pair of best ends of lamb (source: Meat and Livestock Commission)

Rack

A rack of lamb is a prime piece of loin with the bones still attached. The racks shown here are French trimmed, which means the excess fat is trimmed away to reveal clean, white bones.

Shoulder

This is a more basic cut of lamb that is excellent value. Slow cooking the shoulder brings out the flavour and makes it very tender.

Shank

This flavoursome cut is best slow-cooked for several hours, with stock and vegetables. Then it becomes so tender it simply falls off the bone.

Off-cuts

Off-cuts of lamb can be diced and minced to make a tasty alternative to the various cuts of lamb.

Cutlets

Lamb cutlets are usually cut with one rib bone, but for those who prefer the meat underdone, double cutlets can be cut with two rib bones.

Lamb chops

Chops are cut either from the loin (loin chops) or the chump end (chump chops).

A double loin chop is cut approximately 2 cm across a saddle and left on the bone. This is also known as a Barnsley chop.

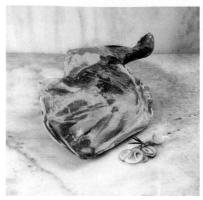
Shoulder of lamb

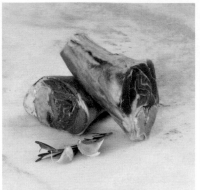
Lamb shank

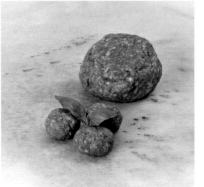
Minced lamb from off-cuts

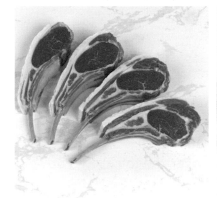
Lamb cutlets

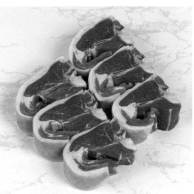
Lamb loin chops

Quality points

- The lean meat should be a dull red colour and have a firm texture.
- There should be an even amount of fat. This should be hard and flaky and a clear white colour.
- In young animals the bones should be pink and fairly soft. As the animals grow older, their bones become harder and white.

> **Food safety note**
>
> Whenever you reheat pre-prepared meat dishes (such as slow-cooked stews), use a meat thermometer to check the core temperature, which should reach 82°C. Only ever reheat once. See also Chapter 8 for more details about safe storage and cooking temperatures.

Cooking lamb

RECIPE

1 Roast rack of lamb

Get ready to cook

See the pictures and captions below, showing how to prepare a rack of lamb for roasting

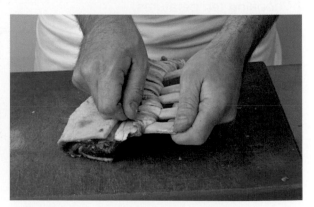

INGREDIENTS
Rack of lamb
Salt
Vegetable oil
Brown stock for gravy (page 127)

Cooking

1 Season the rack lightly with salt and place fat side up on a bed of bones or a metal trivet in a roasting tray.

2 Add a little vegetable oil on top and cook in a hot oven at 175–185 °C.

3 Roast for approximately 20–25 minutes. Baste (spoon fat over the joint) two or three times during cooking.

4 To test if cooked, remove the rack, place on a warm plate and press the lean meat to force out a little juice. If the juice does not show any pinkness (sign of blood) it is cooked right through. If the lamb is to be cooked pink, then reduce the cooking time by approximately 5 minutes.

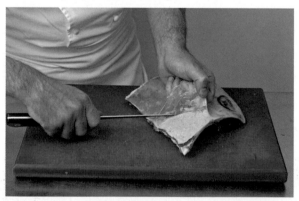

Removing the skin from the joint, leaving plenty of fat behind. Remove the skin from top to bottom (head to tail) and front (breast) to back

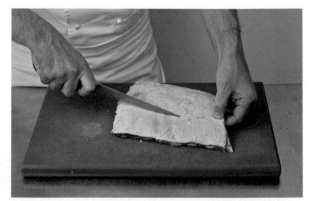

Scoring the fat to about 2 mm deep. Scoring is cutting lightly with the tip of the knife

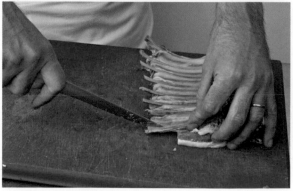

Preparing the rib bones: scoring down the middle of the back of each bone

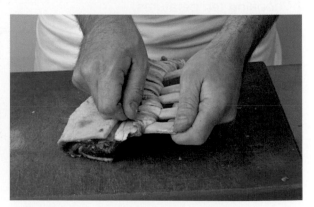

Pulling the skin, fat and meat away from the end of each bone, so that the bones will be visible after cooking, and cleaning away any sinew

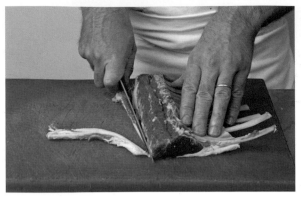

Cutting off the sinew

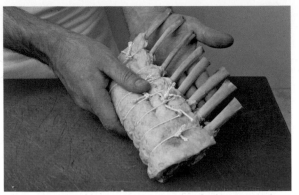

Tying the joint. If necessary, trim the overall length of the rib bones to two and a half times the length of the nut of lean meat. This is the main part, or 'eye' of the meat

To make roast gravy, once the rack is cooked and removed from the tin:

1 Pour off any surplus fat from the roasting tin (retain any juicy sediment) and place the tin on a low heat.

2 Add 60 ml of brown stock (page 127), simmer gently and stir in any sediment or meat juices.

3 Taste, correct seasoning, strain and skim off any fat. The remaining liquid is the roast gravy.

Try something different

For extra flavour in the gravy, add a peeled sliced onion, celery and carrot to the roasting tin with the lamb rack.

There are a number of commercial gravy products that can be used to boost the gravy if it is not tasty enough.

Serving suggestion

In addition to roast gravy, offer mint sauce (see below) and/or redcurrant jelly.

RECIPE

 2 Mint sauce

INGREDIENTS	
Water	125 ml
Caster or demerara sugar	1 tsp
Mint leaves, chopped	2–3 tbsp
Malt vinegar	to taste

Making the sauce

1 Boil the water and dissolve the sugar in it. Allow to cool.
2 Add the chopped mint leaves and enough malt vinegar to give a slightly sharp but pleasant taste.

3 Grilled lamb cutlets

Lamb cutlets

Salt

Vegetable oil

Cooking

1 Lightly season the cutlets with salt and brush them with oil or fat.

2 If you are cooking on a grill preheat it and grease the bars. If you are cooking under a grill preheat the salamander and place the cutlets on lightly greased trays beneath the grill.

3 Cook for approx 5 minutes, then turn them over and cook for a further 3–4 minutes. Do not overcook.

Serving suggestion

You could serve with, for example, deep-fried potatoes and a sprig of watercress.

You could also serve a slice of compound butter for each cutlet. Compound butter is made by mixing the flavouring ingredients (see below) into softened butter. The butter is shaped into a roll 2 cm in diameter, wrapped in damp greaseproof paper or foil, hardened in the refrigerator and cut into ½ cm slices when required. You could use the following flavourings:

- mint butter – chopped fresh mint
- parsley butter – chopped fresh parsley and lemon juice
- herb butter – chopped fresh herbs, e.g. tarragon, parsley, chives
- garlic butter – garlic juice and chopped parsley or other fresh herbs; for garlic juice, peel garlic cloves and press them in a garlic press
- rosemary butter – chopped fresh rosemary.

Activity

1 Suggest two other suitable variations of compound butter to accompany lamb cutlets.

2 Suggest an alternative(s) to fried potatoes.

3 Suggest what you would consider to be a suitable vegetable to accompany the potato.

4 Suggest an alternative to a vegetable.

RECIPE
4 Grilled lamb chops

Get ready to cook

A first-class lamb chop should have a substantial piece of lamb kidney skewered in the centre. The kidney must be skinned, cut in half and the tough centre piece of gristle cut out. The remainder can be cut into four pieces, one for each chop.

1 Skin the loin and remove excess fat and sinew.
2 Cut into even-sized chops approximately 100–150 g in weight.
3 You may need to use a meat chopper to lightly cut through the bones. If so, make sure you use a chopping block and not a cutting surface, as this will damage it.

Cooking

Chops are cooked in exactly the same way as cutlets. The time may need to be varied according to the thickness of the meat.

RECIPE
5 Spicy lamb chops

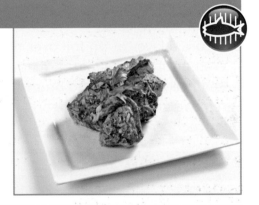

Get ready to cook

1 Make the marinade by chopping the onion, garlic and chilli.
2 Mix these with the dried spices and the lemon juice.

INGREDIENTS	4 portions	10 portions
Lamb chops	4–8, depending on size	10–20, depending on size
Onion, finely chopped	½	1
Garlic, finely chopped (optional)	1 clove	2 cloves
Red chilli, small, deseeded and finely chopped (or a little chilli powder)	1	2
Cumin, ground	½	1 tsp
Coriander, ground	½	1 tsp
Ginger, ground	1 tsp	2 tsp
Lemon juice	1 tbsp	2 tbsp

Cooking

1 Spoon the marinade over the chops.
2 Cover and leave to marinate for 1–2 hours.
3 Grill as for lamb cutlets, but do not add salt.

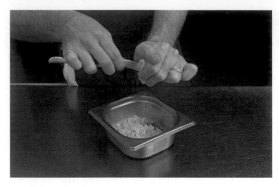

Mixing the ingredients for the marinade

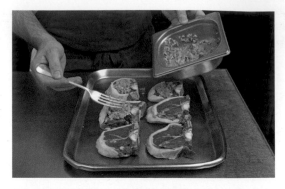

Coating the chops with marinade

Try something different

Instead of grilling the chops you could barbecue them.

1 If possible, use gas rather than charcoal as it is easier to control the temperature with gas. Allow the gas barbecue to pre-heat for 30 minutes.

2 If cooking on charcoal, always wait for the flames to go out and for the embers to start glowing before beginning to cook.

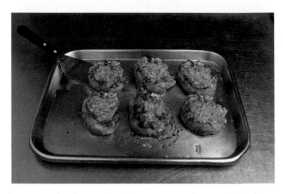

Grilling the chops

3 Secure a layer of tin foil over the barbecue.

4 Wait until the grill bars are hot or the charcoal embers glow.

5 Remove the tinfoil and brush the grill bars with a firm, long-handled wire brush to remove any unwanted debris.

6 Proceed as for grilling chops.

Activity

1 Prepare and cook the spicy lamb chops, then taste, assess and discuss them.

2 Suggest suitable accompaniments.

RECIPE

6 Lamb kebabs

Get ready to cook

1 Cut the meat into squares.

2 Deseed the red pepper and cut into squares.

3 Peel the onion and cut into squares.

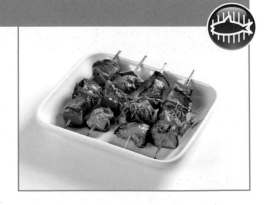

INGREDIENTS	4 portions	10 portions
Lamb, lean meat of the loin or rack	600 g	1½ kg
Red pepper, cut into largish squares	2	5
Onion, cut into largish squares	1	3
Bay leaves	4	10
Thyme, dried	½ tsp	1 tsp
Vegetable oil	2 tbsp	5 tbsp

The ideal cuts of lamb are the nut of the lean meat of the loin or rack.

Kebabs, a dish of Turkish origin, are pieces of food impaled on skewers and cooked on or under a grill or barbecue. There are many variations, and different flavours can be added by marinating the kebabs. This involves soaking the meat, before cooking, in a combination of oil, vinegar, lemon juice, spices and herbs, for two hours at room temperature or four hours in the refrigerator. Kebabs can be made using tender cuts of various meats with pieces of vegetables or fruits in between.

Cooking

1 Push the squares of meat on skewers, alternating these with squares of red pepper, onion and a bay leaf.
2 Brush with oil and lightly sprinkle with dried thyme.
3 Cook over or under a grill.

Serving suggestion

Serve with pilau rice (page 192) and finely sliced raw onion.

Activity

1 Each member of the group should devise their own kebab from a range of ingredients: meat, vegetables, herbs and spices.

2 The group then cooks, serves, tastes and assesses each version.

RECIPE

 7 Shallow-fried lamb cutlets and chops

INGREDIENTS
Lamb cutlets or chops
Salt
Light oil or fat

Both cutlets and chops are equally suitable to cook in this way.

Cooking

1 Place a thick-bottomed frying pan or a sauté pan on a hot stove.
2 Add a little light oil or fat to the pan.
3 Season the meat lightly with salt.

4 When the fat is hot, carefully place the meat in the pan. Put the edge of the meat closest to you in first and lay it away from you. This way, if any hot fat splashes it will splash away from you rather than on to you.

5 Cook on a high heat until lightly browned, then turn over and repeat.

6 Lower the heat by a half and cook for approximately 4–5 minutes in total (depending on the thickness of the meat).

Serving suggestion

Serve as for lamb cutlets or offer a suitable potato and vegetable, e.g. sauté potatoes (with or without onions) and leaf spinach with toasted pine nuts.

Activity

Fry a dish of cutlets or chops and serve with your idea of a suitable garnish or a potato, vegetable and/or salad. Taste, assess and discuss.

RECIPE

8 Brown lamb or mutton stew

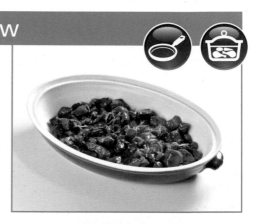

Get ready to cook

1 Trim the meat of any excess fat and bone, and cut into even pieces.

2 Peel and roughly chop the onion and carrot.

3 Prepare a bouquet garni with rosemary.

INGREDIENTS	4 portions	10 portions
Stewing lamb: shoulder, neck end, breast	500 g	1½ kg
Salt		
Oil	2 tbsp	5 tbsp
Onion, roughly chopped	100 g	250 g
Carrot, roughly chopped	100 g	250 g
Flour, white or wholemeal	25 g	60 g
Tomato purée	1 level tbsp	2¼ level tbsp
Brown stock, mutton stock or water	500 ml	1250 ml
Bouquet garni		
Garlic clove (optional)	1	2–3
Parsley, chopped		

Cooking

1 Season the meat lightly with salt. Heat some oil in a suitable pan and fry the meat quickly until just coloured, then add the onion and carrot and continue frying until well browned.

2 Drain off any surplus fat and discard.

3 Mix in the flour with a wooden spoon or heat-proof spatula and cook on a low, heat stirring continuously, for 3–4 minutes.

4 Mix in the tomato purée, then allow the meat mixture to cool slightly.

5 Put it back on the heat and gradually add the stock and stir to the boil.

6 Add the bouquet garni and garlic. Skim and cover with a lid.

7 Simmer gently, in a moderate oven at 180°C or on the side of the stove, for approximately 1½–2 hours.

8 When cooked, pick out the meat and put it into a clean pan.

9 Taste and correct the sauce and pass it through a strainer on to the meat.

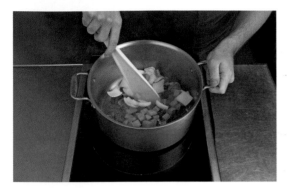

Frying the lamb with the onions and carrots

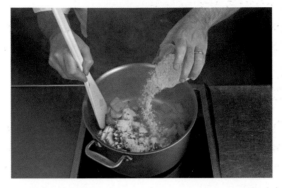

Adding the flour

Serving suggestion

Serve lightly sprinkled with chopped parsley.

Try something different

Either separately or in with the stew, cook a garnish of small, neat vegetables, e.g. carrots, turnips, button onions, potatoes, peas. If cooking them with the stew, add them approximately 30 minutes before the meat is cooked.

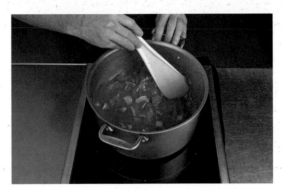

Bringing to the boil after adding the stock

Activity

As a group, prepare, cook, serve, taste and assess the recipe using:

• an ordinary brown stock (page 127)

• a well-flavoured lamb or mutton brown stock

• water.

9 Irish stew

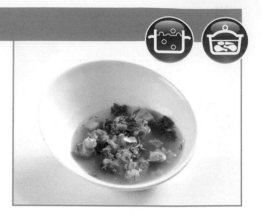

Get ready to cook

Trim the meat of any excess fat and bone, and cut into even pieces.

Some recipes for Irish stew will include carrots.

INGREDIENTS	4 portions	10 portions
Stewing lamb: shoulder, neck end, breast	500 g	1½ kg
Water or white stock	400 g	1 kg
Salt		
Bouquet garni		
Potatoes	100 g	250 g
Onions	100 g	250 g
Celery	100 g	250 g
Savoy cabbage	100 g	250 g
Leeks	100 g	250 g
Button onions (optional)	100 g	250 g
Parsley, chopped		

Cooking

1 Place the meat in a shallow saucepan, cover with water and bring to the boil.
2 Place the meat under running water until meat is clean, then return it to the cleaned pan.
3 Cover with water or white stock, season lightly with salt and add the bouquet garni.
4 Skim, cover with a lid and allow to simmer for 45 minutes to an hour.
5 Peel and wash the vegetables, and cut into neat, small pieces then add to the meat.
6 Simmer for 30 minutes, skimming frequently.
7 Add the button onions and simmer for a further 20–30 minutes.
8 Skim, taste and correct the seasoning.

Serving suggestion

Serve lightly sprinkled with chopped parsley. You could also accompany it with Worcester sauce and/or pickled red cabbage.

10 Braised lamb shanks

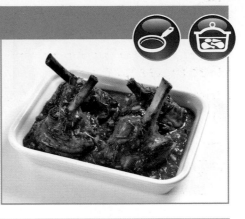

Get ready to cook

1 Peel and chop the onions.
2 Peel and crush the garlic.
3 Drain and chop the tomatoes.
4 Rinse and drain the beans.

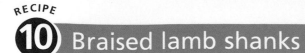

INGREDIENTS	4 portions	10 portions
Lamb shanks	4	10
Oil	3 tbsp	7 tbsp
Red onions, finely chopped	50 g	125 g
Garlic cloves, peeled and crushed	2	5
Plum tomatoes (canned), drained and chopped	400 g	1 kg
Lamb stock	250 ml	625 ml
Flageolet beans (canned), rinsed and drained	400 g	1 kg
Honey, clear	1 tbsp	2½ tbsp
Rosemary, fresh chopped	1 tbsp	2½ tbsp
Salt		
Parsley, chopped		

Cooking

1 Lightly season the shanks.
2 Heat the oil in a suitable braising pan.
3 Quickly fry the shanks on all sides until golden brown. Remove from the pan and set aside.
4 Add the chopped onion and garlic to the pan (if there is insufficient oil, add a little more). Allow to sweat gently over a moderate heat until soft.
5 Stir in the tomatoes and stock.
6 Place the shanks back in the pan.
7 Bring to the boil, then reduce the heat so that the cooking is at a gentle simmer. Cover and put in the oven at 160°C for 1 hour.
8 Check the shanks to see that they are cooked by using a two-pronged fork, which should slide in as far as the bone in the thickest part of the shank.
9 Remove the shanks and stir in the beans, honey and rosemary.
10 Replace the shanks and reheat to a gentle simmer
11 Skim, taste the liquid and correct the seasoning.

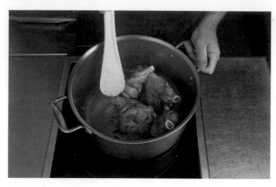

Quickly frying the lamb shanks in the braising pan

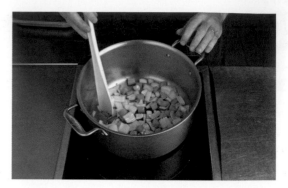

Cooking the vegetables in the pan

Serving suggestion

Serve in an earthenware dish, sprinkled with freshly chopped parsley.

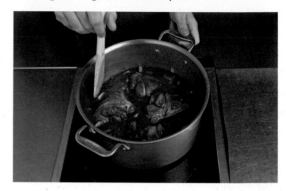

Putting the shanks back into the pan ready for braising

Activity

You can make many variations to this recipe, using different beans, additional vegetables, different herbs, etc.

1 Formulate your own recipe. Then prepare, cook, taste, assess and discuss it.

2 Suggest what accompaniments you would like to serve with the shanks.

RECIPE

11 Shepherd's pie

Get ready to cook

1 Remove all the fat and gristle from the cooked meat and then mince.
2 Peel, cook and mash the potatoes (page 276).
3 Peel and chop the onions.

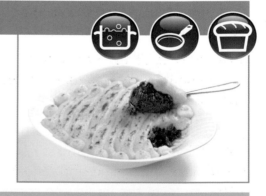

INGREDIENTS	4 portions	10 portions
Onions, finely chopped	100 g	250 g
Oil	35 g	100 g
Cooked lamb or mutton (minced), all fat and gristle removed	400 g	1¼ kg
Salt		
Worcester sauce	2–3 drops	5 drops
Thickened gravy (recipe on page 148 or convenience product)	125–250 ml	300–600 ml
Potato, mashed (page 276)	400 g	1¼ kg
Milk or eggwash		

The ideal lamb joint for this is shoulder cooked by roasting, but any left-over lamb can be used provided all fat and gristle is removed.

This dish can also be prepared from left-over cooked beef or raw minced beef, which would require extra cooking time until the meat is quite soft. This is known as cottage pie.

Cooking

1 Gently cook the onion in the oil in a thick-bottomed pan, without colouring, until soft.
2 Add the cooked meat and season lightly.
3 Add Worcester sauce and sufficient thickened gravy to bind the mixture. This should not be too dry (unappetising) or too sloppy (because the potato would sink in).
4 Bring to the boil, stirring frequently, and simmer for 10–15 minutes.
5 Place into an ovenproof dish.
6 Pipe or neatly arrange the mashed potato on top, and brush with eggwash or milk.
7 Colour to a golden brown in a hot oven or under the salamander.

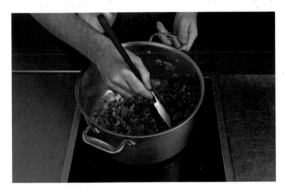

Cooking the onions and meat

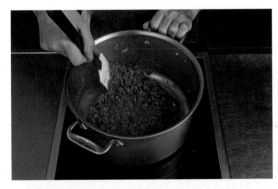

Simmering the meat

Serving suggestion

Serve accompanied with a sauceboat of thickened gravy and a suitable vegetable.

It can also be served with a light sprinkling of garam masala and grilled pitta bread.

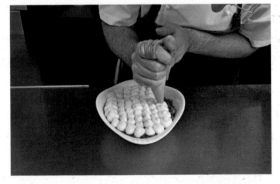

Piping the mashed potato

Try something different

Many variations can be made to this basic dish.

- Cover the meat with canned baked beans before adding the potato.
- Sprinkle with grated cheese before browning.
- Vary the flavour of the meat by the adding herbs or spices.
- Vary the potato topping by mixing in grated cheese or chopped spring onion.

Activity

Prepare, cook, serve and taste your own variation. Assess and discuss.

RECIPE

12 Lamb and vegetable pie

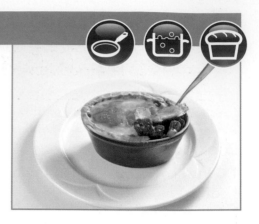

Get ready to cook

1 Dice cut the lamb into 1½ cm dice.
2 Peel the carrots and cut into 1 cm dice.
3 Peel and chop the onions and garlic.
4 Prepare the pastry (page 300).

INGREDIENTS	4 portions	10 portions
Vegetable oil		
Onions, finely chopped	½	1
Garlic, crushed and chopped	1 clove	2 cloves
Shoulder or leg of lamb, diced	300 g	750 g
Margarine or butter	25 g	50 g
Flour	25 g	50 g
Vegetable stock	200 ml	500 ml
Carrots, diced 1 cm	80 g	200 g
Peas	160 g	400 g
Shortcrust pastry	80 g	200 g

Cooking

1 Heat the oil in a suitable pan. Add the onions and garlic and cook without colouring.

2 Add the diced lamb with a little stock. Cover with a lid and cook for 10 minutes, stirring occasionally.

3 Make a blond roux with the margarine and flour (page 145). Allow to cool.

4 Add the boiling stock to make a velouté (page 145). Strain.

5 Add the velouté to the lamb and cook until tender.

6 Add the diced carrots and peas and cook for a further 5 minutes.

7 Place into a pie dish and allow to cool.

8 Cover with short pastry and eggwash. Stand the dish on an oven tray and bake at 180°C for approximately 15 minutes until golden brown.

Try something different

- Use puff pastry for the top.
- Other vegetables may also be used, e.g. parsnips, turnips, red and green peppers, sweetcorn.
- Add chopped fresh herbs to the velouté, e.g. rosemary, coriander, sage, oregano, mint or a little chilli powder.

RECIPE

13 Tagine of lamb with prunes and almonds

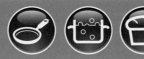

Get ready to cook

1 Dice the lamb.
2 Peel the carrots and cut into ½ cm dice.
3 Peel and chop the onions and garlic.
4 Prepare the spices by blending together the coriander, cumin, chilli powder, paprika, turmeric, garlic and 3 tablespoons of oil.
5 Add the spice mixture to the lamb, cover all over and allow to marinate overnight.
6 Toast the blanched almonds.

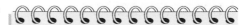

Tagine is a traditional Moroccan dish cooked in a clay or earthenware pot, which is known as a tagine.

INGREDIENTS	4 portions	10 portions
Coriander seeds	2 tsp	5 tsp
Cumin seeds	2 tsp	5 tsp
Chilli powder	2 tsp	5 tsp
Paprika	1 tbsp	2½ tbsp
Ground turmeric	1 tbsp	2½ tbsp
Garlic, crushed and chopped	4 cloves	10 cloves
Vegetable oil	4 tbsp	10 tbsp
Shoulder or leg of lamb, diced	1 kg	2½ kg
Carrot, diced	1	2½
Onions, finely chopped	2	5
Brown stock	1 litre	2½ litres
Prunes, stones removed	250 g	625 g
Cinnamon sticks	3	7
Bay leaves	4	10
Ground almonds	50 g	125 g
Ground black pepper		
Button onions	8	20
Honey	1 tbsp	2½ tbsp
Blanched almonds, toasted	50 g	125 g

Cooking

1 In a suitable pan, heat a little oil. Add the carrots and onions and shallow fry without colouring. Remove and reserve.
2 In the same pan, shallow fry the lamb until it is browned all over.
3 Remove the lamb and deglaze the pan with a little brown stock to remove all the sediment.
4 Put the carrots and onions back in the tagine and add half the prunes. Add the brown stock, cinnamon sticks, bay leaves, ground almonds and lamb. Season with ground black pepper.
5 Cover with a lid or foil and cook in an oven at 170°C for approximately 1½–2 hours until the lamb is tender.
6 Shallow fry the button onions in vegetable oil, then add the honey. Cook to golden brown and glazed. Add these to the lamb 30 minutes before the lamb is cooked.

7 When the lamb is cooked, remove from the dish and keep warm.

8 Bring the sauce to the boil and reduce to a syrupy consistency.

9 Place the lamb back into the sauce with the remaining prunes.

Serving suggestion

Serve in the tagine or a suitable dish garnished with toasted almonds. Sprinkle with flat parsley and coriander. Serve with hot couscous.

RECIPE

(14) Lamb biryani

Get ready to cook

1 Dice the lamb.

2 Peel and chop the onions and garlic.

3 Peel and grate the ginger.

4 Deseed and slice the chillies.

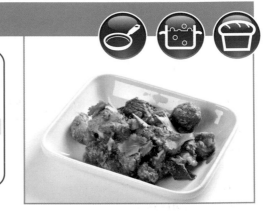

INGREDIENTS	4 portions	10 portions
Vegetable oil	2 tbsp	5 tbsp
Onions, finely chopped	1	2½
Garlic, crushed and chopped	1 clove	2½ cloves
Cardamom, ground	2 tsp	5 tsp
Ginger root, grated	1 tsp	2½ tsp
Chilli powder	1 tsp	2½ tsp
Coriander seeds, ground	2 tsp	5 sp
Cumin, ground	2 tsp	5 tsp
Turmeric	2 tsp	5 tsp
Shoulder or leg of lamb, diced	500 g	1¼ kg
Natural yoghurt	150 g	375 g
Basmati rice	225 g	450 g
Bay leaves	2	5
Green chillies, deseeded and finely chopped	2	5
Lemon juice	½ lemon	1 lemon
Coriander leaves		

Cooking

1 Heat the oil in a suitable ovenproof pan. Add the onion and garlic and cook without colouring.

2 Add the spices, lamb and yoghurt and stir continuously to set the meat.

3 Remove from the heat, cover and leave to infuse the spices for 30 minutes.

4 Cook the basmati rice for 5 minutes in boiling water with the bay leaves.

5 Drain the rice and add it to the lamb.

6 Sprinkle with chillies and add the lemon juice.

7 Cover tightly with a lid and bake for 1 hour at 170°C.

8 Before serving, stir well to combine the lamb and rice.

Serving suggestion

Sprinkle with coriander leaves before serving.

RECIPE

(15) Kashmiri lamb

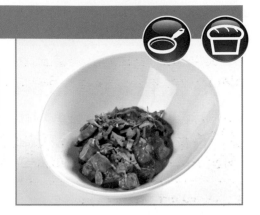

Get ready to cook

1 Dice the lamb.

2 Drain and chop the tomatoes.

INGREDIENTS	4 portions	10 portions
Blanched almonds	100 g	250 g
Vegetable oil	2 tbsp	5 tbsp
Fennel seeds, crushed	1 tbsp	2½ tbsp
Shoulder or leg of lamb, diced	600 g	1½ kg
Kashmiri curry paste	90 g	225 g
Paprika, ground	1 tbsp	2½ tbsp
Plum tomatoes (canned), chopped	400 g	1 kg
Fresh coriander		

Cooking

1 Quickly fry half the almonds in the vegetable oil until golden brown. Drain and put to one side.

2 Purée the remaining the almonds in a food processor. Alternatively, use ground almonds.

3 Add the fennel seeds to the oil and fry for one minute.

4 Add the lamb dice and fry on all sides.

5 Add the curry paste, paprika and ground almonds. Continue to fry, stirring frequently, for approximately 5 minutes.

6 Place the lamb in an ovenproof dish with the other ingredients, including the chopped tomatoes. Deglaze the pan with a little water and add this to the lamb.

7 Cover and place in the oven to cook at 180°C for 30 minutes.

8 Add the chopped coriander and continue to cook until tender.

Serving suggestion

Serve on suitable plates, garnish with the toasted almonds and more chopped coriander.

Serve with steamed basmati rice, and a dish of natural yoghurt with diced cucumber and chopped onion.

Try something different

To make the dish fiery, add 1 tsp of red chilli powder for four portions and 2½ tsps for ten portions.

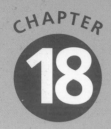
Beef

A butcher's guide to beef cuts and joints

A side of beef is divided into various joints for cooking.

Images and text courtesy of Donald Russell (www.donaldrussell.com).

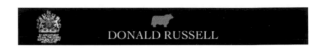

Shin

This old-fashioned cut is lighter in fat and mellower in flavour than the rib trim (see 'Rib', below). Shins are cut from superior hindquarter and are perfect for casseroles and stews.

Oxtail

As the name suggests, this cut is from the tail of the animal. The thicker top part of the tail, where the meat is most plentiful, is best. This is a delicious, old-fashioned cut that benefits from long, slow braising to release its full flavour.

Rump

Rump has a rich, beefy taste and a firm, juicy bite. It is suitable for cutting into steaks, or for roasting or pot roasting as a joint.

Sirloin

Sirloin is one of the most flavoursome steaks and it is almost as tender as fillet, which is why it is so popular. Lightly marbled, with a thin strip of fat on one edge, sirloin can be cut into steaks or roasted whole as a joint.

Fillet

The fillet is the muscle least used by the animal and is therefore the most tender part. It is also the most expensive. The meat is lean. It can be cut into steaks, the centre cut can be roasted as a joint, or the tail of the fillet can be cut into strips and stir fried.

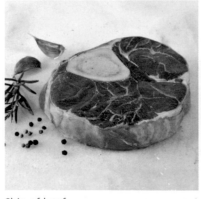

Shin of beef

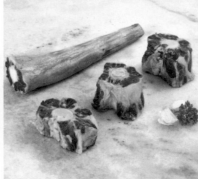

Oxtail

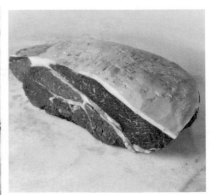

Rump

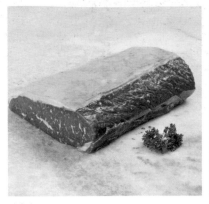

Sirloin

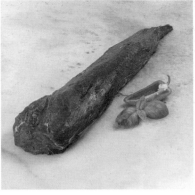

Fillet

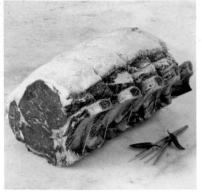

5-bone rib

5-bone rib

A popular choice at carveries, this magnificent joint is unbeatable for special family meals.

Ribeye

This heavily marbled cut has a ribbon of fat at its core, which melts during cooking, making the meat juicy. It can be roasted as a joint or cut into steaks.

Brisket

Cut from the breast of the animal, top-quality brisket can be hand rolled and tied to keep its shape during cooking. It is suitable for braising or boiling.

Rib

The meat between the rib bones is very heavily marbled and, as such, is full of flavour. It needs long, slow cooking to break down the fat, but the reward is an intense flavour. It can be used for slow cooking, or as whole beef back rib racks for roasting, pot roasting or barbecuing.

Ox tongue

A favourite from days gone by, unsalted ox tongue tastes delicious served hot or cold. It has a rich, beefy flavour and is best cooked for several hours to tenderise the meat.

Off-cuts

Off-cuts of beef can be used for kebab cubes, minced steak, diced steak and burgers.

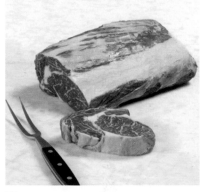

Ribeye

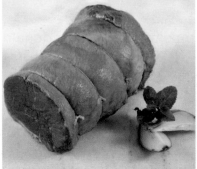

Brisket

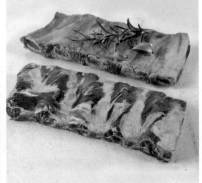

Rib

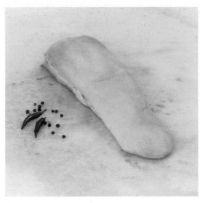

Ox tongue

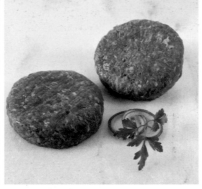

Burgers made from beef off-cuts

Cuts of beef

The cuts of beef vary considerably from the very tender fillet steak to the tough brisket or shin, and there is a greater variety of cuts of beef than for any other type of meat.

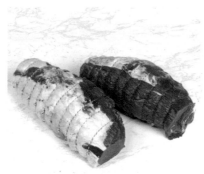

Rolled topside of beef

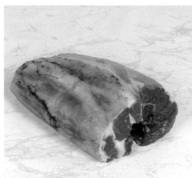

Boned shin of beef

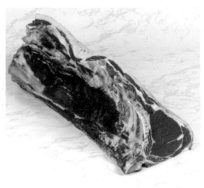

Fillet and loin of beef

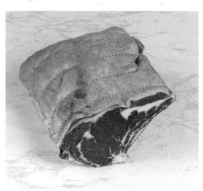

Forerib of beef

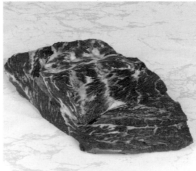

Beef, chuck steaks

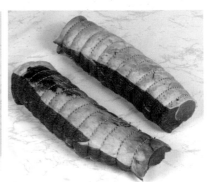

Beef, silverside (rolled)

Steaks

Images and text courtesy of Donald Russell (www.donaldrussell.com).

Fillet	**Fillet is the most tender, lean and mild-flavoured of all the steaks**

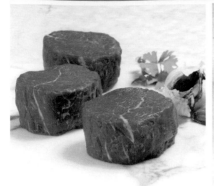 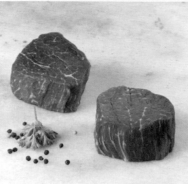 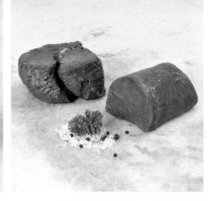

Classic fillet steak	**Fillet medallion**	**Fillet double-steak**
Minimum weight: 170 g	Minimum weight: 70 g	Minimum weight: 340 g
Recommended cooking: pan frying or grilling	Recommended cooking: pan frying or grilling	Recommended cooking: pan-to-oven

Sirloin	**Sirloin is tasty and tender with good marbling and a covering of fat on the outside**

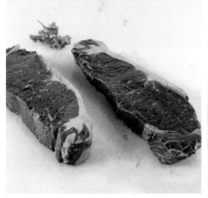 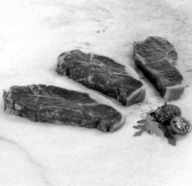 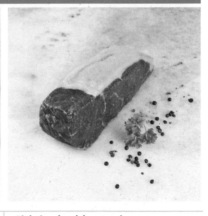

Sirloin steak	**Minute sirloin steak**	**Sirloin double-steak**
Minimum weight: 210 g	Minimum weight: 110 g	Minimum weight: 430 g
Recommended cooking: pan frying or grilling	Recommended cooking: pan frying or grilling	Recommended cooking: pan-to-oven or grilling

Ribeye	Ribeye is juicy and richly flavoured with a rugged appearance, generous marbling and firm texture

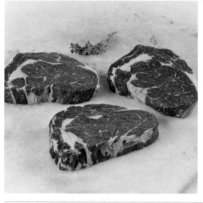 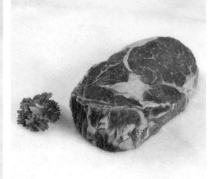

Ribeye steak	**Minute rib-eye steak**	**Ribeye double-steak**
Minimum weight: 210 g	Minimum weight: 110 g	Minimum weight: 430 g
Recommended cooking: pan frying or grilling	Recommended cooking: pan frying or grilling	Recommended cooking: pan-to-oven or grilling

Rump	Traditional rump steaks are very sinewy, but your butcher can cut round the sinews; this thicker cut, popular on the continent, is called 'pavé'

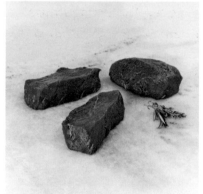 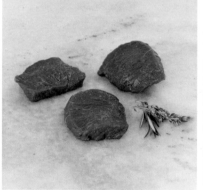 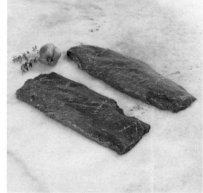

Pavé rump steak	**Pavé rump medallion**	**Minute rump steak**
Minimum weight: 170 g	Minimum weight: 70 g	Minimum weight: 170 g
Recommended cooking: pan frying or grilling	Recommended cooking: pan frying or grilling	Recommended cooking: pan frying or grilling

Quality points

- The lean meat should be bright red with small flecks of white fat (brown or marbled).
- The fat should be firm and easy to break. It should be a creamy-white colour and should not smell of anything.

- The fat in older animals and dairy breeds (milking cattle) is usually a deeper-yellow colour.

Safety note

Whenever you reheat pre-prepared meat dishes (such as slow-cooked stews), use a meat thermometer to check the core temperature, which should reach 82°C. Only ever reheat once. See also Chapter 8 for more details about safe storage and cooking temperatures.

Roasting beef

Timings and testing

Roasting time, in a hot oven at 200–220°C, is approximately 15 minutes per ½ kg plus 15 minutes.

To test whether a joint is cooked

1 If you do not have a temperature probe:
  - remove the joint from the oven and place on a dish or plate
  - firmly press the meat surface to force out some meat juice
  - check the colour of the juice
    red – indicates that the meat is underdone
    pink – indicates that the meat is medium done
    clear – indicates that the meat is cooked through.

2 If you are using a temperature probe, set the required internal temperature and insert the probe horizontally into the centre of the meat. Leave the probe inside the joint during cooking. It will set off a beeper alerting you when your meat is cooked to perfection.

3 When using a meat temperature thermometer, insert it into the part of the joint that was the thickest before it was placed in the oven. The internal temperature reached should be as follows:
  - rare or underdone meat 52–55°C
  - medium done (pinkish) 66–71°C
  - just done (slightly pink) 78–80°C.

1 Traditional roast beef and gravy

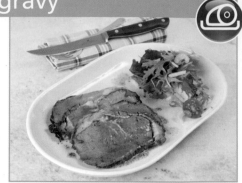

Get ready to cook

1 Trim the joint to remove sinew, excess fat and any bones that may make carving difficult. Depending on the joint and the way you prepare it, you may want to tie it with string to keep its shape.
2 Wash, peel and roughly chop the vegetables.
3 Prepare a brown stock (page 127).
4 Preheat the oven to 250 °C.

Suitable roasting joints are:

- first class – sirloin, wing ribs, fore ribs, fillet
- second class – middle ribs, topside.

INGREDIENTS
Joint of beef of your own choice and size
Salt
Dripping or oil
Roughly chopped onion, carrot and celery
Brown stock

Cooking

1 Season the joint lightly with salt and place on a trivet (metal or bones) in a roasting tray.
2 Place a little dripping or oil over the meat and cook it in a hot oven at 230–250°C for around 15 minutes, then reduce the heat to 200–220°C, depending on the size of the joint. Time the cooking as per the guidance given above.
3 Baste frequently and, for large joints, gradually reduce the heat by 5–10°C (depending on the size of the joint).
4 Roughly chopped onion, carrot and celery can be added to the roasting tray approximately 30 minutes before the joint is cooked, to give extra flavour to the gravy.
5 Remove the tray from the oven and place the joint onto a dish or plate to check whether it is cooked (see above).
6 Once you are happy that the meat is cooked, cover it with foil and leave to rest in a warm place for at least 15 minutes. This allows the meat to set and become tender for carving.

Making the gravy

7 While the meat is resting you can make the gravy by carefully pouring off as much fat as possible, leaving any meat juice or sediment and vegetables in the tray.
8 Place this over a low heat, add sufficient brown stock for the amount of gravy required and allow it to simmer for 5 minutes, scraping off all the sediment and meat juice from the joint with a non-metal spoon.
9 Taste the gravy and correct the seasoning. Pass it through a fine strainer and skim off any remaining fat. If the gravy is lacking in flavour, a little commercial product can be added (see Chapter 11, page 127).

Serving suggestion

- Carve the meat against the grain; see the carving guidance given in Chapter 10 (page 116).
- Serve with Yorkshire pudding, gravy and a selection of roast and steamed vegetables.

RECIPE

2 Yorkshire pudding

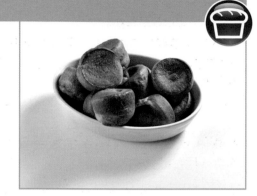

Yorkshire pudding is the traditional accompaniment to roast beef

INGREDIENTS	4 portions	10 portions
Plain flour	85 g	215 g
Eggs	2	5
Milk	85 ml	215 ml
Water	40 ml	100 ml
Salt		
Beef dripping from the joint or a light oil	20 g	50 g

Cooking

1 Place the flour and eggs into a mixing bowl and mix to a smooth paste.
2 Gradually add the milk and water, beating strongly to incorporate air, which should start to appear in small bubbles on the surface. Add the salt and allow the mixture to rest for 1 hour.
3 Heat the pudding trays in a hot oven at 190°C. Add a little dripping in each tray, preferably from the meat as this will give flavour. Otherwise, use oil.
4 Ladle in the mixture so each tray is two-thirds full.
5 Place in the oven for 20–30 minutes. When checking, only open the oven door sufficiently to glance at the puddings, and then close it slowly without banging.
6 For the last 10 minutes of cooking, take the trays out, turn the puddings over and return them to the oven to dry out and complete cooking. Serve immediately.

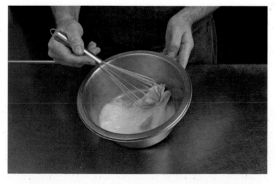

Mixing the milk in with the eggs

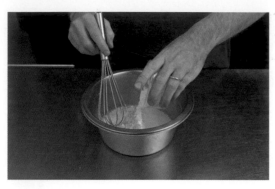

Adding the flour

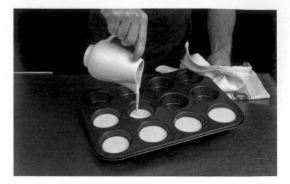

Placing the mixture into a hot pudding tray

RECIPE

3 Horseradish sauce

Horseradish sauce is the traditional sauce offered with roast beef.

INGREDIENTS	4 portions	10 portions
Horseradish, grated	25 g	65 g
Cream, lightly whipped	120 ml	300 ml
Malt vinegar or lemon juice	1 tbsp	2½ tbsp
Salt		

Making the sauce

1 Thoroughly wash the horseradish, peel and grate finely.
2 Mix all the ingredients, season lightly with salt and taste.

RECIPE

4 Pan-to-oven roast beef

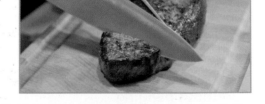

Get ready to cook
Preheat your oven to 230°C.

INGREDIENTS
Joint of beef of your own choice
Olive oil

This method is perfect for medium-sized cuts weighing 250 g–1 kg as it helps the meat stay particularly juicy and succulent. It also gives a better colour than oven roasting alone.

Images and text courtesy of Donald Russell (www.donaldrussell.com).

Cooking

1 Heat the frying or griddle pan on the stove. Once it is very hot, add a little olive oil to the pan, or brush the oil directly onto the meat to avoid using too much.

2 Place the meat into the pan – you should hear a sizzle. Sear the meat for between 4 and 10 minutes, depending on the size of your joint. Searing browns and caramelises the outside of the meat and enhances the flavour.

3 Place the meat uncovered on a trivet (metal or bones) in a roasting tin, and put it in the preheated oven.

4 Cook for the recommended time (see page 231) or use a meat thermometer. Be careful not to overcook the meat, as this will make it dry and tough.

5 Once you are happy that the meat is cooked, remove it from the oven and leave to rest in a warm place for at least 15 minutes. Use this time to warm plates, prepare vegetables or make a sauce.

Serving suggestion

This is the same as for a traditional roast (pages 232–3).

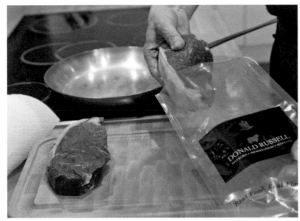
Bringing the meat to room temperature

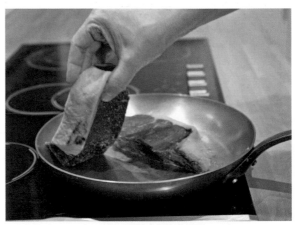
Adding the meat to a pre-heated pan

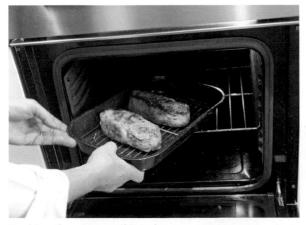
Cooking the meat until it is done

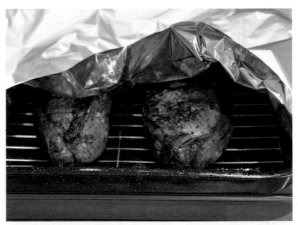
Resting the meat after cooking

5 Low-temperature roasting

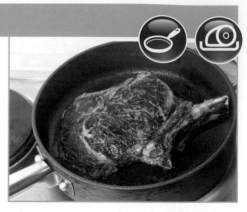

Get ready to cook

Preheat the oven (with the fan turned off) to 80°C and place a roasting tray in the oven to heat up. Always preheat the roasting tray as a cold one increases the cooking time.

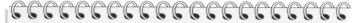

Low-temperature cooking can be used for just about every naturally tender cut of beef, even something as small as a steak.

A meat thermometer is essential for good results.

INGREDIENTS

Cut of beef of your own choice

Olive oil

Images and text courtesy of Donald Russell (www.donaldrussell.com).

Cooking

1 Heat a griddle or frying pan to a high temperature. Add a little olive oil to the pan, or brush the oil directly onto the meat to avoid using too much.

2 Sear the meat on all sides for the recommended time to brown it all over. This will vastly improve both the flavour and appearance of your meat.

3 Season the meat with salt and pepper. (Do not season before searing as salt can suck the moisture out of the meat.) Place the meat on the preheated roasting tray. Do not be tempted to transfer the meat to the oven in the same pan used for searing, as this will make the meat cook too quickly.

4 Set the meat thermometer to the desired internal temperature and insert the probe horizontally into the centre of the meat. Place the meat in the preheated oven with the thermometer cord through the door (the main unit remains outside).

5 Keep the oven door closed during cooking. Opening the door lets heat escape and increases the cooking time.

6 When the thermometer beeps or shows the correct temperature, your meat is ready to serve straight away. There is no need to rest your meat as it has rested during the cooking process. The lower temperatures allow the meat juices to

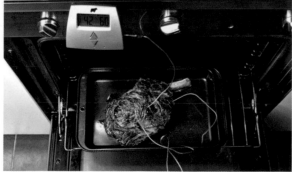

The meat thermometer probe is inserted into the meat and stays in place during cooking. The main part of the thermometer stays outside the oven.

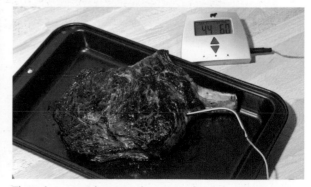

There is no need to rest the meat after low-temperature cooking

circulate continually during cooking so the meat stays incredibly soft and the joint is cooked more evenly.

7 You can keep the meat warm at 60°C for up to an hour for large joints and 30 minutes for smaller cuts. If your oven does not have a setting as low as 60°C, simply switch off the oven.

Cooking steaks

There are ten beef steaks that can be cooked by grilling. Four of the most popular are the sirloin, fillet, ribeye (see pages 229–30) and T-bone.

Cooking the perfect steak can be a challenge, even for top chefs. That's because smaller cuts of meat can dry out easily or cook too quickly, so they become dry, tough or leathery.

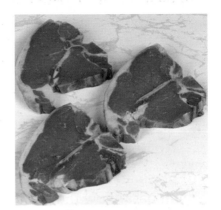

T-bone steaks (Source: Meat and Livestock Commission)

Degrees of cooking and testing

Customers may request their steak to be cooked to different degrees:

- very rare (or blue) – cooked over a fierce heat for only a few seconds each side to give a good brown colour
- rare – the cooked meat has a reddish tinge
- medium – the cooked meat is slightly pinkish
- well done – thoroughly cooked with no sign of pinkness.

Testing without a temperature probe

Use finger pressure and the springiness of the meat, together with the amount of blood that comes from it, to check how well it is cooked. This requires experience, but if you put the meat on a plate and press firmly then the more underdone the steak, the more springy it is and the more blood will appear on the plate.

Testing with a temperature probe

1 Insert the probe into the thickest part of the meat.
2 The internal reading should be:
   - rare 45–50°C
   - medium 55–60°C
   - well done 75–77°C

RECIPE

6) Grilled beef steak

Get ready to cook
Preheat the grill.

INGREDIENTS
Steaks
Oil

If you barbecue your steaks you can marinate them using a good oil, seasoning and/or herbs before cooking.

Cooking

1 Season the steaks lightly with salt and brush both sides with oil.
2 Place on hot, preheated, greased grill bars.
3 Turn the steaks over halfway through cooking and brush occasionally with oil.
4 Cook to the degree ordered by the customer (see guidance above).

Serving suggestion

Serve garnished with a small bunch of well-washed and dried watercress, chips (pommes frites) and a suitable sauce, e.g. a compound butter sauce (page 212).

Try something different

Instead of grilling the steaks you could barbecue them.

1 If possible, use gas rather than charcoal as it is easier to control the temperature with gas. Allow the gas barbecue to preheat for 30 minutes.
2 Secure a layer of tin foil over the barbecue.
3 Wait until the grill bars are hot or the charcoal embers glow. (If cooking on charcoal, always wait for the flames to go out and for the embers to start glowing before beginning to cook.)
4 Remove the tinfoil and brush the grill bars with a firm, long-handled wire brush to remove any unwanted debris
5 Proceed as for grilling steaks.

RECIPE

7 Pan-fried steak

> ### Get ready to cook
> Preheat the grill.

INGREDIENTS
Steaks
Oil

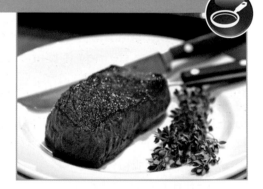

This method is perfect for small to medium-sized cuts.

You can use a meat thermometer to check the internal temperature of your steaks.

Images and text courtesy of Donald Russell (www.donaldrussell.com)

Cooking

1 Preheat a heavy frying pan or griddle (ridged pan) to a high heat. It should be hot enough to sizzle when you place the meat into the pan. If your pan is not hot enough this can make the meat tough.
2 Put a little oil in the pan or brush oil directly onto the steaks (do the latter if you are using a griddle).

3 Fry the steaks for the recommended time for rare, medium or well done (see above).

4 Cook one side first and then the other. Turn your steaks gently and only once to avoid letting out precious juices and drying out the meat. Be careful not to overcook, as this can make your meat dry and tough.

5 Use the press test (page 237) to check if your steaks are done, and then rest them. Place the steaks on a rack so they do not lie in their own juice, cover with foil and leave in a warm place. It is always better to over-rest than under-rest steaks.

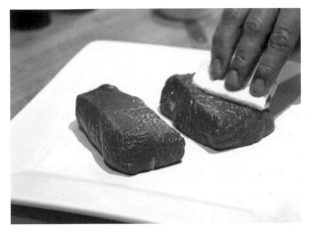

Patting some defrosted meat with kitchen paper to dry it

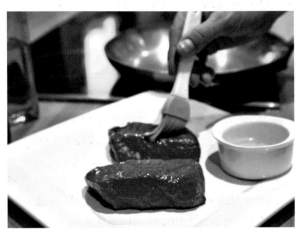

Brushing oil onto the steaks

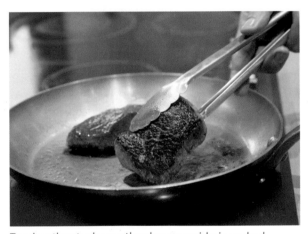

Turning the steaks gently when one side is cooked

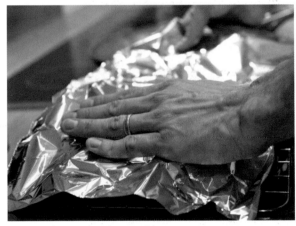

Resting the steaks after cooking

Boiling beef

Before cooking, the prepared joint should be pre-soaked in a brine tub (a salty solution used to preserve and flavour the meat). This will often be done by the butcher, but you may want to do this yourself.

RECIPE

8 Boiled silverside of beef with carrots and dumplings

Get ready to cook

1 Peel the onions and carrots and leave whole.

2 Soak the meat in cold water to remove excess brine.

INGREDIENTS	4 portions	10 portions
Boiled silverside		
Silverside, salted (pre-soaked)	400 g	1¼ kg
Small onions, peeled and left whole	200 g	500 g
Small carrots, peeled and left whole	200 g	500 g
Suet paste for dumplings		
Flour (soft) or self-raising	100 g	250 g
Baking powder	10 g	25 g
Salt – season lightly		
Beef suet, prepared	100 g	250 g
Water	125 ml	300 ml

If you are cooking a large joint of silverside (approximately 6 kg), soak it overnight and allow a cooking time of 25 minutes per ½ kg plus 25 minutes.

Cooking

1 Place the meat in a saucepan and cover with cold water.
2 Bring to the boil, skim and simmer for 45 minutes.
3 Meanwhile, make the dumplings. Sieve the flour, baking powder and salt.
4 Rub the suet into this mixture.
5 Make a well in the mixture and add the water.
6 Mix lightly to a fairly stiff paste, then put to one side.
7 Add the onions and carrots to the pan with the meat and continue simmering until the vegetables are cooked.
8 Divide the suet paste into even pieces and mould loosely into balls.
9 Add the dumplings to the meat and simmer for 15–20 minutes.

Serving suggestion

1 Serve by carving the meat across the grain.
2 Garnish with the carrots, onions and dumplings, and moisten with a little of the cooking liquor.

Stewing and braising

Brown beef stew can be made by using the recipe for brown lamb stew (page 216) and substituting prepared stewing beef cut into 2 cm pieces in place of the lamb.

9 Traditional braised beef

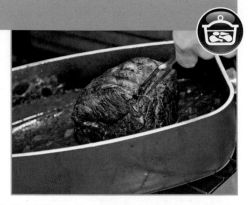

Get ready to cook

1 Pre-heat the oven to 140–160°C.
2 Wash, peel and chop the onions, carrots, celery and leeks.

Braising involves cooking meat in liquid (often stock or wine, or a mixture), at a low temperature in the oven or on the hob (see Chapter 10, page 111).

About one-third of the meat weight gives you the weight of vegetables needed.

Images and text courtesy of Donald Russell (www.donaldrussell.com)

INGREDIENTS
Oil
Cut of beef of your own choice (e.g. brisket, shin, oxtail, etc.)
Onions, roughly chopped
Carrots, roughly chopped
Celery, roughly chopped
Leeks, roughly chopped
Wine, stock or a mixture
Herbs (e.g. bay leaf, peppercorns or cloves)

Cooking

1 Heat a large ovenproof pan on a high heat, add a little oil and sear the meat until nicely browned all over. If you are using small pieces of meat (for stews and casseroles), sear these in batches to make sure they are evenly browned all over. Do not burn the meat as it makes this taste bitter.
2 Remove the meat and sear the vegetables in the same pan until nicely caramelised.
3 Place the meat back in the pan. Add wine, stock or a mixture of both, and the herbs. Make sure that the liquid covers at least a third to a half of the meat.
4 Bring gently to the boil on the hob. Avoid boiling too quickly as this can make the meat stringy.
5 Cover with a lid and transfer into the preheated oven, or continue to simmer gently on the hob at a very low temperature. The oven method is preferable as it is more gentle and the meat does not stick to the bottom of the pot as it can with the hob method.
6 Check from time to time and top up with liquid if needed.
7 Cooking times vary depending on the cut and your oven. As a rule of thumb, you should check casseroles after 1 hour and at regular intervals thereafter. Test stews and casseroles by simply taking a piece out and tasting it. The easiest way to check joints is to insert a meat fork into the thickest part of the meat. It should go in and come out again easily.

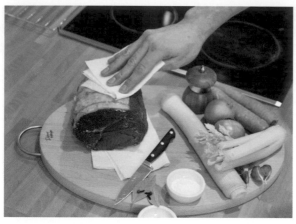

Patting defrosted meat with kitchen paper to dry it before cooking

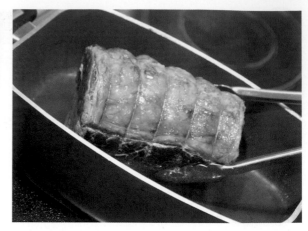

Searing the meat

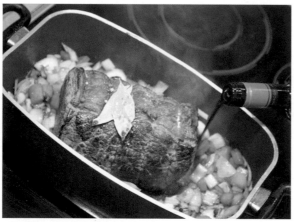

Adding wine to the pan

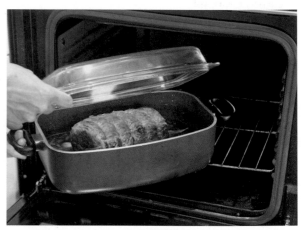

Covering the pan and transferring it to the preheated oven

RECIPE
10 Beef olives

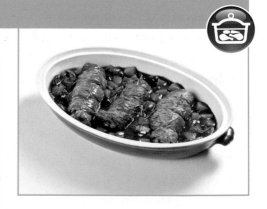

Get ready to cook

1 Cut the meat into four thin slices across the grain and, using a meat bat, carefully thin out the slices.
2 Trim the slices to approximately 10 cm × 8 cm and chop the trimmings.
3 Peel and chop the onions and carrots.
4 Prepare a bouquet garni.
5 Prepare and chop the suet.

Beef olives are thin slices of beef filled with stuffing and rolled up before being cooked. They resemble a stuffed olive!

INGREDIENTS	4 portions	10 portions
Stuffing		
White or wholemeal breadcrumbs	50 g	125 g
Parsley, chopped	1 tbsp	3 tbsp
Thyme, a small pinch		
Suet, prepared and chopped	5 g	25 g
Onion, finely chopped and lightly sweated in oil	25 g	60 g
Salt		
Egg	½	1
Olives		
Lean beef, topside	400 g	1¼ kg
Salt		
Dripping or oil	35 g	100 g
Carrot, chopped	100 g	250 g
Onion, chopped	100 g	250 g
Flour	25 g	60 g
Tomato purée	25 g	60 g
Brown stock	500–700 ml	1¼–1½ litres
Bouquet garni		

Cooking

1 Combine all the stuffing ingredients.
2 Add the meat trimmings and make sure the stuffing is thoroughly mixed.
3 Season the meat lightly with salt.
4 Spread a quarter of the stuffing down the centre of each slice. Neatly roll up each slice and tie with string.
5 In a thick-bottomed pan, heat a little dripping or oil and fry the rolls to a light golden brown on all sides.
6 Add the chopped carrots and onions halfway through.
7 Place the olives and vegetables into a suitable ovenproof pan or casserole.
8 Drain off any remaining fat into a clean pan and if necessary add more to make it up to 25 ml. Mix in the flour and, stirring continuously, brown lightly.
9 Mix in the tomato purée, then cool and mix in the boiling stock.
10 Bring to the boil, skim and pour onto the olives.
11 Add the bouquet garni, cover and simmer gently, preferably in a moderate oven at 160°C, for approximately 1½–2 hours.
12 Once cooked, remove the meat and cut off the strings.
13 Skim, taste and correct the sauce. Pass through a fine strainer onto the meat and serve.

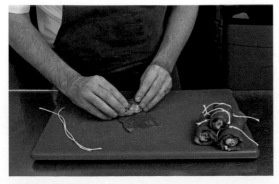

Stuffing the meat

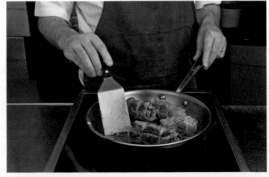

Frying the rolls

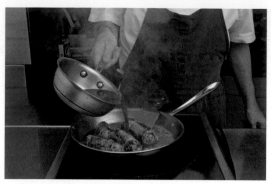

Adding stock to the pan

Activity

As a group, use four variations to the stuffing of your choice. Prepare one without salting the meat then taste, assess and discuss.

Pies and puddings

RECIPE

11 Steak pie

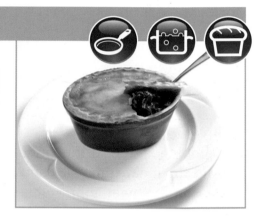

Get ready to cook

1 Make your pastry (page 300).
2 Cut the meat into 2 cm strips and then into squares.

INGREDIENTS	4 portions	10 portions
Oil or fat	50 ml	125 ml
Prepared stewing beef, preferably chuck steak	400 g	1½ kg
Onion, chopped (optional)	100 g	250 g
Worcester sauce	3–4 drops	8–10 drops
Parsley, chopped	1 tsp	3 tsp
Stock or water	125 ml	300 ml
Salt		
Cornflour	10 g	25 g
Short pastry (page 300)		

Cooking

1 Heat the oil in a frying pan, add the meat and quickly brown on all sides.
2 Drain the meat in a colander.
3 Lightly sweat the onion.
4 Place the meat, onion, Worcester sauce, parsley and the liquid in a saucepan. Season lightly with salt.
5 Bring to the boil, skim and allow to simmer gently until the meat is tender.
6 Dilute the cornflour with a little water and stir in to the simmering meat.
7 Re-boil, taste, correct seasoning.
8 Place the mixture in a pie dish – add a pie funnel in the centre of the meat if necessary. Allow it to cool.
9 Cover with pastry. Stand the dish on an oven tray and bake at 200°C for approximately 30–45 minutes.

(12) Steamed steak pudding

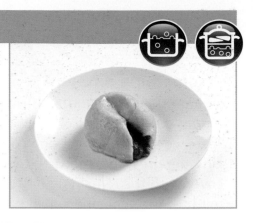

Get ready to cook

1 Cut the meat into 2 cm strips and then into squares.
2 Peel and chop the onion.
3 Grease a half-litre basin.

INGREDIENTS	4 portions	10 portions
Suet paste		
Flour, self-raising	200 g	500 g
Salt, pinch		
Suet, shredded	100 g	250 g
Water	125 ml	300 ml
Flour to roll out		
Filling		
Prepared stewing beef – chuck steak	400 g	1½ kg
Worcester sauce	3–4 drops	8–10 drops
Parsley, chopped	1 sp	2½ tsps
Onion, chopped (optional)	50–100 g	200 g
Water	125 ml approx	300 ml
Salt		

If you do not have self-raising flour, use soft flour with 10 g/25 g baking powder.

If you would like to thicken the gravy in the pudding, lightly toss the meat in flour at the beginning.

Cooking

1 Make the pudding mixture by sieving the flour, baking powder (if needed) and salt.
2 Mix in the suet, then make a well in the mixture and add the water.
3 Mix lightly to a fairly stiff paste.
4 Lightly flour the rolling surface and rolling pin.
5 Roll out three-quarters of the suet paste and use this to line a greased half-litre basin or small individual basins.
6 Mix all the filling ingredients except the water. Season lightly with salt.
7 Place in the lined basin and add the water so that the basin is filled to within 1 cm of the top.
8 Moisten the edge of the paste at the top of the basin. Roll out the remaining paste, cover the filling with this and seal firmly.
9 Cover with greased greaseproof paper or foil or a pudding cloth tied securely with string.
10 Cook in a steamer for at least 3½ hours for a large basin, or 2 hours for individual, one-portion basins.

Serving suggestion

When serving, offer extra thickened gravy separately.

Try something different

1 Simmer the meat (floured if thick gravy is required) in brown stock with chopped onion, Worcester sauce, chopped parsley and a little salt until tender.
2 Taste, correct seasoning and cool quickly.
3 Line the greased basin with the suet paste mixture, add the cooked, cold filling and cover with the remaining paste. Steam for 1–1½ hours for a large basin, or 45 minutes for small, individual basins.

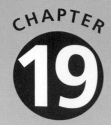

CHAPTER 19

Pork and bacon

Introduction

Pork and bacon both come from pigs. Some pigs are reared to provide **bacon** or **gammon** instead of pork. They are raised to be the right shape and size for good joints of bacon.

Pork does not keep as long as other meat, so it must be stored, handled, prepared and cooked with great care. Pork should always be well cooked.

When a piglet is 5–6 weeks old, with a weight between 5 and 10 kg, it is known as a suckling pig.

A butcher's guide to pork cuts and joints

Images and text courtesy of Donald Russell (www.donaldrussell.com).

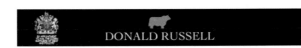

Loin
Equivalent to the sirloin in beef, pork loin is sweet, moist and tasty. Loin steaks can be cut to different thicknesses. Extra-thick steaks stay juicy during cooking. Or you can have a loin roast.

Fillet medallions
A very lean, tender and mild-tasting cut, which tastes delicious pan fried. Because it is so lean, it also works well with creamy sauces.

Mini-steaks
Pork mini-steaks are an innovative cut from the loin, available from some butchers. The meat is very lean, cooks in minutes and stays juicy and tender.

Chops
Pork chops are cut from the loin, but with the rib bone still attached, which gives them a delicious meaty flavour. Like loin steaks, these can be cut extra thick to help them stay moist and succulent.

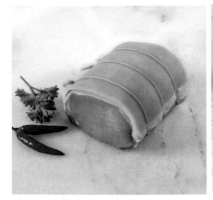

Pork loin for roasting

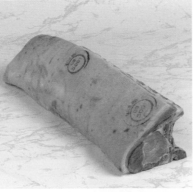

Pork loin on the bone (Source: Meat and Livestock Commission)

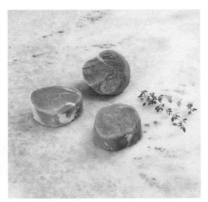

Pork fillet medallions

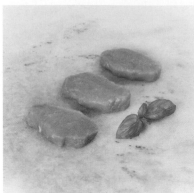

Pork mini-steaks

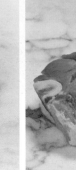
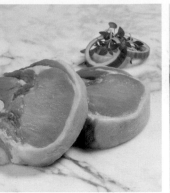

Pork chops

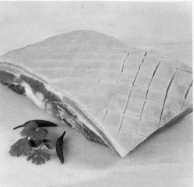

Pork belly

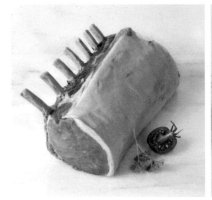

Pork rib

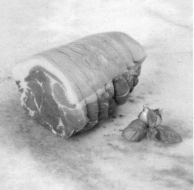

Shoulder of pork

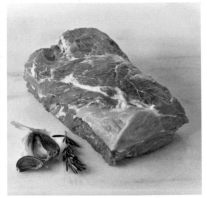

Rindless shoulder of pork

Belly
This traditional cut has rich seams of fat that make it ideal for slow roasting. The fat gives a good savoury flavour and makes the meat very tender. It also makes good crackling (crisped skin), if the skin is scored (as shown here).

Rib
Pork rib roast may have seven highly trimmed bones; it has a fat covering to keep the meat moist.

Shoulder
This is a boneless cut with a good firm texture and lots of flavour. It is suitable for roasting or pot roasting, and is a good-value cut for everyday meals.

Rindless shoulder
Lean and meaty, this joint has a good firm texture and is easy to roast or pot roast. It has a strong flavour that goes well with aromatic herbs.

Quality points
- Lean flesh should be pale pink, firm and with a fine texture or grain.
- There should not be too much fat, and what there is should be white, firm and smooth.
- Bones should be small, fine and pinkish.
- Skin (rind) should be smooth.

Cooking pork

1 Roast loin of pork with apple and onion sauce

Get ready to cook

1 Use a loin that is on the bone. Saw down the chine bone to make it easier to carve. The chine bone is the bone along the back of the loin that attaches the two loins together.
2 Trim off all sinew and excess fat.
3 Score the skin (cut deep with the point of a small sharp knife) in the direction that the loin will be carved. Season lightly with salt.
4 Secure it by tying a string through the chine bone, then place it in the roasting tray, skin side up.
5 Peel, core and quarter the apples, and peel and quarter the onion.
6 Preheat the oven to 250 °C.

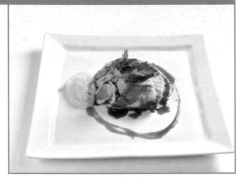

A loin of pork on the bone

INGREDIENTS	4 portions	10 portions
Loin of pork on the bone	950 g	2¾ kg
Salt		
Oil		
Cooking apples, peeled, de-cored and quartered	2	5
Onion, peeled and quartered	1	2–3
Cider	60 ml	150 ml

Cooking

1 Heat some oil in a frying pan. Place the pork into the oil and seal it on all sides.
2 Remove the pork from the pan. Cook the apples and onions in the same pan.
3 Deglaze the pan with some of the cider.
4 Place the meat, apples and onions in a roasting tin. Add the rest of the cider and roast at 200°C for 25 minutes, then reduce the temperature to 170°C and continue to cook until done, approximately 45 minutes.
5 Remove the joint from the tray and put on a plate or dish.
6 Check that it is cooked by pressing the lean meat – no signs of blood should be in the juice.
7 Cover the joint loosely with foil and allow it to rest for 10–15 minutes before carving.
8 Purée the apples and onions in a processor, then reheat. This should be a thickish consistency – if too thick, adjust with cider.

Pork and bacon

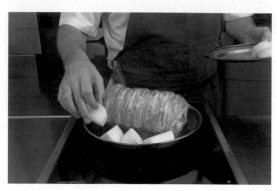
Sealing the meat

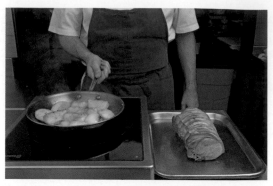
Cooking the vegetables in the pan used to seal the meat

Serving suggestion

Slice the pork and serve with sauce and roast gravy. A piece of the crisp skin (crackling) should be served with each portion of pork.

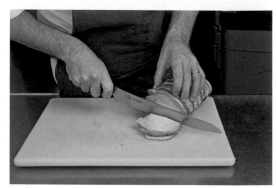
Carving the joint

RECIPE

2 Roast stuffed loin of pork with sage and onion stuffing and apple sauce

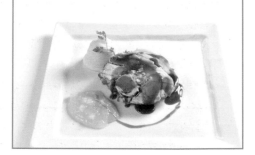

Get ready to cook

1 Use a boned loin, or if it is on the bone then bone it out completely.
2 Remove any sinew and excess fat.
3 Chop the bones into small pieces.
4 Make pork dripping by cutting up the fat trimmings from the pork, putting them into a small roasting tin with a little water and cooking slowly in a moderate oven or on the stove. Once the water has evaporated and the pork fat is browned, carefully strain into a basin.
5 Peel, core and wash the apples. Cut into pieces.
6 Peel and chop the onion.
7 Preheat the oven to 200°C.

If the sage and onion mixture is cooked separately from the joint, it should be called a dressing.

INGREDIENTS	4 portions	10 portions
Loin of pork, boned	950 g	2.75 kg
Sage and onion stuffing		
Onion, chopped	50 g	125 g
Pork dripping	50 g	125 g
White breadcrumbs	100 g	250 g
Parsley, chopped – a pinch	1	3
Sage, dried – a good pinch	1	3
Salt		
Apple sauce	**8 portions**	
Cooking apples (Bramleys)	400 g	
Sugar	50 g	
Margarine or butter	25 g	

Cooking

1 Mix together all the stuffing ingredients to the correct consistency.
2 Place the chopped bones in a roasting tray along with the meat trimmings.
3 Lay the joint out flat and season lightly with salt. Make a line of the stuffing on the opened loin then roll this up, ensuring that the stuffing is fully enclosed, and tie in two or three places with string.
4 Score the skin on the meat lightly with a small, sharp knife in the direction in which the loin is to be carved and lightly rub with salt.
5 Lay the loin on the bones in the roasting tray. Brush lightly with oil.
6 Place in the preheated oven for 25 minutes, basting occasionally.
7 Meanwhile, cook the apples to a purée in a covered pan with the other sauce ingredients and a tablespoon of water.
8 Liquidise or pass through a sieve.
9 Reduce the oven heat to 170 °C and continue cooking for approximately a further 20–25 minutes.
10 Remove loin onto a plate or dish. Press the lean meat to force out some juice and check that it is clear, with no signs of blood.
11 Allow the meat to rest, lightly covered with foil while making the gravy.
12 Pour off any surplus fat from the roasting tray and return the tray to a low heat on the stove.
13 Add sufficient brown stock to make the required amount of gravy and simmer, gently scraping in all the sediment from the tray with a non-metal scraper.
14 Taste, correct the season the gravy and pass it through a fine strainer.

Serving suggestion

Carve the meat into thick slices and serve with roast gravy, hot apple sauce and a suitable potato and vegetable.

Activity

As a group, prepare, cook and serve four loins, each accompanied by a different potato and vegetable. Taste, assess and discuss preferences, giving reasons.

RECIPE

3 Grilled pork chops

Get ready to cook

Preparing a chop from a loin:

1 Remove the skin, excess fat and sinew.
2 Cut, saw or chop through the loin in approximately 1 cm slices.
3 Remove any excess bone and trim neatly.

INGREDIENTS

Pork chops
Salt
Oil

You can buy chops ready prepared, or you can prepare them from a loin as described above.

Cooking

1 Season the chops lightly with salt.
2 Brush with oil or fat and cook on both sides on or under a moderately hot grill or salamander for approximately 10 minutes, until cooked through.

Serving suggestion

Serve with hot apple sauce

RECIPE

4 Stir-fried pork fillet

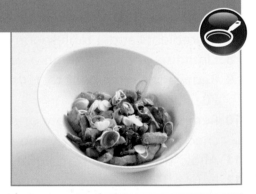

Get ready to cook

1 Peel and finely chop the shallots.
2 Finely slice the mushrooms.
3 Cut the pork into thin strips or slices.

INGREDIENTS	4 portions	10 portions
Oil	2 tbsp	5 tbsp
Shallots, finely chopped	2	6
Garlic (optional)	1	2
Button mushrooms, finely sliced	200 g	400 g
Pork fillet	400 g	2 kg
Salt		
Chinese five spice powder	1 pinch	2 pinches
Soy sauce	1 tbsp	2 tbsp
Honey, clear	2 tbsp	3 tbsp
White stock	2 tbsp	5 tbsp

Cooking

1 Heat the oil in a wok or frying pan.
2 Add the shallots and sweat gently for 1 minute.
3 Add the mushrooms and cook gently until softened.
4 Increase the heat and add the pork fillet strips or slices.
5 Season lightly with salt, add the spice powder and cook for 3–4 minutes, tossing continuously.
6 Reduce the heat, add the soy sauce, honey and white stock, and reduce for 2–3 minutes.
7 Taste, correct seasoning and serve.

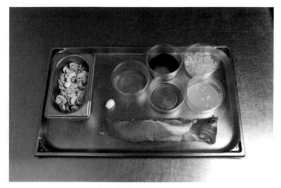

All the ingredients, ready to cook

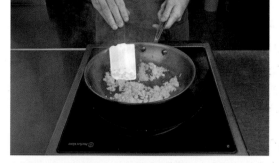

Adding the shallots to the hot pan

Serving suggestion

Serve with noodles, braised rice (page 192) or fried mixed vegetables (page 281), or a combination of these.

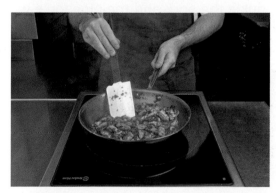

Stir frying

RECIPE

5 Noisettes of pork with spiced pineapple served with steamed rice

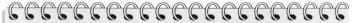

When loin chops are boned and trimmed they are called noisettes.

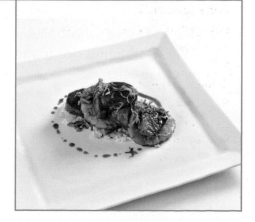

INGREDIENTS	4 portions	10 portions
Vegetable oil	1 tbsp	2 tbsp
Boned pork loin	4 × 100 g	10 × 100 g
Pepper		
White stock or pineapple juice	125 ml	200 ml
Light muscovado sugar	25 g	60 g
Tomato purée	1 tsp	2½ tsp
Pineapple slices, fresh or canned	50 g	50 g
Chilli powder	½ tsp	1¼ tsp
Chinese five spice powder	1 tsp	2½ tsp
Dark soy sauce	1 tbsp	2½ tbsp
Coriander leaves, roughly chopped		

Cooking

1 Heat the oil in a frying pan.

2 Lightly season the pork chops with milled pepper. Gently fry in the oil until golden brown and almost cooked.

3 Place the white stock or pineapple juice in a thick-bottomed pan. Add the sugar and tomato purée.

4 Add the pineapple slices to the pork in the frying pan and allow them to caramelise a little.

5 Sprinkle the pork and the pineapple with the chilli and five spice powder. Allow to fry for a minute to extract the flavour.

6 Add the soy mix to the pork. Bring to the boil and allow to reduce slightly.

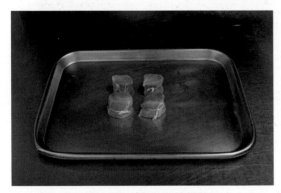

Raw noisettes of pork, ready to cook

Stir-frying after adding the spices

Serving suggestion

Sprinkle the pork with roughly chopped coriander and serve with boiled rice (page 192) or steamed rice (page 108) and Chinese greens.

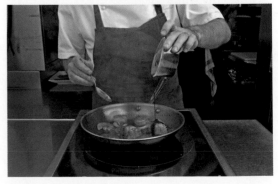

Adding the soy mixture

6 Egg and crumbed pork escalopes

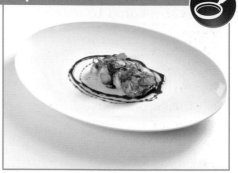

Get ready to cook

1 Trim and remove any sinew from the meat.
2 Using a little water, bat out with a meat hammer as thinly as possible to ½ cm at least.

INGREDIENTS	4 portions	10 portions
Pork fillet or nut from the loin, 75–100 g	4	10
Flour, seasoned	25 g	60 g
Egg	1	2
Fresh white breadcrumbs	50 g	125 g
Oil for frying	60 ml	150 ml

Cooking

1 Pass the escalopes through seasoned flour, eggwash and breadcrumbs (pané).
2 Shake off any surplus crumbs and pat each side firmly with a palette knife.
3 Shallow fry in hot fat or oil on both sides until they are golden brown and crisp.

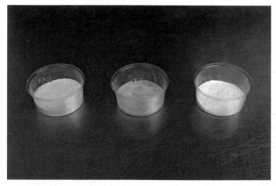

Flour, egg and breadcrumbs ready to be used as a coating

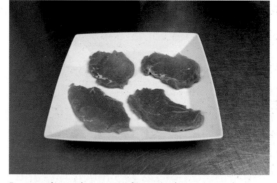

Raw pork escalopes, ready to cook

Serving suggestion

Drain on kitchen paper and serve with a suitable sauce, e.g. thickened gravy (page 148) with the addition of some thinly sliced small gherkins, or an apple purée thinned down with cream or yoghurt.

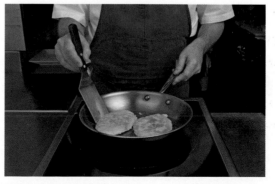

Frying the coated meat

Pork and bacon

A butcher's guide to bacon

The meat is **cured** to make bacon. This means that it is **salted** and then **smoked**.

Ham is very similar to bacon but it is not the same. It comes from a different breed of pig, and it is cured in different ways. Make sure you know the difference.

One of the most popular ways of cooking bacon is in rashers. Rashers are thin slices with the rind removed.

There are three types of rasher:

1 Streaky – cut from the belly
2 Back – cut from the loin
3 Gammon – cut from the gammon.

Rashers can be cooked in the following ways.

- Shallow fry in a little light oil
- Grill on a lightly greased tray
- Cook in a hot oven on a lightly greased tray

Cook them on both sides until they are crisp and golden brown.

Rashers can be served for breakfast or at any time of day. They are often served with accompaniments such as:

- Toast
- Fried, scrambled or poached eggs
- Sausages or black pudding
- Mushrooms and tomatoes
- Baked beans.

Quality points

- There should be no sign of stickiness.
- There should be a pleasant smell.
- The rind should be thick and smooth.
- There should not be too much fat, and what there is should be white and smooth.
- The lean meat should be a deep-pink colour and firm.

Cooking bacon

RECIPE

7 Boiled bacon (hock, collar or gammon)

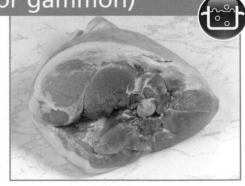

Get ready to cook

You can use a hock, collar or gammon joint for this recipe. Prepare them as follows.

- Hock: cook it whole, or bone it and tie it with string.
- Collar: remove the bone and tie the joint with string.
- Gammon: cook it whole or cut it into 2 or 3 pieces and tie it with string if necessary.

> *Depending on how salty the bacon joint is, you may need to soak it in cold water for 2–3 hours (or longer) before cooking.*

Cooking

1 Place the joint in a suitably sized pan and cover with water.
2 Bring to the boil, skim and simmer gently. The cooking time will depend on the size and weight of the joint: simmer for approximately 25 minutes per ½ kg plus another 25 minutes.
3 Remove the pan from the heat and allow the joint to cool in the liquid.
4 Remove the rind and brown skin, and any excess fat.

Serving suggestion

Carve into thick slices and serve with a little of the cooking liquor. It can be accompanied by a traditional dish of puréed peas, known as pease pudding (see below), and a suitable sauce, e.g. parsley or mustard (see page 145).

RECIPE

8 Pease pudding

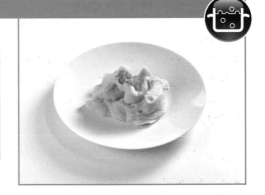

Get ready to cook

1 Soak the split peas overnight and then drain.
2 Peel the onion and then push a clove into it, sharp end first, so the round end is on the outside of the onion.

INGREDIENTS	4 portions	10 portions
Yellow split peas (dried), soaked	200 g	500 g
Water	½ litre	1¼ litres
Onion, studded with a clove	50 g	125 g
Carrot	50 g	125 g
Bacon trimmings	50 g	125 g
Salt		
Butter or margarine	50 g	125 g

Cooking

1 Place all the ingredients except the butter in a thick-bottomed saucepan. Cover with a tight-fitting lid.
2 Bring to the boil and skim the water.
3 Allow the peas to cook, preferably in an oven at 180–200°C, for 2 hours.
4 Remove the onion, carrot and bacon, and either pass the peas through a sieve or use a food processor.
5 Return the peas to a clean pan and mix in the butter. Taste and correct the consistency, which should be firm.

Poultry

A butcher's guide to poultry

The word 'poultry' means all domestic fowl (birds) bred for food. It includes chickens, turkeys, ducks, geese and pigeons. Chickens and turkeys are the two that are used most in cooking, and the recipes in this chapter are for chicken and turkey.

Cuts of chicken

You can buy chicken in ready cut pieces such as breasts (suprêmes), thighs and drumsticks. These can be roasted, grilled, poached, steamed, shallow fried (sautéed) or deep fried.

Alternatively, you can cut up a whole chicken into different pieces yourself. A medium-sized chicken weighing 1–2 kg is suitable for this.

Quality points

- The breasts should be plump and firm.
- The wishbone should easy to bend between your fingers and thumb.
- The skin should be white and unbroken. Broilers (birds that are 3–4 months old) have a faint bluish tint.

Old birds have coarse leg scales, large spurs on their legs and long hairs on their skin.

Cooking chicken and turkey

RECIPE

 1 Boiled or poached chicken with suprême sauce and pilau rice

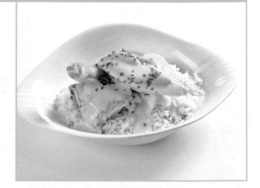

Get ready to cook

1 Wash and peel the carrot and celery. Leave them whole.
2 Peel the onions for the chicken and stud with one clove per onion.
3 Prepare a bouquet garni.
4 Peel and chop the onion for the rice.
5 Wash the chicken and truss it. Trussing is a way of tying the chicken to hold and improve its shape so that it is easier to carve.

INGREDIENTS	4 portions	10 portions
Chicken		
Boiling fowl, 2–2½ kg, trussed	1	2–3
Onion studded with a clove	50 g	125 g
Carrot	50 g	125 g
Celery	50 g	125 g
Bouquet garni	50 g	125 g
Salt, pinch		
Sauce		
Butter, margarine or oil	75 g	180 g
Flour	75 g	180 g
Chicken stock	1 litre	1½ litres
Cream or non-dairy cream	4 tbsps	10 tbsps
Lemon juice – a few drops		
Salt		
Rice		
Onion, chopped	50 g	125 g
Butter, margarine or oil	50 g	125 g
Rice, long grain	200 g	500 g
Chicken stock	500 ml	1¼ litres

Cooking

1 Place the prepared chicken into a saucepan. Cover it with cold water. Bring to the boil and skim.

2 Add the peeled whole vegetables, bouquet garni and a little salt.

3 Simmer gently until cooked (approximately 1–1½ hours).

4 While the chicken is cooking, prepare the suprême sauce as per the velouté recipe on page 145, and the pilau rice as per the recipe on page 192.

5 Cook the velouté for 30–45 minutes.

6 Once the sauce is cooked, taste it and correct the seasoning.

7 Pass it through a fine chinois and mix in the cream.

8 To check that the chicken is cooked, insert a two-pronged fork between a drumstick and a thigh and remove the chicken from the stock. Hold it over a plate and allow the juices to come out. There should be no trace of blood in the juices. Also pierce the drumstick with a trussing needle or a skewer, which should easily slide in as far as the bone.

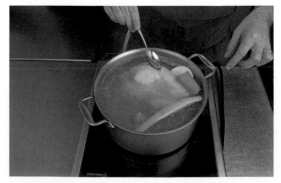

Placing the chicken into the water

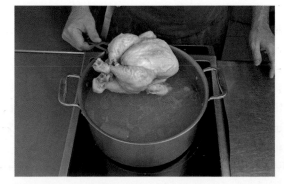

Removing the chicken from the stock

Serving suggestion

1 Remove the legs and cut each leg into two (drumstick and thigh).
2 Remove the breasts and cut each one in two.
3 A portion for one person is one piece of leg and one piece of breast.
4 Place the rice and chicken portions carefully on plates. The chicken can be placed on top of the rice or beside it. Coat the chicken with the sauce.

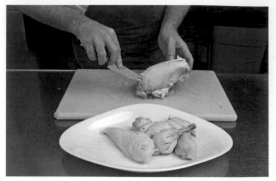

Cutting up the chicken after the skin has been removed

RECIPE

2 Sauté of chicken

Get ready to cook

1 If you are using a whole chicken (or chickens), cut this into pieces.
2 Prepare the thickened gravy (page 148).

INGREDIENTS	4 portions	10 portions
Chicken – 1¼–1½ kg – or ready cut: 2 drumsticks, 2 thighs and 2 suprêmes (breasts cut into 2 pieces)	1	2½
Butter, margarine or oil	50 g	125 g
Thickened gravy (page 148)	250 ml	625 ml
Parsley, freshly chopped		

If using a whole chicken, chop up the carcass and any trimmings and use these when you are making the gravy.

Cooking

1 Place the fat in a sauté pan over a hot stove.
2 Season the chicken pieces lightly with salt. Place them in the pan in the following order: drumsticks, thighs, breasts (you put in the tougher pieces first as they take longer to cook).
3 Cook to a golden brown on both sides. Cover with a lid.
4 Reduce the heat and cook gently until the chicken is tender.
5 Remove the chicken pieces and drain off the fat from the sauté pan.
6 Return the pan to a moderate heat. Add the thickened gravy and bring it to the boil.
7 Taste the gravy and correct the seasoning. Pass it through a fine strainer onto the chicken.
8 Lightly sprinkle with chopped parsley and serve.

Try something different

You can make lots of variations to this simple basic recipe, such as adding:

- sliced mushrooms
- tomato concassé or tomato purée halfway through the cooking time
- freshly chopped soft herbs, e.g. chives, chervil, tarragon
- light spices, e.g. curry powder, five spice powder, garam masala.

> ### Activity
>
> In groups, prepare a selection of variations of chicken sauté. Use your own ideas. Taste each other's dishes and discuss.

RECIPE

3 Chicken Kiev

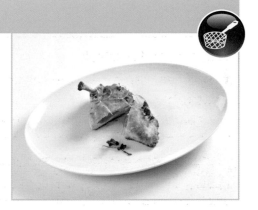

> ### Get ready to cook
> 1 Season the flour.
> 2 Beat the eggs to make the eggwash.

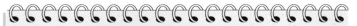

The butter in a chicken Kiev can be flavoured with garlic and/or herbs.

INGREDIENTS	4 portions	10 portions
Chicken suprêmes, skin removed, 150 g	4	10
Butter	100 g	250 g
Flour, lightly seasoned with salt	25 g	65 g
Eggwash (beaten eggs)	1	2
Fresh, white breadcrumbs	100 g	250 g

Cooking

1 Carefully make an incision (cut) in the top of each suprême with a sharp knife.
2 Pipe 25 g of softened butter into each incision. Press down the opening to keep the butter inside.
3 Pané the chicken. This means pass it through the seasoned flour, beaten egg (eggwash) and breadcrumbs. Make sure the chicken is well coated. Pass it through the eggwash and crumbs twice if necessary.
4 Shake off any surplus crumbs. Pat the suprêmes with a palette knife to make the coating as firm as possible. Loose crumbs that come off during frying will burn and spoil the appearance and flavour of the chicken and the oil.
5 Deep fry the suprêmes at a temperature of approximately 175 –180°C and serve.

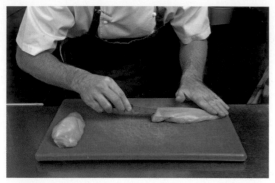
Carefully making an incision in the top of the suprême

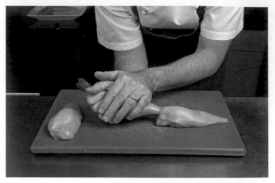
Stuffing the suprême with softened butter

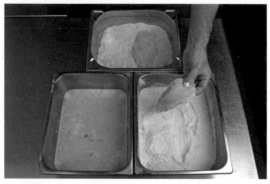
Coating the chicken with breadcrumbs

RECIPE

4 Turkey escalopes

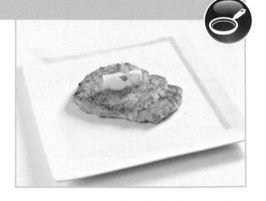

Get ready to cook

1 Season the flour.
2 Beat the eggs to make the eggwash.

You can buy turkey breasts whole or cut into portion-sized pieces known as escalopes.

INGREDIENTS

| Turkey escalopes |
| Flour, seasoned or seasoned and spiced |
| Oil or butter |

Cooking

1 Pass the escalopes through seasoned flour.
2 Heat the oil or butter in a frying pan.
3 Place the turkey in the pan and shallow fry to a golden brown on both sides.

Try something different

Rather than coating the escalopes in flour, you can pané them (coat with flour, eggwash and fresh white breadcrumbs). Gently shallow-fry them on both sides in a sauté pan until a light golden brown.

You can also cook turkey escalopes by:

- gently roasting them with a little oil, butter or margarine – baste frequently so they do not dry out
- grilling them – brush them frequently with oil, butter or margarine.

Activity

In groups, prepare a selection of the above and serve them with a suitable garnish of two items of your own choice. Discuss and vote on your favourites.

RECIPE

5 Breadcrumbed turkey escalopes with ginger and lemon grass, served with mixed leaves and plum tomato salad

Get ready to cook

1 Season the flour.
2 Beat the eggs to make the eggwash.
3 Chop the lemon grass and grate the ginger.

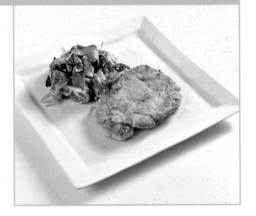

INGREDIENTS	4 portions	10 portions
Ginger, grated	1 tsp	2½ tsp
Lemon grass, chopped	½ tsp	1 tsp
Wholemeal breadcrumbs	200 g	450 g
Turkey escalopes, 100 g	4	10
Flour, seasoned	100 g	250 g
Eggs	2	4
Cooking oil	2 tbsp	5 tbsp
Mixed leaves		
Olive oil	2 tbsp	5 tbsp
Fresh lime juice	2	5
Plum tomatoes	4	10
Radicchio lettuce	1	2
Lamb's lettuce	2 bunches	4½ bunches
Cos lettuce	½	1

Cooking

1 Add the grated ginger and the chopped lemon grass to the breadcrumbs.
2 Pass the escalopes through the flour, then through the egg and coat with the breadcrumbs.
3 Heat a little oil in a shallow frying pan. Place the escalopes in the pan and lightly fry until cooked and golden brown on both sides.

4 Mix the olive oil with the lime juice.

5 Cut the tomatoes into quarters.

Serving suggestion

- Dress on plates with the mixed leaves and tomato quarters.
- Drizzle the dressing over the leaves and the escalopes.

RECIPE

6 Turkey fajita

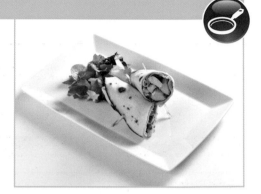

Get ready to cook

1 Cut the turkey into 2 cm dice.

2 Peel and chop the garlic and shred the onion.

3 Wash the peppers and dice finely.

4 Chop the tomatoes.

INGREDIENTS	4 portions	10 portions
Oil for frying	50 ml	125 ml
Onions, shredded	100 g	250 g
Garlic cloves, crushed and chopped	2	5
Turkey, raw, diced	450 g	1125 g
Cajun seasoning	½ tsp	1½ tsp
Green peppers, finely diced	100 g	250 g
Red peppers, finely diced	100 g	250 g
Plum tomatoes (canned), chopped	500 g	1250 g
Black pepper		
Flour tortillas	4	10

Cooking

1 Heat the oil in a suitable pan. Add the onions and garlic and cook for 2 minutes.

2 Add the diced turkey, Cajun seasoning and diced peppers and fry for another 5 minutes.

3 Add the chopped tomatoes and black pepper.

4 Cook until the turkey is tender and thoroughly cooked.

5 Lay the tortillas out flat. Spoon a portion of the mixture in the centre and roll up.

Serving suggestion

Serve on a suitable plate garnished with flat parsley or a tossed salad.

7 Chicken breasts with mango, peas and rice

Get ready to cook

1 Peel and chop the onion and garlic.
2 If you are using dried beans (rather than tinned), you will need to soak these overnight and then cook them.

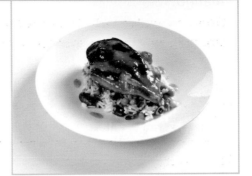

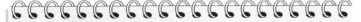
You can use dried or beans or canned beans.

INGREDIENTS	4 portions	10 portions
Vegetable oil	4 tbsp	10 tbsp
Onion, finely chopped	50 g	125 g
Garlic cloves, crushed and chopped	2	5
Long grain rice	200 g	500 g
Kidney beans, cooked	300 g	750 g
Black eyed beans, cooked	300 g	750 g
Vegetable stock	500 ml	1¼ litres
Coconut milk	200 ml	½ litre
Black pepper		
Mango chutney	200 g	500 g
Lemon zest and juice	2	5
Chicken breasts, 150 g, boneless	4	10
Thyme, fresh leaves	¼ tsp	1 tsp
Peas	175 g	440 g

Cooking

1 Heat half the oil in a frying pan and lightly fry the onion until lightly brown.
2 Add the garlic and stir in the rice. Cook for 1 minute.
3 Add the beans, boiling vegetable stock and coconut milk. Season with a little ground pepper.
4 Bring to the boil and gently simmer until the rice is cooked – approximately 25–30 minutes.
5 Mix the mango chutney and lime zest and juice with the remaining oil.
6 Brush the mango mix over the chicken breasts.
7 Heat a little oil in a frying pan. Place the chicken breast in the pan and fry gently until cooked.
8 When cooked, remove the chicken from pan and keep it warm. Add the remainder of the mango mix to the frying pan and heat through.
9 Add the thyme and peas 2 minutes before the rice is cooked and served.

Serving suggestion

- Place the cooked rice in the centre of individual plates.
- Place the chicken breasts on top of the rice and nap (coat or cover) with the mango.

RECIPE

8 Spiced chicken balti with quinoa

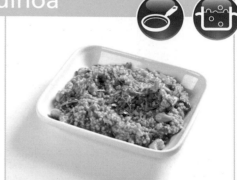

You can use dried or beans or canned beans.

Get ready to cook

1 Blanch, peel and dice the tomatoes.
2 Peel and shred the onion.

INGREDIENTS	4 portions	10 portions
Vegetable oil	1 tbsp	2½ tbsp
Onion, shredded	50 g	125 g
Chicken suprêmes, 150 g	4	10
Balti paste	4 tbsp	10 tbsp
Quinoa	200 g	500 g
Plum tomatoes, blanched, peeled and diced	400 g	1 kg
Chicken stock	1 litre	2½ litres
Roasted salted cashew nuts (optional)	50 g	125 g
Coriander leaves, chopped		

Quinoa is a small, round grain similar to millet. It is pale brown and high in protein.

Balti paste is a commercial product made from a mixture of spices.

Cooking

1 Heat the oil in a frying pan. Add the onions and sweat them for 5 minutes until lightly coloured. Remove them from the pan.
2 Put the chicken breasts in the pan and brown on each side.
3 Remove the chicken and clean the pan. Add a little fresh oil and stir in the balti paste, quinoa and then the onions.
4 Add the tomatoes and stock and mix well.
5 Put the chicken back in the pan with the other ingredients. Simmer for approximately 25 minutes until the chicken breasts are cooked and the quinoa is tender.
6 Add the cashew nuts (if using) and coarsely chopped coriander leaves. Stir these in and then serve the dish on suitable plates.

9 Jerk chicken

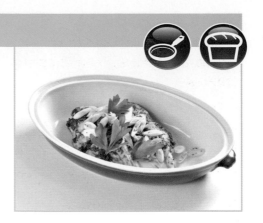

Get ready to cook

1 Mix together all the spices, herbs, sugar and tomato purée.
2 Place the chicken pieces on a suitable tray. Rub the herb/spice mixture into the pieces of chicken and leave to marinate for at least 1 hour or overnight in the refrigerator.
3 Peel and chop the onion and garlic, and chop the spring onions.

INGREDIENTS	4 portions	10 portions
Chicken, either boned chicken legs or boned breasts	4	10
Onions, finely chopped	60 g	150 g
Thyme, chopped	¼ tsp	½ tsp
Garlic cloves, crushed and chopped	1	2
Oregano	½ tsp	1 tsp
Chilli powder	½ tsp	1 tsp
Brown sugar	½ tsp	1 tsp
Cinnamon	½ tsp	1 tsp
Black pepper	¼ tsp	½ tsp
Tomato purée	½ tsp	1 tsp
Spring onions, chopped	20 g	50 g

Cooking

1 Heat the oil in a suitable pan and fry the pieces of chicken until lightly browned.
2 In a separate pan, fry the finely chopped onion until lightly coloured.
3 Add the onion and spring onion to the chicken pieces.
4 Cook the chicken in the oven at 200°C until it is cooked through. Turn it once while it is cooking.

Serving suggestion

Place the chicken in a serving dish. Garnish with spring onions and flat parsley.

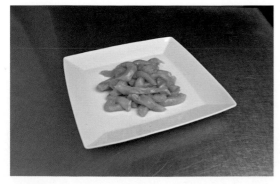

Pieces of chicken, ready to be marinated

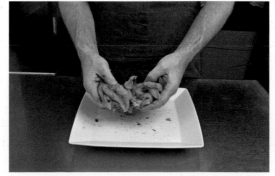

Rubbing herbs and spices into the chicken

Poultry

267

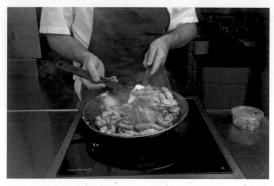

Frying the chicken

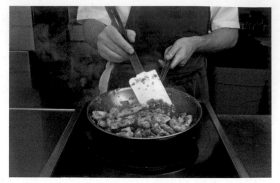

The finished dish, ready to serve

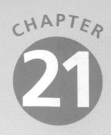

Vegetables and vegetarian food

Introduction

Vegetables are plants, or parts of plants, that you can eat. Broadly speaking, vegetables can be divided into three groups:

1 root vegetables
2 green vegetables
3 pulses.

Some plants that we think of as vegetables (e.g. tomatoes, avocados, peppers) are actually fruits, but they are used as vegetables because they are not sweet. Also, mushrooms are actually fungi but, again, they are commonly considered as vegetables.

Quality points

Root vegetables (e.g. potatoes, carrots, turnips, parsnips) must be:

- clean, with no soil on them
- firm, not soft or spongy (we say that firm vegetables are 'sound')
- free from blemishes (marks and dark patches)
- of an even size and shape.

Green vegetables (e.g. cabbage, Brussels sprouts, cauliflower) must:

- be absolutely fresh
- have bright, crisp leaves that are not wilted, damaged or discoloured.

Pulses (e.g. beans, peas, lentils) must be:

- a good colour (no discolouration)
- free of foreign bodies (e.g. small stones or grit)
- odourless – they should not have an unpleasant smell.

Root vegetables and tubers

Root vegetables grow underground and include carrots, parsnips, radishes and turnips. Potatoes also grow underground but are called tubers because of the way they grow. They are some of the most widely used vegetables and several varieties are grown in Britain. They all have different characteristics and some are more suitable for certain methods of cooking than others.

Choosing potatoes

Make sure that you inspect potatoes and select the ones you want before buying them or accepting a delivery.

- Choose firm, smooth ones.
- Avoid wrinkled, withered, cracked potatoes and do not buy any that have green patches or are sprouting small shoots.

You can buy ready-prepared potatoes in many convenience forms – peeled and prepared in various shapes.

- Chips are available fresh, frozen, chilled or vacuum packed.
- Mashed potato powder is also available.

Portions of potato

The different types of potato will also yield (give) different portions:

- ½ kg of old potatoes will yield approximately 3 portions
- ½ kg of new potatoes will yield approximately 4 portions
- 1 kg of old potatoes will yield approximately 4–6 portions
- 1 kg of new potatoes will yield approximately 8 portions.

Green vegetables

Green vegetables must be used fresh, with bright green leaves that have no blemishes and are not withered.

Take care not to prepare green vegetables too far in advance or overcook them as they will lose some of their nutritive value. Cook them by boiling them briefly in lightly salted water, or steaming them, to retain their colour.

Pulses

Pulses are the dried crop from a wide variety of beans and peas. Pulses are highly nutritious and can make a good contribution to our diet. There are 21 varieties altogether, including:

- black-eyed beans
- soy beans
- dried peas – blue (also known as marrowfat), split green and split yellow, chickpeas
- lentils – orange, yellow, red, Indian brown.

You should store dried pulses in clean airtight containers off the floor in a dry store.

Some pulses need to be soaked in cold water before cooking. The length of time they need to be soaked for will vary according to their type, quality and how long they have been stored.

Do not add salt before or during the cooking of pulses as this can make them tough. You may add a little salt when the pulses are almost cooked, if required.

Preparing and cooking vegetable dishes

Cutting vegetables

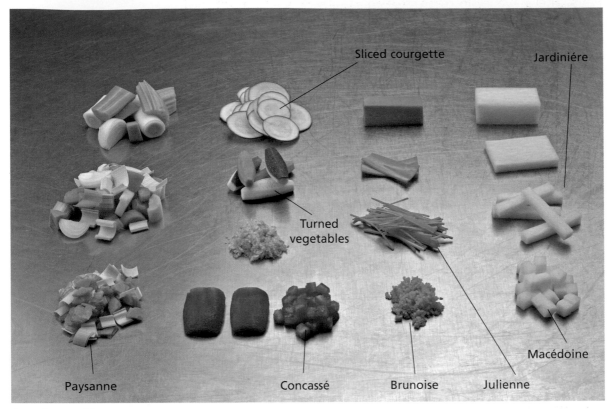

Cuts of vegetables

The size to which you cut vegetables may vary according to what you are using them for, but the shape does not change. There are different ways of cutting them.

Julienne (strips)

- Cut the vegetables into 2 cm lengths (short julienne).
- Cut the lengths into thin slices.
- Cut the slices into thin strips.
- Double the length (4 cm) is a long julienne. This is used for garnishing (e.g. salads, meats, fish, poultry dishes).

Brunoise (small dice)

- Cut the vegetables into convenient-sized lengths.
- Cut the lengths into 2 mm slices.
- Cut the slices into 2 mm strips.
- Cut the strips into 2 mm squares.

Macédoine (½ cm dice)

- Cut the vegetables into convenient lengths.
- Cut the lengths into ½ cm slices.
- Cut the slices into ½ cm strips.
- Cut the strips into ½ cm squares.

Jardinière (batons)

- Cut the vegetables into 1½ cm lengths.

- Cut the lengths into 3 mm slices.
- Cut the slices into batons (3 × 3 × 18 mm).

Paysanne

There are at least four accepted methods of cutting paysanne:

- 1 cm-sided triangles
- 1 cm-sided squares
- 1 cm-diameter rounds
- 1 cm-diameter rough-sided rounds.

The method you use will depend on the shape of the vegetables. Always cut them thinly.

Concassé

Roughly chop the vegetables (e.g. skinned and deseeded tomatoes are roughly chopped for many food preparations).

Cooking times

The times given in the recipes in this chapter are approximate. The quality, age, freshness and size all affect the length of time for which the vegetables need to be cooked. Cook young, freshly picked vegetables for a shorter time than vegetables that may have been allowed to grow older and may have been stored for a while.

Fresh vegetables are an important source of nutrition. In order to preserve their goodness they should always be cooked as quickly as possible – overcooking can destroy their nutritional value.

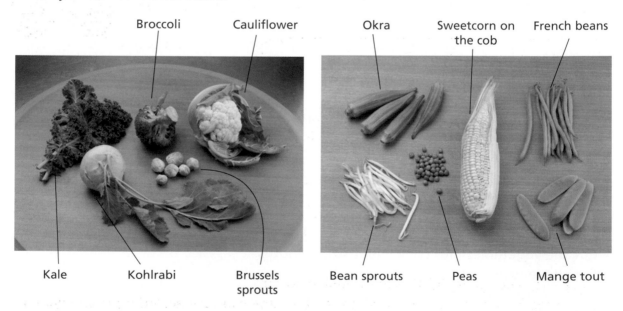

Broccoli Cauliflower Okra Sweetcorn on the cob French beans

Kale Kohlrabi Brussels sprouts Bean sprouts Peas Mange tout

Boiling and steaming

All vegetables that can be boiled can also be steamed. The vegetables are prepared in the same way for boiling and steaming.

- Boil green, leafy vegetables in the smallest possible amount of lightly salted boiling water until slightly crisp. Do not let them go mushy.
- Just cover root vegetables with lightly salted cold water. Bring the water to the boil and cook the vegetables until they are slightly firm. Again, do not let them go

mushy. The one exception to this is potatoes that you are boiling to mash, which should be allowed to cook until they are a bit softer but not mushy.

- To steam vegetables, place them in steamer trays and salt lightly. Steam them under pressure for as short a time as possible. The less time they are cooked for, the more nutritional value and colour they will keep.

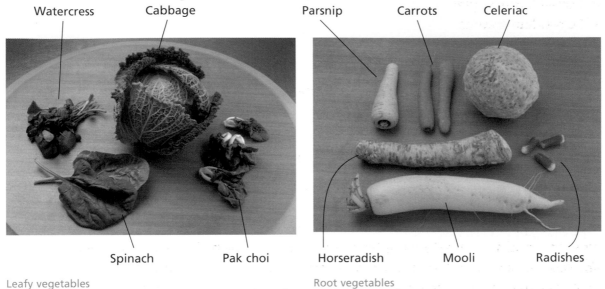

Watercress   Cabbage   Parsnip   Carrots   Celeriac

Spinach   Pak choi   Horseradish   Mooli   Radishes

Leafy vegetables   Root vegetables

Vegetable and vegetarian recipes

RECIPE

1 Boiled/steamed cabbage

Get ready to cook

1 Remove the outer leaves.
2 Cut the cabbage into quarters.
3 Remove the hard stalk in the centre.
4 Using a large knife, shred (finely chop) the cabbage and then wash it well.

INGREDIENTS	4 portions	10 portions
Cabbage, prepared	½ kg	1¼ kg

Cooking

1 Place the cabbage in lightly salted boiling water.
2 Boil steadily or steam for 5–10 minutes – the time will vary according to the type of cabbage. Do not overcook it.
3 Drain well in a colander before serving.

Try something different

In order to make cabbage more interesting, you can add various things to the cooked cabbage, such as:

- some lightly sautéed shredded onions with chopped ginger
- some chopped fresh herbs, e.g. basil, coriander, chives
- some soaked sultanas and flaked almonds.

273

2 Boiled/steamed cauliflower

Get ready to cook

1 Remove the outer leaves.
2 Trim the stem.
3 Cut into florets and wash.

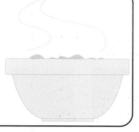

INGREDIENTS	4 portions	10 portions
Cauliflower, prepared	1 medium sized	2 large

Cooking

1 Place the cauliflower in lightly salted water. Bring the water to the boil.
2 Boil or steam for approximately 3–5 minutes. Do not overcook.
3 Drain well before serving.

Serving suggestion

- Serve plain or lightly coated with melted butter.
- Serve with a cream sauce (page 145).
- Place the cauliflower on a tray or dish. Coat it with cream sauce and sprinkle with grated Cheddar or Parmesan cheese. Lightly brown the topping under the salamander or in a hot oven.

3 Boiled/steamed broccoli

Get ready to cook

Break the broccoli into florets, removing the main stem.

INGREDIENTS	4 portions	10 portions
Broccoli, prepared	½ kg	1¼ kg

Cooking

1 Place the broccoli in lightly salted water. Bring the water to the boil.
2 Boil or steam for approximately ½–1 minute. This should leave the broccoli slightly crisp and not mushy. Do not overcook. As they are in florets they require very little cooking.
3 Drain well and serve as for any of the cauliflower recipes.

4 Boiled/steamed spinach

Get ready to cook

1 Remove the stems from fully grown spinach. You do not need to remove them from young or baby spinach.

2 Wash the leaves carefully in deep water, several times if the spinach feels gritty. When washing, lift the spinach out of the deep water into a colander with your hands.

INGREDIENTS	4 portions	10 portions
Spinach, prepared	2 kg	5 kg

Cooking

1 Place the spinach into a saucepan and season lightly with salt. If you are cooking the spinach immediately after washing it there should be no need for extra water. If it is dry add a little water.

2 Cover it with a lid and cook for 1–3 minutes (according to its age), over a fierce heat.

3 Tip it into a colander over the sink and press it several times to remove all the water.

4 Squeeze the spinach into portion-sized balls ready for service.

Serving suggestion

● Reheat the spinach in a steamer. Use a two-pronged fork to separate the leaves loosely.

● Or you could heat the spinach in a thick-bottomed pan containing 25 g butter per portion.

Try something different

● Make spinach purée by passing the cooked spinach through a sieve or mouli (vegetable puréeing mill), or using a food processor. Reheat in 25 g butter per portion. Try adding a little freshly grated nutmeg.

● You can halve the amount of butter you use and add a tablespoonful of cream instead.

● You can also serve young spinach leaves raw as a salad, e.g. with bread croûtons, fried cubes of bacon and a vinaigrette.

5 Boiled/steamed potatoes

Get ready to cook

1 Wash, peel and re-wash the potatoes.
2 Cut into evenly sized pieces, 2–3 pieces per portion.

INGREDIENTS

Potatoes, washed, peeled and cut; quantities as per page 270.

Cooking

1 Place the potatoes in a pan of lightly salted cold water and bring it to the boil.
2 Cook carefully for approximately 15–20 minutes. When they are cooked, they will feel tender when you insert a small knife into the centre.
3 Drain well and serve.

Try something different

- You can steam the potatoes rather than boiling them.
- Brush 10 g melted butter per portion onto the potatoes.
- Sprinkle lightly with freshly chopped parsley.

6 Mashed potatoes

Get ready to cook

1 Wash, peel and re-wash the potatoes.
2 Cut into evenly sized pieces.

INGREDIENTS

Potatoes, washed, peeled and cut; quantities as per page 270.
Salt
Butter; 25 g per ½ kg of potatoes
Milk, warm; 30 ml

Cooking

1 Cook the potatoes in lightly salted water, or steam them.
2 Drain off the water, cover the pan and return it to a low heat to dry out the potatoes.
3 Pass the potatoes through a medium sieve or a potato masher.
4 Return the potatoes to a clean pan.
5 Using a wooden spoon, mix in 25 g of butter per ½ kg of potatoes.
6 Gradually mix in 30 ml of warm milk until the potato is smooth and creamy.
7 Taste, correct the seasoning, taste again and serve.

7 Sauté potatoes

Get ready to cook

Scrub the potatoes well (do not peel). Leave them whole.

INGREDIENTS

Potatoes, scrubbed, whole; quantities as per page 270.
Oil for sautéing
Salt, pinch

Cooking

1 Plain boil or steam the potatoes for approximately 15 minutes.
2 Cool them slightly and then peel them.
3 Cut them into 3 mm slices.
4 Toss the slices in hot shallow oil in a frying pan until nicely browned.
5 Season *lightly* with salt.

Serving suggestion

Serve sprinkled with freshly chopped parsley.

8 Roast potatoes

Get ready to cook

1 Wash, peel and re-wash the potatoes.
2 Cut into evenly sized pieces, 3–4 pieces per portion.
3 Dry the potatoes well *or* par-boil or partly steam them, then drain them well.
4 Preheat the oven to 230–250 °C.

INGREDIENTS

Potatoes, washed, peeled and cut; quantities as per page 270.
Oil or dripping for roasting
Salt, pinch

Cooking

1 Heat a good measure of oil or dripping in a roasting tray.
2 Add the well-dried potatoes and lightly brown on all sides.
3 Season *lightly* with salt and cook for ¾–1 hour in a hot oven (230–250°C).
4 Turn the potatoes halfway through cooking.
5 Cook to a crisp, golden brown, then drain off the fat and serve.

Vegetables and vegetarian food

9 Baked jacket potatoes

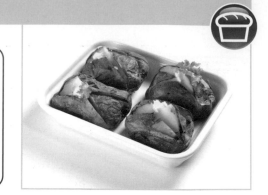

Get ready to cook

1 Select good, evenly sized potatoes and scrub well.
2 With the point of a small sharp knife, cut an incision skin deep around the potatoes.
3 Preheat the oven to 230–250°C.

INGREDIENTS

Potatoes, scrubbed; quantities as per page 270.

Cooking

1 Place the potatoes on a tray in a hot oven (230–250°C) for about an hour.
2 Turn the potatoes after 30 minutes.
3 Test by holding the potato in a clean teacloth (in case it bursts) and squeezing gently. If it is cooked, it should feel soft.

If you use a microwave to cook the potatoes, be sure to prick the skins first, otherwise they could burst open in the oven.

Serving suggestion

Cut in halves, season lightly with salt and add 25 g butter per potato.

Try something different

There are numerous filling you can add to make the potato into a substantial snack meal, e.g. grated cheese, baked beans, cream cheese and chives.

Activity

Within the group, suggest as many different fillings as possible.

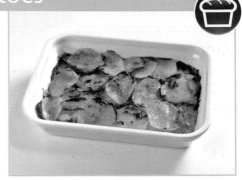

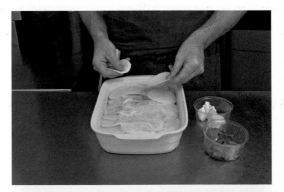

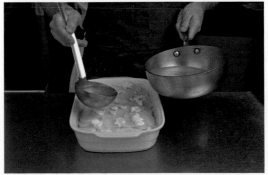

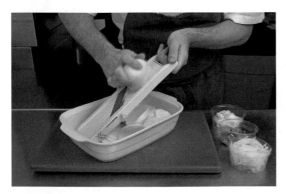

10 Savoury (boulangère) potatoes

Get ready to cook

1 Using a mandolin, and taking great care, cut the potatoes into 2 mm slices.
2 Using a large knife, peel, halve and finely slice the onions.
3 Preheat the oven to 230–250°C.

INGREDIENTS	4 portions	10 portions
Potatoes, peeled and washed	400 g	1¼ kg
Onions, peeled and sliced	100 g	250 g
Salt		
White stock	½ litre	1¼ litres
Butter, margarine or oil	25–50 g	60–100 g
Parsley, chopped		

Cooking

1 Put the neatest slices of potato to one side. Mix the remainder with the onions.
2 Season lightly and place in a well-greased shallow earthenware dish or a roasting tin. Just cover with stock.
3 Neatly arrange the rest of the slices of potatoes overlapping on top.
4 Brush lightly with oil or butter.
5 Cook in a hot oven (230–250°C) for approximately 20 minutes, until lightly coloured.
6 Reduce the heat to 180°C and continue to cook for approximately another ¾–1¼ hours. Press down the potatoes from time to time with a clean, flat-bottomed pan.
7 When cooked, all the stock should have been absorbed.
8 If cooked in an earthenware dish, clean the edges with a damp cloth dipped in salt.

Serving suggestion

Sprinkle with freshly chopped parsley and serve.

Vegetables and vegetarian food

279

11 Chips

Get ready to cook

1 Peel and wash the potatoes.
2 Cut into slices 1 cm thick and 5 cm long.
3 Cut the slices into chips 5 cm × 1 cm × 1 cm.
4 Wash well and dry in a cloth.
5 Preheat the oil in a deep fat fryer to 165 °C.

INGREDIENTS

Potatoes, scrubbed; quantities as per page 270.

Cooking

1 Place the chips in a frying basket, and slowly and carefully immerse in moderately hot (165°C) deep oil.
2 When they are almost completely cooked, drain them and place them on kitchen paper on trays until they are needed.
3 When required, raise the temperature in the fryer to 185 °C. Put the required amount of chips in a frying basket and immerse them in the deep oil.
4 Cook until crisp and golden brown.

Serving suggestion

Drain well, lightly season with salt and serve.

12 Arlie potatoes

Get ready to cook

Bake the potatoes in their jackets (recipe 9).

INGREDIENTS	per 500 g of potatoes
Potatoes, baked in their jackets	
Soft butter	50 g
Salt and pepper	
Chopped parsley	
Cheese, grated	

Cooking

1 Cut off the top of each potato, about one-third of the way down.
2 Scoop out the flesh from the potatoes and place it in a bowl. Keep the jackets. Mash or purée the flesh.
3 Add the butter and a little parsley. Season with salt and pepper. Mix.
4 Use a piping bag and star tube to pipe the mixture into the empty jackets.
5 Sprinkle with grated cheese and cook in the oven at 200°C until golden brown.

13 Fried mixed vegetables with coconut milk

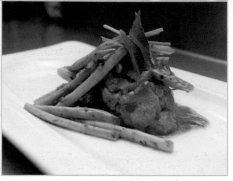

Get ready to cook

1 Cut the French beans into 4 cm lengths.
2 Cut the cauliflower into florets.
3 Deseed and coarsely chop the tomatoes.
4 Julienne the carrots.
5 Slice the shallots lengthwise.
6 Chop the garlic.

INGREDIENTS	4 portions	10 portions
Vegetable oil	½ tsp	1 tsp
Mustard seeds	6	10
Curry leaves	½ tsp	1 tsp
Shallots, sliced lengthwise	3	8
Garlic cloves, chopped	2	5
Chilli powder diluted with 1 tsp water	¼ tsp	¾ tsp
Turmeric powder diluted with 1 tsp water	¼ tsp	¾ tsp
Tomatoes, deseeded and coarsely chopped	50 g	125 g
Coconut milk	½ tsp	1 tsp
French beans, cut into 4 cm lengths	100 g	250 g
Cauliflower, cut into florets	75 g	185 g
Carrots, julienne	50 g	125 g
Salt	125 ml	310 ml

Cooking

1 Heat the oil in a wok and fry the mustard seeds and curry leaves for 1–2 minutes. Keep stirring until the seeds pop.
2 Add the shallots and garlic and fry until soft and fragrant.
3 Stir in the chilli and turmeric paste, and add the tomatoes. Fry till heated through.
4 Add the coconut milk and bring to a boil. Stir in all the vegetables.
5 Cook for 4–5 minutes until the vegetables are cooked but still crisp. Season lightly with salt and simmer for another 1–2 minutes. Serve immediately.

Vegetables and vegetarian food

RECIPE 14 Leek and mustard mash

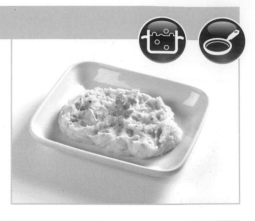

Get ready to cook

1 Peel and wash the potatoes. Cut into evenly sized pieces.
2 Wash and shred the leeks.

INGREDIENTS	4 portions	10 portions
Floury potatoes	1 kg	2½ kg
Butter or margarine	25 g	60 g
Leeks, washed and shredded	200 g	500 g
Milk	3 tbsp	7 tbsp
Wholegrain mustard	1 tbsp	2½ tbsp

Cooking

1 Cook the potatoes in boiling water. Remove from the heat and drain thoroughly.
2 Dry the potatoes quickly over the heat for 2 minutes.
3 Melt the butter in a saucepan and add the shredded leeks. Cook for five minutes until they lose their colour.
4 Purée the potatoes. Stir in the leeks, milk and wholegrain mustard.

RECIPE 15 Bengali-style potatoes

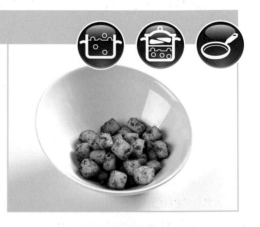

Get ready to cook

1 Peel and wash the potatoes. Cut into 1½ cm dice.
2 Crush the garlic, peel and grate the ginger, and chop the chilli.

INGREDIENTS	4 portions	10 portions
Potatoes	1½ kg	3¾ kg
Ghee or vegetable oil	1 tbsp	2½ tbsp
Panch phora	1 tbsp	2½ tbsp
Garlic cloves, crushed	3	7½
Fresh ginger, grated	1 tbsp	2½ tbsp
Red chilli, chopped	1	2
Cumin, ground	1 tbsp	2½ tbsp
Ghee or vegetable oil, extra	3 tbsp	7½ tbsp
Cracked black pepper	1 tsp	2½ tsp
Lemon juice	60 ml	150 ml
Fresh coriander leaves, chopped	1 tsp	2½ tsp

Panch phora is a combination of five aromatic seeds — cumin, fennel, mustard, fenugreek and kulonji (black onion) fried in hot oil. It is used in various meat and vegetable dishes.

Cooking

1 Boil or steam the potatoes and then drain well.
2 Heat the ghee or vegetable oil in a suitable pan and add the panch phora. Stir until fragrant.
3 Add the garlic, ginger, chilli and cumin and cook for 1 minute. Remove from the heat.
4 Heat half the extra ghee or vegetable oil in a large pan and add the potatoes. Stir gently for 5 minutes.
5 Add the spice mixture, pepper and lemon juice. Stir well.

Serving suggestion

Sprinkle with fresh, chopped coriander leaves and serve.

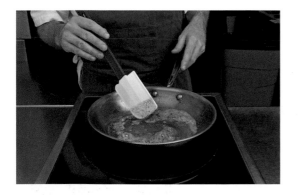 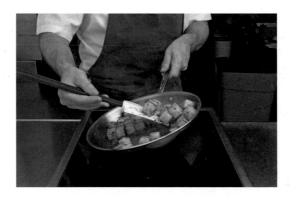

RECIPE
 Bergedil kentang (Asian potato cakes with minced beef)

Get ready to cook

1 Wash the potatoes and boil them in their skins.
2 When the potatoes are cooked, allow them to cool and then remove the skins and mash the potatoes.
3 Shallow fry the minced beef.
4 Lightly beat the egg.
5 Slice the shallots and chop the spring onions and parsley.

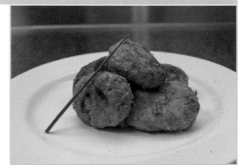

INGREDIENTS	4 portions	10 portions
Vegetable oil	1 litre	2½ litres
Shallots, thinly sliced	50 g	125 g
Potatoes, peeled, boiled and mashed	300 g	750 g
Chinese parsley, chopped	30 g	75 g
Spring onions, chopped	30 g	75 g
Cooked minced beef	50 g	125 g
Salt and pepper to taste		
Plain flour	80 g	200 g
Egg, lightly beaten	1	3

Cooking

1 Heat up half of the vegetable oil on a medium heat and fry the sliced shallots until slightly brown. Drain on a paper towel and set aside.

2 Combine the mashed potatoes, fried shallots, Chinese parsley, spring onions, beef, salt and pepper. Mix thoroughly.

3 Divide the mixture into 40 g balls and shape them into patties.

4 Dredge the potato patties in the flour, then the beaten eggs.

5 Heat up the remaining oil and shallow fry the patties until golden brown. Drain.

Serving suggestion

Serve with green salad.

Try something different

- For a spicier version, you could also add two chopped bird's eye chillies into the patties.
- You could replace the minced beef with dried shrimps.

RECIPE

(17) Braised bean curd (tofu) with garlic and pepper

Get ready to cook

1 Crush the marinade ingredients in a mortar and pestle or processor to form a paste.

2 Cut the bean curd into squares and place in a suitable dish. Cover with marinade and leave overnight.

INGREDIENTS	4 portions	10 portions
Bean curd		
Bean curd (tofu)	400 g	1 kg
Vegetable oil	90 ml	225 ml
Vegetable stock	150 ml	375 ml
Soy sauce	2 tbsp	5 tbsp
Tomato purée	1 tbsp	2½ tbsp
Rice vinegar or white wine vinegar	1 tbsp	2½ tbsp
Arrowroot	1 tsp	2½ tsp
Sesame oil	2 tsp	5 tsp
Ground black pepper		
Marinade		
Garlic cloves	3	7
Coriander root, chopped	2 tsp	5 tsp
Soy sauce	2 tsp	5 tsp
Brown sugar	1 tsp	2½ tsp
Vegetable oil	4 tbsp	9 tbsp
Sesame oil	1 tsp	2½ tsp

Cooking

1 Heat the oil and fry the marinated bean curd until golden brown on both sides. Remove and drain well.

2 Remove the excess oil from the pan. Add the vegetable stock, soy sauce, tomato purée and vinegar. Bring to the boil. Stir in the diluted arrowroot and re-boil.

3 Return the bean curd to the pan and simmer for 1 minute.

Serving suggestion

Serve on suitable plates and season with ground black pepper.

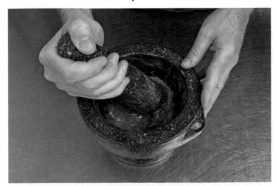
Crushing the marinade ingredients

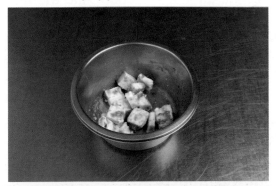
Marinating the bean curd

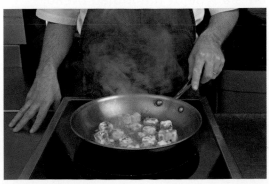
Frying the bean curd

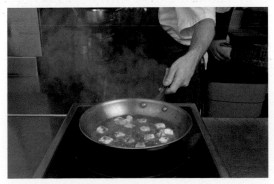
Simmering all the ingredients

RECIPE

18 Aloo gobi

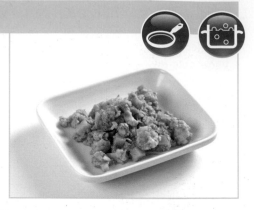

Get ready to cook

1 Peel and wash the potatoes and cut into 1 cm cubes.
2 Finely chop the onion.
3 Cut the cauliflower into small florets.

INGREDIENTS	4 portions	10 portions
Oil for frying	1 tbsp	2 tbsp
Onions, chopped	120 g	300 g
Potatoes, diced	150 g	350 g
Cauliflower, medium, cut into florets	1	2
Cumin, ground	½ tsp	1 tsp
Garam masala	½ tsp	1 tsp
Turmeric	½ tsp	1 tsp
Chilli powder	½ tsp	1 tsp
Ginger, ground	½ tsp	1 tsp
Black pepper	½ tsp	1 tsp
Chickpeas (tinned)	250 g	600 g
Vegetable stock	200 ml	500 ml
Lemon, juice of	½	1
Naan bread		

Cooking

1 Heat the oil in a saucepan. Add the finely chopped onion and cook without colouring.
2 Add the diced potatoes and cook for 10 minutes.
3 Add the cauliflower florets, all the herbs and spices and the drained chickpeas. Cook for 5 minutes.
4 Add the vegetable stock and bring to the boil. Simmer until the potatoes and cauliflower are cooked.
5 Stir in the lemon juice.

Serving suggestion

Serve in a suitable dish with hot naan bread. Naan is a type of flat Indian bread traditionally cooked in a tandoori oven.

19 Vegetable casserole with herb dumplings

Get ready to cook

1 Peel and chop the onion.
2 Peel the carrots, parsnip, swede, turnip and Jerusalem artichokes and cut into ½ cm pieces.
3 Clean the mushrooms and cut into quarters.
4 Chop all of the fresh herbs.

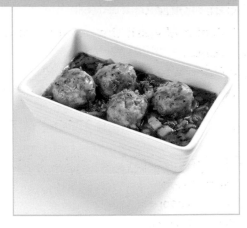

INGREDIENTS	4 portions	10 portions
Casserole		
Vegetable oil	2 tbsp	5 tbsp
Onion, chopped	50 g	125 g
Garlic cloves, crushed	2	5
Carrots, diced	100 g	250 g
Parsnip, diced	100 g	250 g
Swede, diced	100 g	250 g
Turnip, diced	100 g	250 g
Jerusalem artichokes, diced (optional)	60 g	150 g
Fresh thyme, chopped	1 tsp	2½ tsp
Fresh parsley, chopped	1 tsp	2½ tsp
Button mushrooms, quartered	100 g	250 g
Vegetable stock	1 litre	2½ litres
Yeast extract	1 tsp	2½ tsp
Ground pepper		
Dumplings		
Plain flour	200 g	500 g
Baking powder	10 g	25 g
Vegetable suet	100 g	250 g
English mustard	½ tsp	1¼ tsp
Water	125 ml	300 ml
Herbs, freshly chopped:		
Parsley	1 tsp	2½ tsp
Chervil	1 tsp	2½ tsp
Tarragon	1 tsp	2½ tsp
Oregano	1 tsp	2½ tsp
Rosemary	1 tsp	2½ tsp
Basil	1 tsp	2½ tsp

Cooking

1 Shallow fry the onion, garlic, carrots, parsnips, swede, turnip and artichoke for 5–10 minutes. Stir continuously.

2 Sprinkle with the fresh herbs. Add the mushrooms and cook for a further 5 minutes.

3 Add the vegetable stock and yeast extract, and season with ground pepper. Simmer until the vegetables are tender.

4 Prepare the dumplings by sifting the flour with the baking powder.

5 Mix in the shredded suet.

6 Dilute the mustard powder in the water and add this and the herbs. Mix well.

7 Add the water to the flour and suet, and mix to a soft dough. Knead and form into small dumplings. These may be cooked in the casserole or separately in vegetable stock. Cook for 10–15 minutes.

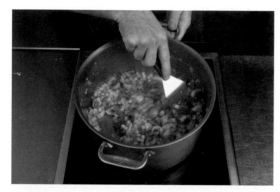

Shallow frying the vegetables and garlic

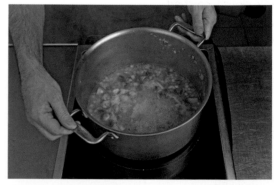

Simmering the vegetables

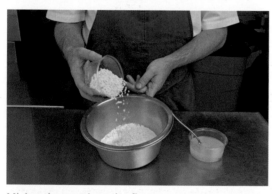

Mixing the suet into the flour

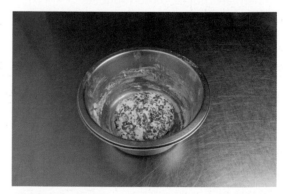

The mixed dough

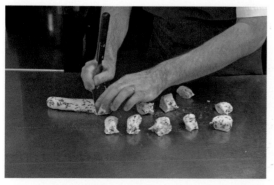

Forming the dumplings

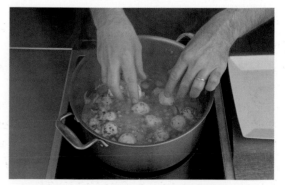

Cooking the dumplings in the casserole

Serving suggestion

Serve the casserole with the dumplings in a suitable dish.

20 Vegetable couscous

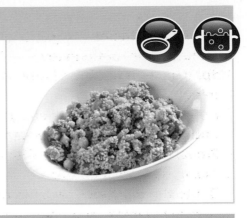

Get ready to cook

1 Peel and chop the onion and crush the garlic.
2 Deseed the peppers, and cut these and the aubergine and courgette into ½ cm pieces.

INGREDIENTS	4 portions	10 portions
Vegetable oil	3 tbsp	7 tbsp
Onion, chopped	50 g	125 g
Garlic cloves, crushed	2	5
Aubergine, diced	1	2½
Courgettes, diced	2	5
Red pepper, deseeded and diced	1	2½
Cumin, ground	1 tsp	2½ tsp
Paprika	1 tsp	2½ tsp
Ginger, ground	½ tsp	1¼ tsp
Allspice	½ tsp	1¼ tsp
Plum tomatoes (canned)	600 g	1½ kg
Chickpeas (canned)	175 g	450 g
Vegetable stock	125 ml	300 ml
Apricots (dried), diced	50 g	125 g
Couscous	200 g	500 g
Harissa paste	2 tsp	5 tsp
Coriander, fresh	2 tbsp	5 tbsp

Couscous is a type of fine semolina that comes from wheat.

Harissa is a spice mix of dried red chillies, coriander seeds, garlic, olive oil, cumin seeds and salt.

Cooking

1 Heat the oil in a pan and gently fry the onion and garlic until soft and golden brown.
2 Add the aubergine, courgettes and red pepper, and gently fry, stirring occasionally.
3 Add the spices and cook for 1 minute.
4 Add the chopped tomatoes and stock and bring to the boil.
5 Stir in the chickpeas and apricots. Simmer until the vegetables are tender.
6 Place the couscous in a colander lined with a cloth and steam for 1–2 minutes. Separate the grains and fluff up the couscous.
7 Mix the harissa paste into the sauce.

Serving suggestion

Place the couscous on suitable plates. Serve the vegetables with the couscous and sprinkle with coriander.

RECIPE
21 Vegetable pakoras

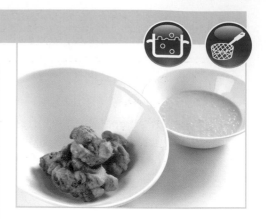

Get ready to cook

1 Peel and crush the garlic.
2 Sift the chickpea flour, the self-raising flour and spices into a bowl. Add the crushed garlic.
3 Whisk in sufficient water to make a thick batter. Cover and refrigerate for 30 minutes.
4 Wash the broccoli and cauliflower, and cut into florets.
5 Slice the courgettes and aubergine into 2 mm slices.

INGREDIENTS	4 portions	10 portions
Pakoras		
Broccoli florets	100 g	250 g
Cauliflower florets	100 g	250 g
Water	180 ml	450 ml
Courgettes	2	5
Aubergine, medium	1	2
Chickpea flour (besan)	100 g	250 g
Self-raising flour	35 g	85 g
Cumin, ground	2 tsp	5 tsp
Garam masala	1 tsp	2½ tsp
Chilli powder	½ tsp	1¼ tsp
Turmeric, ground	¼ tsp	⅝ tsp
Garlic cloves, crushed	2	5
Vegetable oil		
Yoghurt mint dipping sauce		
Mint jelly	2 tbsp	5 tbsp
Yoghurt	180 ml	450 ml
Red chilli, finely chopped	1	2½

A batter made with besan will not absorb the fat, so the fat will not get through to the food inside.

Cooking

1 Cook the broccoli and cauliflower and lightly refresh under cold water. Dry well.
2 Dip these and the courgette and aubergine into the batter. Remove any excess batter with your fingers.
3 Deep fry in vegetable oil at approximately 180°C until crisp and golden brown. Drain on kitchen paper.
4 For the dipping sauce, place all ingredients in a bowl and mix well. Refrigerate until ready to serve.

Serving suggestion

Serve with the yoghurt dipping sauce.

22 Grilled vegetable bake

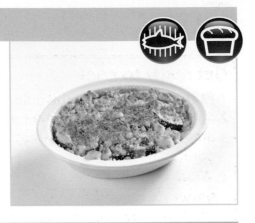

Get ready to cook

1 Peel and crush the garlic.
2 Cut the aubergine and courgettes into 5 mm slices and the peppers into 1 cm dice.
3 Preheat the oven to 150–180°C.

INGREDIENTS	4 portions	10 portions
Aubergines, sliced	250 g	725 g
Courgettes, sliced	400 g	1 kg
Red peppers, deseeded and diced	3	8
Vegetable oil	90 ml	225 ml
Pesto	1 tbsp	2½ tbsp
Garlic cloves, crushed	2	5
Breadcrumbs	60 g	150 g
Parsley, chopped	1 tbsp	5 tbsp
Basil, chopped	1 tbsp	5 tbsp
Cheshire cheese, grated	80 g	200 g

Pesto is a green sauce made from fresh basil leaves, garlic, toasted pine nuts, Parmesan cheese and olive oil. It can be bought ready made.

Cooking

1 Sprinkle the vegetables with oil, pesto, and the crushed and chopped garlic.
2 Lightly grill the vegetables on a griddle pan.
3 Line a suitable shallow dish with half the breadcrumbs and chopped parsley and basil.
4 Arrange in the dish the courgettes and the aubergines overlapping in rows with the peppers.
5 Add the rest of the breadcrumbs to the grated cheese. Sprinkle this mixture over the vegetables.
6 Bake in a moderate oven (150–180°C) for approximately 20 minutes.

Serving suggestion

Serve with a suitable salad, e.g. mixed leaves with rice noodles seasoned with soy sauce, garnished with tomato, chopped onion and avocado.

Vegetables and vegetarian food

RECIPE

23 Aubergine and lentil curry

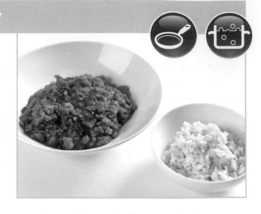

Get ready to cook

1 Peel and finely chop the onion.
2 Cut the aubergine into 2 cm dice.
3 Chop the tomatoes.

INGREDIENTS	4 portions	10 portions
Vegetable oil	2 tbsp	5 tbsp
Aubergines, large, diced	2	5
Onion, finely chopped	1	2½
Curry paste	2 tbsp	5 tbsp
Plum tomatoes (canned), chopped	1 kg	2½ kg
Stock		
Red lentils	150 g	375 g
Spinach leaves	200 g	250 g
Fresh coriander, finely chopped	1 tsp	2½ tsp
Greek yoghurt, low-fat	2 tbsp	5 tbsp

Cooking

1 Heat the oil in a suitable pan. Add the aubergine and fry until golden brown. Remove from the pan and keep warm.
2 In the same pan, lightly fry the onion. Add the curry paste and cook for 2 minutes.
3 Add the tomatoes, stock, lentils and the fried aubergines. Bring to the boil. Simmer for 20–25 minutes until the lentils are cooked.
4 Tear the spinach leaves in half and add these, the coriander and the yoghurt.

Serving suggestion

Serve the curry in suitable bowls. Serve boiled rice (page 192) separately.

RECIPE

24 Chickpea stew (dhal)

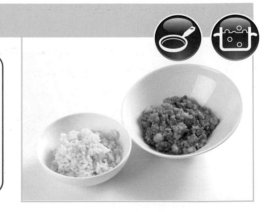

Get ready to cook

1 Peel and finely chop the onion and garlic.
2 Peel the potatoes and carrots and cut into ½ cm cubes.
3 Chop the tomatoes.
4 Deseed and finely dice the green peppers.

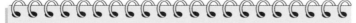

Dhal is the Hindi word for dried peas and beans.

INGREDIENTS	4 portions	10 portions
Lentils	160 g	400 g
Potatoes, diced	100 g	250 g
Chickpeas, canned	240 g	600 g
Oil for frying	20 ml	50 ml
Onion, finely chopped	60 g	150 g
Garlic cloves, crushed and chopped	1	2
Cumin, ground	½ tsp	1 tsp
Coriander, chopped	½ tsp	1 tsp
Green peppers, finely diced	40 g	100 g
Carrots, diced	80 g	200 g
Plum tomatoes (canned), chopped	200 g	500 g

Cooking

1 Wash and cook the lentils.
2 Place the peeled, diced potatoes into cold water. Bring to the boil and cook until tender, then drain.
3 Drain and wash the chickpeas.
4 Heat the oil in a suitable pan and cook the onions without colouring them. Add the garlic, cumin and coriander, diced peppers and carrots.
5 Add the chopped tomatoes. Bring to the boil and simmer for 5 minutes.
6 Stir in the potatoes and chickpeas, and season with black pepper.
7 Simmer until everything is cooked.

Serving suggestion

Serve in a suitable dish with naan bread and plain boiled rice (see page 192).

RECIPE

 Bean quesadillas

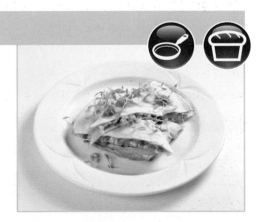

Get ready to cook

1 Peel and finely chop the onion and garlic.
2 Drain and wash the kidney beans.
3 Cut the peppers in half. Deseed and cut into ½ cm dice.
4 Blanch and skin the tomatoes. Remove the seeds and cut into small cubes.

Quesadillas originate in Mexico. To make them, the ingredients are cooked inside a corn or wheat tortilla or a wrapping of masa (cornmeal) dough.

INGREDIENTS	4 portions	10 portions
Vegetable oil for frying	20 ml	60 ml
Onions, finely chopped	½	1
Garlic cloves, crushed and chopped	1	2
Green peppers	1	2
Tomatoes, large and ripe, skinned, deseeded and diced	1	10
Sweetcorn, cooked	40 g	100 g
Kidney beans (canned)	200 g	500 g
Flour tortillas	8	20
Cheddar cheese	60 g	150 g
Vegetable oil	5 ml	15 ml

Cooking

1 Heat the oil for frying in a suitable pan. Lightly fry the chopped onion and garlic, and cook without colouring.

2 Add the diced pepper and diced tomatoes to the onion and garlic. Cook for a few minutes.

3 Add the sweetcorn and kidney beans. Stir well.

4 Spread the tortillas with the vegetable mixture.

5 Top with the remaining tortillas to form quesadillas and sprinkle with equal amounts of grated cheese.

6 Line a baking sheet with silicone paper. Place the tortillas on the tray and brush with oil. Bake in a preheated oven at 180°C until the cheese has melted and the tortillas are lightly browned. Cut in half and serve on a suitable dish.

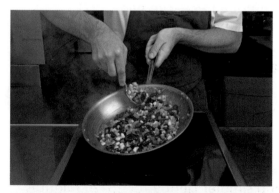

Cooking the mixture

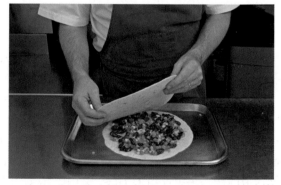

Filling the quesadilla

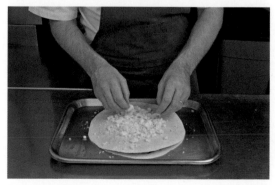

Sprinkling with grated cheese

26 Red Dragon pie with aduki beans

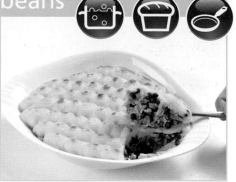

Get ready to cook

1 Wash the beans and rice.
2 Wash, peel and dice the carrots.
3 Peel the onion and chop it finely.
4 Peel, cook and mash the potatoes.
5 Preheat the oven to 180°C.

The Chinese call aduki beans 'red dragon' or 'red wonder' beans as they have found them to be so full of goodness. This is where the name 'red dragon' comes from.

INGREDIENTS	4 portions	10 portions
Aduki beans, washed	100 g	250 g
Rice, long grain, washed	50 g	125 g
Oil	1 tbsp	2½ tbsp
Onion, finely chopped	1	2–3
Carrot, peeled and cut into small dice	200 g	500 g
Tomato purée	1 tbsp	2½ tbsp
Soy sauce	1 tbsp	2½ tbsp
Mixed dried herbs	1 level tsp	2½ level tsp
Potatoes, cooked and mashed	400 g	1 kg
Butter	25 g	70 g

Cooking

1 Cook the aduki beans in plain water until soft. Drain the beans and keep the stock.
2 Cook the rice in lightly salted water until soft, then drain.
3 Heat the oil in a thick-bottomed pan and gently sweat the onions for 3–4 minutes.
4 Add the carrots and cook for 2–3 minutes.
5 Mix in the tomato purée, soy sauce and the aduki bean stock.
6 Mix in the beans and rice. Bring to the boil and simmer gently for 15–20 minutes.
7 Mix in the herbs, season lightly and taste to check the seasoning.
8 The mixture should be moist but not sloppy, and can be adjusted with a little stock if necessary.
9 Place the mixture into a suitably sized, greased, ovenproof dish or tray.
10 Spread the mashed potatoes over the beans and vegetables.
11 Bake in a hot oven at 180°C until the potatoes are brown and crisp.

Vegetables and vegetarian food

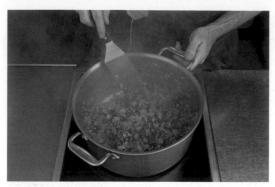

Cooking the mixture

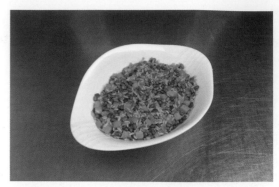

Placing the mixture in a pie dish

Serving suggestion

You can serve a tomato sauce with some sliced mushrooms with this dish.

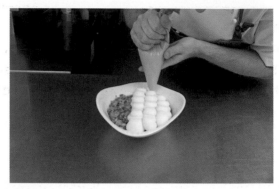

Piping the mashed potato on top

RECIPE

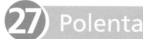 Polenta

Polenta is a golden-yellow cornmeal made from ground maize. It is also the name given to the savoury cornmeal porridge that is made from it. It is used in a wide variety of Italian recipes.

INGREDIENTS	
Water	1 litre
Salt	
Maizemeal	300 g
Hot water	1½ litres

Cooking

1 Bring the litre of water and salt to the boil.
2 Sprinkle in the maizemeal, stirring continuously.
3 As the mixture thickens, gradually add a ladleful of the hot water. This is the secret of good polenta. Harden it over the heat and soften it by *gradually* adding the hot water.
4 Continue cooking and stirring for between 15 and 30 minutes, until the mixture comes cleanly away from the sides of the pan.
5 Pour the polenta onto a clean surface or stainless steel tray and allow it to set.
6 Cut into portions.

Serving suggestion

Polenta can be eaten on its own, with butter and/or cheese, or as a substitute for bread.

Try something different

Once the polenta has set it can be grilled on a barbecue.

28 Mushrooms fried with a polenta crust

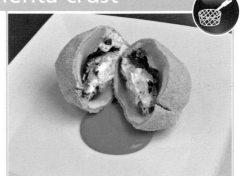

Get ready to cook

1 Remove the stalks from the mushrooms.
2 Trim the mushrooms, stalk side up, so that two mushrooms can be pressed together.

INGREDIENTS	4 portions	10 portions
Cream cheese	150 g	375 g
Chives, chopped	1 tsp	2½ tsp
Black pepper to taste		
Closed cup mushrooms	32	80
Sesame seeds	3 tbsp	7½ tbsp
Polenta (maizemeal)	75 g	187 g
Eggs	2	5
Vegetable oil	2 tbsp	5 tbsp

Cooking

1 Season the cream cheese with chives and black pepper.
2 Sandwich two mushrooms together with the cream cheese filling and make sure they fit snugly together.
3 Add the sesame seeds to some polenta. Pass the mushrooms through beaten egg and the polenta and sesame seed mixture.
4 Chill well.
5 Deep fry the mushrooms in hot oil until golden brown all over.
6 When cooked, drain on absorbent paper.

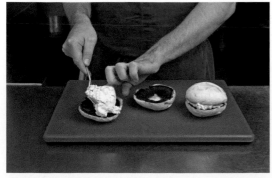

Sandwiching the mushrooms together with the cheese filling

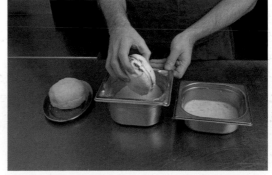

Passing the mushrooms though egg and flour

Serving suggestion

Serve hot with a tomato sauce (page 150).

Try something different

You could add a little chopped chilli or paprika to the cream cheese.

RECIPE

(29) Chickpea and vegetable protein curry with coconut rice

Get ready to cook

1 Reconstitute the vegetable protein in cold vegetable stock.
2 Peel and finely chop the onion.
3 Peel, crush and chop the garlic.
4 Chop the chillies and tomatoes.

Textured vegetable protein is made from soya flour that has had the fat removed. It is processed and dried to give a sponge-like texture, which is often flavoured to resemble meat. It is often used in recipes as a meat substitute. It is also available unflavoured.

INGREDIENTS	4 portions	10 portions
Onion, finely chopped	1	2
Vegetable oil	2 tbsp	5 tbsp
Garlic cloves, crushed and chopped	1	3
Fresh ginger, grated	1 tbsp	2½ tbsp
Lemon grass	1 stalk	3 stalks
Thai chilli peppers, chopped	2	5
Thai curry paste	2 tbsp	5 tbsp
Coriander, finely chopped	½ tsp	1 tsp
Textured vegetable protein, dried	120 g	300 g
Chickpeas, cooked	180 g	450 g
Kaffir lime leaves	3	7
Plum tomatoes (canned), chopped	350 g	875 g
Tomato purée	50 g	125 g
Button mushrooms	100 g	250 g
Sesame seeds, toasted	30 g	70 g

Cooking

1 Shallow fry the chopped onion in the vegetable oil without colouring it. Add the garlic, ginger and lemongrass.
2 Add the Thai peppers. Continue to shallow fry for 1 minute.
3 Add the curry paste and stir in the coriander. Stir well.
4 Add all other ingredients except the sesame seeds. Simmer for 5–10 minutes.
5 The sauce may require a little extra moisture. Adjust with water or vegetable stock.

Serving suggestion

Serve with pilaff rice (page 192), substituting three-quarters of the vegetable stock with coconut milk.

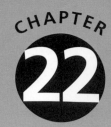
Pastry

Introduction

In addition to being one of the most important sections of the kitchen, pastry work can also be particularly enjoyable and rewarding. Although it is called 'pastry work', it actually includes making breads, desserts, sweets and more, not just goods made from pastry.

Basic ingredients

- **Flour** is probably the most important ingredient in pastry cooking. Wheat flour is the type mainly used. There are many other types of flour but in this chapter we use either soft flour for most pastry goods or strong flour for bread and dough.
- **Fats** include butter, margarine, pastry margarine, cake margarine, shortening and lard.
  - Butter is the most complete fat. It has a delicate flavour that enhances many soft products.
  - Margarine is made from a blend of oils.
  - Shortening is another name for any fat used in pastry making that is made from oils and is 100% fat.
  - Lard is a type of shortening made from rendered pork fat.
- **Sugar** is extracted from sugar cane or sugar beet. It is refined (processed) and sieved into several grades (sizes), e.g. granulated sugar, caster sugar, icing sugar.
- **Baking powder** is a raising agent (an ingredient used in pastry to make a product rise) that contains baking soda and an acid.
- **Eggs** are important and versatile ingredients.
- **Cream** is the concentrated milk fat that is skimmed off the top of the milk when it has been left to sit. Cream must contain at least 18 per cent butterfat (the fatty part of the milk). Cream for whipping must contain more than 30 per cent butterfat.
- **Salt** is another very important ingredient. It must be used carefully and in small amounts. It improves the flavour of many pastry products.

Making pastry, pies and tarts

Pastry is the basis for most pies and tarts. There are several varieties of pastry (for details refer to *Practical Cookery**), but in this book we will consider only two:

1 short pastry – this is made from soft flour and half as much fat (butter, margarine or lard), which gives the pastry a crumbly, 'short' texture
2 sweet pastry – this is made from soft flour and butter and margarine; there is more fat than in short pastry. Caster sugar is added and whole egg is used instead of water, to give it a rich, crisp texture.

*John Campbell, David Foskett and Victor Ceserani, *Practical Cookery*, 11th edition (Hodder Education, 2008)

Plain pastry can be used for fruit pies, Cornish pasties, treacle tart, apple dumplings, etc.

Sweet pastry can be used for flans, tartlets, tarts, etc.

At this level you are not expected to be able to make puff pastry. You can buy ready-made frozen puff pastry, and this is commonly used to make items that require puff pastry.

Troubleshooting in making short or sweet pastry

If you find that your pastry is not of the right texture, or is otherwise not quite right, there are various reasons why this might be the case.

If your pastry is too hard, you may have:

- added too much water or egg
- added too little fat
- not rubbed in the fat sufficiently
- handled and rolled it too much
- over-baked it.

If your pastry is too soft and crumbly, you may have:

- added too little water or egg
- added too much fat.

If your pastry is blistered, you may have:

- added too little water or egg
- added the water unevenly or not mixed the egg enough
- rubbed in the fat unevenly.

If your pastry is soggy, you may have:

- added too much water or egg
- had the oven too cool
- not baked it for long enough.

If your pastry is shrunken, you may have:

- handled and rolled it too much
- stretched it while handling it.

RECIPE

1 Short pastry

Get ready to cook
Ensure that your hands are well scrubbed, rinsed under cold water and dried.

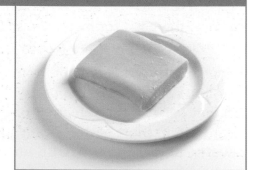

- The amount of water required can vary according to the type of flour (a very fine soft flour can absorb more water).

- The amount of heat the pastry is subjected to (e.g. warm weather conditions, prolonged contact with hot hands) will affect its quality.

INGREDIENTS	5–8 portions	10–16 portions
Flour, soft	200 g	500 g
Salt	Pinch	Large pinch
Lard or vegetable fat	50 g	125 g
Butter or margarine	50 g	125 g
Water	2–3 tbsp	5–8 tbsp

Preparation

1 Sieve the flour and salt into a bowl or onto a cool surface.

2 Using your fingertips, lightly rub in the fat to the flour until it is a sandy texture.

3 Make a well in the centre of the mixture.

4 Add enough water to make a fairly firm paste. Mix it together, handling it as little and as lightly as possible.

5 Ideally, allow the pastry to rest, covered with a damp teacloth, in a cool place (refrigerator) before using. This allows the pastry to relax, which means there is less chance of it shrinking when it has been pinned out (rolled out using a rolling pin) and moulded into shape.

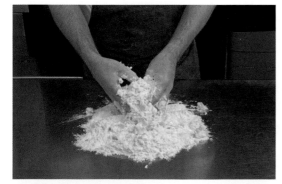

Rubbing the fat into the flour

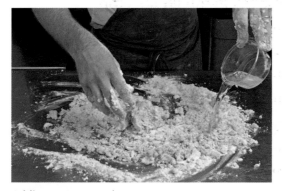

Adding water to make a paste

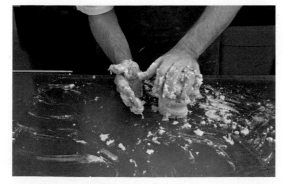

Mixing the dough

Preparing fruit for pies and tarts

- Apples – peel, quarter, core, wash and slice. Bramleys are an ideal apple for cooking.
- Cherries – remove stalks and wash.
- Gooseberries – remove stalks and tails, and wash.
- Damsons – pick and wash.
- Rhubarb – remove leaves, root and any stringy fibres. Cut into 2 cm pieces and wash.

RECIPE

 Fruit pies

Get ready to cook

1 Prepare and wash the fruit.
2 Make the pastry and keep refrigerated until you need it.
3 Preheat the oven to 220°C.

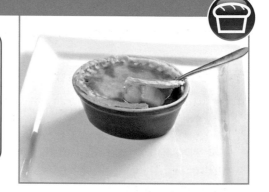

INGREDIENTS	4 portions	10 portions
Fruit of your choice	400 g	500 g
Sugar, granulated	100 g	250 g
Water	2 tbsp	5 tbsp
Short pastry using flour weight of	100 g	250 g

Cooking

1 Place the fruit in a half-litre pie dish.
2 Add the sugar and water (for an apple pie, add a clove).
3 Roll out the pastry ½ cm thick to the shape of the pie dish. Use as little dusting flour as possible on the table surface, the pastry and rolling pin. Allow the pastry to relax for a few minutes.
4 Dampen the rim of the pie dish with water or milk and press a thin strip of pastry onto it.
5 Carefully roll the pastry onto the rolling pin and then unroll it over the top of the fruit, being careful not to stretch it.
6 Seal the pastry onto the dish rim firmly, and cut off any extra pastry.
7 Brush the pastry with milk and sprinkle with sugar.
8 Place the pie on a baking sheet and bake in a hot oven at 180°C for about 10 minutes.
9 Reduce the heat to 180°C and cook for a further 20–30 minutes (if the pastry colours too quickly, cover it with greaseproof paper or foil).

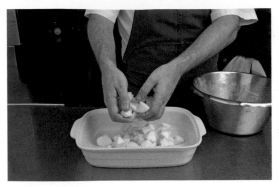
Placing the fruit into a pie dish

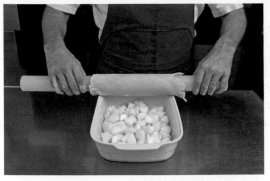
Covering the pie with pastry

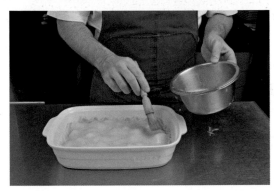
Brushing the pastry with milk

Serving suggestion

Serve with custard, cream or ice cream.

Try something different

You could use a combination of fruit. Combinations that work well in pies include:

- apple and blackberry
- apple and damson
- apple and gooseberry.

RECIPE

Sweet pastry

INGREDIENTS	4 portions	10 portions
Eggs, medium sized	1	2–3
Caster sugar	50 g	125 g
Butter or margarine	125 g	300 g
Flour, soft	200 g	500 g
Salt	Pinch	Large pinch

Preparation

1 Thoroughly mix the egg and sugar in a bowl.
2 Mix in the fat until completely combined.
3 Sieve the flour and salt, and mix in lightly.
4 Allow to rest in a cool place covered with clingfilm or a damp cloth.

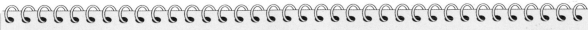

You could rub the fat in, as described in recipe 1.

4 Pastry cream

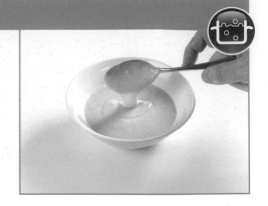

INGREDIENTS	
Eggs, medium sized	2
Caster sugar	100 g
Flour	50 g
Custard powder	10 g
Milk	½ litre
Vanilla (pods or essence)	

Pastry cream is also known as confectioner's custard. It is used in many tarts and other pastry items.

Vanilla pods can be re-used to make vanilla sugar. After you have used them, wash them off in warm water, dry well and keep them in sealed glass jars filled with caster sugar. The sugar will then become vanilla flavoured.

Cooking

1 Whisk the eggs and sugar in a bowl until almost white.
2 Mix in the flour and custard powder.
3 Boil the milk in a thick-bottomed pan.
4 Pour the milk onto the eggs, sugar and flour, whisking continuously until it is thoroughly mixed.
5 Pour out the mixture, clean the pan and then return the mixture to it.
6 Stirring continuously, bring to the boil.
7 Add a few drops of vanilla essence or a vanilla pod.
8 Remove from the heat and pour into a basin.
9 Place clingfilm over the top and press down to prevent a skin forming.

Try something different

Pastry cream is a good base for many flavour variations, e.g. chocolate, orange, almond.

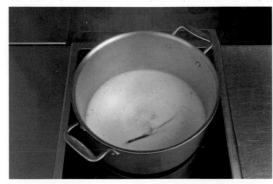

Boiling the milk

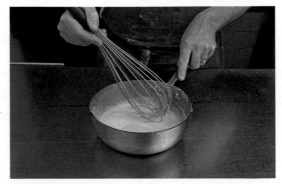

Mixing the milk into the eggs

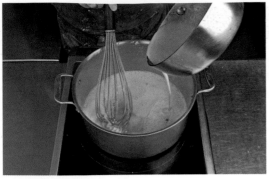

Pouring the mixture back into the pan

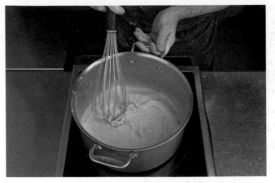

Stirring the mixture continuously

5 Fruit tartlets

Get ready to cook

1 Prepare the sweet pastry as per Recipe 3.
2 Prepare the pastry cream as per Recipe 4, or prepare custard.
3 Preheat the oven to 200–220°C

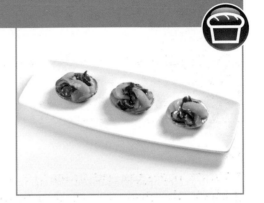

Soft fruits (e.g. strawberries, raspberries) and tinned fruits (e.g. pineapple, peaches, pears) are popular for these tartlets. Strawberries should be well washed and completely dried, then, depending on their size, either neatly arranged whole or cut into slices.

The pastry cases are cooked 'blind', which means that they are cooked before the filling is added.

INGREDIENTS	4 portions	10 portions
Sweet pastry	100 g	250 g
Pastry cream or custard	4 tbsp	10 tbsp
Fruit, fresh or tinned, approximately	100 g	250 g
Arrowroot for glaze (optional)		

Cooking

1 Roll out the sweet pastry 3 mm thick.
2 Using a fluted (wavy) cutter, cut out rounds.
3 Place the pastry rounds in lightly greased tartlet moulds.
4 Neaten them carefully to shape, using a light coating of flour on the fingers only if necessary.
5 Prick the bottoms gently with a fork in 2–3 places.
6 Cut rounds of greaseproof paper to fit comfortably in each lined tartlet case.
7 Place the paper on top of the pastry and fill the centres with dried peas, baking beans or pieces of stale bread. Place the tartlets on a baking sheet.
8 Bake at 200–220°C for approximately 20 minutes until cooked and nicely browned.

9 Remove from the oven onto a cooling rack.

10 When cooled, remove the papers and beans.

11 Place a thin layer of pastry cream or thick custard in the bottom of each tartlet case.

12 Neatly arrange the fruit on top.

13 If you have used tinned fruit, dilute some arrowroot in a basin with a little of the fruit juice (10 g arrowroot to ¼ litre of the juice).

14 Boil the remainder of the juice in a small pan and gradually stir in the diluted arrowroot, stirring continuously until it re-boils. Allow the glaze to cool before use.

15 Use this glaze to thinly mask (coat or cover) the fruit in the tartlets.

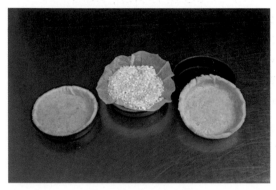

The pastry cases have been baked with a lining of greaseproof paper and a filling of dried rice

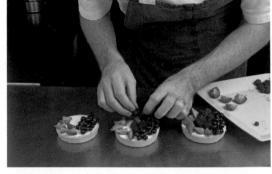

Arranging fruit on top of the pastry cream filling

Try something different

For soft fruits, a red glaze can be made by diluting a matching jam with a little water or syrup, heating it gently until mixed, then passing it through a fine strainer.

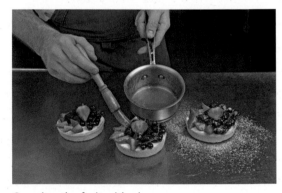

Covering the fruit with glaze

Making bread, buns and scones

Bread making – a simple guide

Bread made without yeast or baking powder is known as 'unleavened' bread. Unleavened bread is flat, e.g. some pitta bread. Most bread today is leavened (made to rise) by yeast or baking powder (bread made with baking powder is called soda bread). Leaven is a substance that makes a dough ferment and rise.

Yeast is a living plant (a type of fungus). There are many types of yeast. Yeast produces carbon dioxide by fermentation. This happens when it is given:

- food – usually in the form of sugar
- warmth – ideally 25–29°C; it is destroyed at higher temperatures and is slow acting at lower temperatures
- moisture – usually milk or water; milk improves the nutritive value and water acts more quickly.

In bread making, the carbon dioxide collects in small bubbles throughout the dough. Together, these raise the dough.

Types of yeast
- **Compressed or fresh yeast** is the most widely used. It is packed and sold in blocks. It crumbles easily and has a fresh, fruity smell. It keeps in a cold place (refrigerator) for one week.
- **Dried yeast** can be stored for a long time. Always follow the directions on the packet.
- **Instant yeast** is dried in a fine powder. It is added directly to flour.

Choice of flour
For bread, strong flour is needed. Strong flour produces lots of gluten, which is a strong substance that can absorb water. When the flour mixes with water during bread making, the gluten becomes elastic (stretchy) and can be pushed up by the carbon dioxide gas produced by the yeast. The gluten traps the bubbles of carbon dioxide gas. When it is heated it sets, giving the bread its typical open texture. Soft flour is unsuitable for bread because it contains less gluten.

Proportions of yeast to flour
It is important to use the right amount of yeast with the right amount of flour:

- for less than 300 g flour use 15 g yeast
- for 300 g–1.5 kg flour use 25 g yeast
- for 1½–3 kg flour use 50 g yeast.

More yeast is needed for quick fermentation methods, if you need to speed up the process.

Steps in bread making
There are nine steps in the traditional process of bread making: creaming, sponging, mixing, kneading, rising, re-kneading, shaping, proving and baking.

Throughout the process the dough must be kept warm (at approximately body temperature) but must not be overheated. Dough can, however be stored, if necessary, for up to 24 hours in mild refrigeration. It must then be allowed to soften in a warm place, and be shaped and proved before baking. Flour and utensils must also be kept warm before starting.

Creaming is when the yeast is mixed with the sugar. Not much fermentation occurs at this stage.

Sponging is when liquid is added to the yeast and sugar mixture. Rapid fermentation occurs at this stage.

Mixing is when the flour is mixed in well with the liquid. This thoroughly mixes the yeast throughout the dough so that it can get the maximum amount of food. The protein in the flour absorbs water to form gluten, which can be stretched by the carbon dioxide gas produced by the yeast.

Kneading helps to spread the yeast throughout the dough.

During **rising** the steady process of fermentation continues. The dough is left in a warm place so that the yeast can grow. The gluten stretches more quickly, becoming soft and more elastic. It resembles a honeycomb sponge, but will collapse if it rises too much.

Re-kneading breaks down the large bubbles of carbon dioxide into small, evenly sized bubbles. It also allows air to get in to help the yeast to do its job.

Shaping is when the dough is cut and shaped.

During **proving** the dough continues to expand, but it does it more evenly than during the rising. The gluten recovers from the strain of shaping.

During **baking** the dough rises rapidly at first, when gluten is pressed up by the gases and then sets. The yeast is then killed by the heat and no more carbon dioxide gas is produced. The baking temperature must be hot at first to destroy the yeast, and then lower if required.

Important points in bread making

- Yeast must be fresh and in the correct proportion to the amount of flour.
- Flour must be strong.
- Yeast must be worked at an even temperature, i.e. body temperature.
- Draughts must be avoided.
- Mixing and kneading must be thorough to incorporate the yeast. The second kneading should not be too heavy or too much gas will be lost.
- Proving must be done carefully. If proving is too short, the bread will not be light. If over-proved, the bread will be tough and sour. If too hot, the yeast will be destroyed.

Storage

Uncooked bread and dough products should be kept in the refrigerator until ready for baking. Always keep frozen bread and dough products in the deep freeze until ready for baking.

RECIPE

6 Simple basic white loaf

INGREDIENTS	10 portions
Yeast, dried or fresh	10 g dried, 25 g fresh
Water, warm	125 ml
Caster sugar	2 tsp
Strong flour, plain	375 g
Salt	1 tsp
Melted butter, margarine or vegetable oil	30 g
Milk, warm	125 ml

Cooking

1 Combine the yeast, water and sugar in a bowl and whisk until the yeast is dissolved. Cover and stand in a warm place to ferment (bubble) for about 10 minutes or until the mixture is frothy.

2 Sift the flour and salt into a large bowl. Stir in the melted butter, milk and yeast mixture. Mix to form a dough.

3 Place the dough on a floured surface. Knead for about 10 minutes, working the dough until smooth and elastic.

4 Place the dough into a lightly oiled bowl. Stand in a warm place covered with a damp cloth and allow to prove (rise and increase in size) until it has doubled in size. This may take up to 1 hour.

5 Turn the dough out onto a floured surface and knock it back (re-knead) to its original size and until it is smooth.

6 Roll the dough into a rectangle 18 cm × 35 cm. Roll this up like a Swiss roll. Place it in a greased bread tin 14 cm × 21 cm. Cover and stand in a warm place for about 20 minutes until it has doubled in size.

7 Brush the top of the loaf with milk to give a rich brown colour. Place it in a preheated hot oven (180–200°C) for approximately 45 minutes.

8 Turn out the bread onto a wire rack. Check that it is cooked by tapping the bottom of the loaf. It should make a hollow sound.

Try something different

For brown bread, substitute half the plain flour with wholemeal plain flour. The mixture may require a little more warm milk.

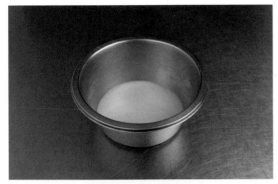
Combining the yeast, water and sugar

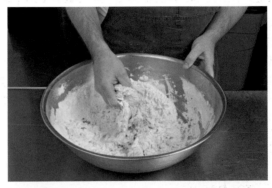
Making the dough

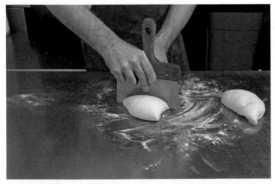
Dividing the dough

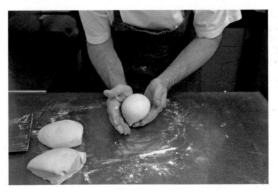
Forming the dough

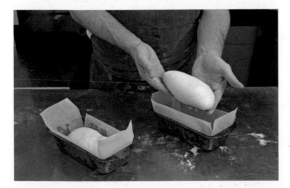
Placing the dough into a loaf tin

RECIPE 7 Gluten-free bread

Some people are allergic to gluten, a protein found in wheat. Coeliac disease is caused by a reaction to gluten. Gluten-free is a safe alternative to ordinary bread for coeliacs and those allergic to gluten.

INGREDIENTS	
Gluten-free plain flour	450 g
Baking powder	2 tsp
Salt	1½ tsp
Oat bran	180 g
Sunflower seeds	160 g
Butter, margarine or vegetable oil	70 g
Egg	2
Milk	375 ml
Poppy seeds	2 tsp

Cooking

1 Sift the flour, baking powder and salt into a large bowl. Add the oat bran and stir well. Mix in the sunflower seeds.
2 Rub in the butter or mix in the vegetable oil.
3 Beat the eggs and milk. Add this to the mixture.
4 Mix to a dough.
5 Press the dough into a greased loaf tin measuring 14 cm × 21 cm. Brush with milk. Sprinkle with poppy seeds.
6 Bake in a preheated oven at 160–180°C for approximately 1 hour.
7 When baked, allow the bread to stand in the loaf tin for 10 minutes. Turn it out onto a wire rack. Check that it is cooked by tapping the bottom. It should make a hollow sound. Leave to cool.

RECIPE 8 Focaccia – an Italian bread

INGREDIENTS	
Yeast	50 g
Sugar	1 tsp
Water, lukewarm	330 ml
Extra virgin olive oil, plus extra to drizzle on the bread	70 g
All-purpose flour, unbleached	725 g
Salt	½ tsp
Coarse salt for the topping	
Rosemary, picked, for the topping	

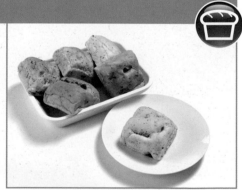

Cooking

1 Dissolve the yeast and sugar in one-third of the lukewarm water in a bowl. Leave to ferment.
2 In another bowl add the olive oil and the rest of the water. Pour this into the yeast mixture.
3 Blend in the flour and salt, a quarter at a time, until the dough combines.
4 Knead the dough on a floured board for 10 minutes, adding flour as needed, to make it smooth and elastic.
5 Lightly oil a bowl and put the dough in it. Turn the dough so that it is oiled all over. Cover with a cloth.
6 Leave the dough to prove in a warm place until it has doubled in size – about 1 hour.
7 Knock back (re-knead) the dough and knead for 5 minutes. Gently roll it out to 2 cm thick on a large baking sheet.
8 Cover and allow to rise for 15 minutes.
9 Oil your fingers and make dents with them 3 cm apart in the dough.
10 Leave to prove for 1 hour.
11 Drizzle the loaf with olive oil, sprinkle with coarse salt and picked points of rosemary.
12 Bake at 220°C for approximately 10–15 minutes until golden brown.

Serving suggestion

Cut into squares and serve warm.

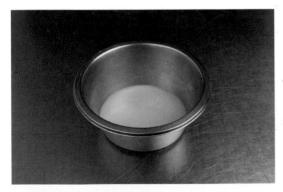

Combining the yeast, sugar and water

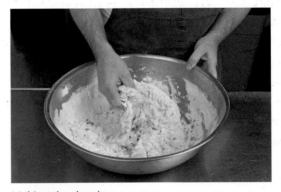

Making the dough

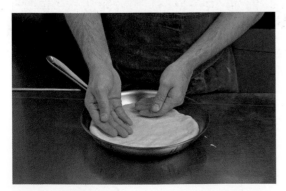

Moulding the dough

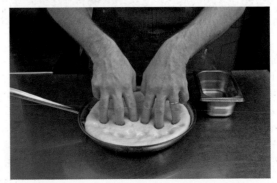

Making dents in the dough after proving

9 Bun dough – basic recipe

INGREDIENTS	8 buns	20 buns
Bun dough		
Flour, strong	200 g	500 g
Yeast	15 g	40 g
Milk and water (approximately)	60 ml	150 ml
Egg, medium sized	1	2–3
Butter or margarine	50 g	125 g
Caster sugar	25 g	60 g
Bun wash		
Sugar	100 g	
Water or milk	125 ml	

Cooking

1 Sieve the flour into a bowl and warm.
2 Cream the yeast in a basin with a little of the liquid.
3 Make a well in the centre of the flour.
4 Add the dispersed yeast, sprinkle a little flour over it, cover with a cloth and leave in a warm place until the yeast ferments (bubbles).
5 Beat together the egg, fat, sugar and the remainder of the liquid, and add this to the yeast mixture.
6 Knead well to form a soft, slack dough.
7 Continue kneading until smooth and not sticky.
8 Keep covered in the bowl and allow to prove. Knock back gently.
9 Mould the dough into balls. Place these on a lightly greased baking tray. Cover with a cloth and allow to prove again.
10 Bake in a hot oven (220°C) for 15–20 minutes.
11 Boil together the ingredients for the bun wash until it is a thick syrup.
12 Remove the buns from the oven and brush liberally with bun wash.
13 Remove onto a cooling rack.

10 Fruit buns

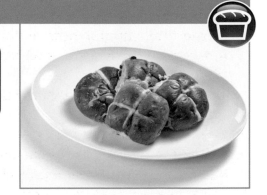

> **Get ready to cook**
> 1 Prepare the bun dough as per Recipe 9.
> 2 Prepare the bun wash as per Recipe 9.

INGREDIENTS
Bun dough (see recipe 9)
Bun wash (see recipe 9)
Washed dried fruit (e.g. currants, sultanas) 50 g
Mixed spice, pinch

Cooking

1 Add 50 g of washed dried fruit (e.g. currants, sultanas) and a pinch of mixed spice to the basic bun dough recipe.
2 Mould the dough into round balls. Place these on a lightly greased baking sheet.
3 Cover with a cloth and allow to prove.
4 Bake in a hot oven (220°C) for 15–20 minutes.
5 Remove from oven and brush liberally with bun wash.
6 Remove onto a cooling rack.

Try something different

To make hot cross buns, as shown on the previous page:

1 Make fruit buns as above, but use a little more spice.
2 When moulded, make a cross on top of each bun with the back of a knife.
3 Alternatively, make a slack mixture of flour and water in a greaseproof paper cornet and pipe on neat crosses.

RECIPE

11 Bread rolls

INGREDIENTS	8 rolls	20 rolls
Flour, strong	200 g	500 g
Yeast	5 g	12 g
Liquid – ½ water, ½ milk	125 ml	300 ml
Butter or margarine	10 g	25 g
Caster sugar	¼ tsp	½ tsp
Salt	Small pinch	Large pinch
Egg, beaten for eggwash	1	2

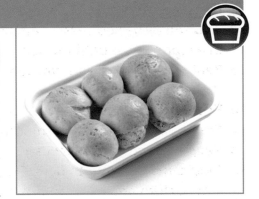

Cooking

1 Sieve the flour into a bowl and warm in the oven or on the stove.
2 Cream the yeast in a basin with a quarter of the liquid.
3 Make a well in the flour and add the dissolved yeast.
4 Sprinkle over a little of the flour, cover with a cloth and leave in a warm place until the yeast ferments (bubbles).
5 Add the remainder of the warmed liquid, the fat, sugar and salt.
6 Knead firmly until smooth and free from wrinkles.
7 Return to the basin, cover with a cloth and leave in a warm place to prove (double in size).
8 Knock back (lightly knead) the dough to remove the air and bring it back to its original size.
9 Mould the dough in a roll and cut into even pieces.
10 Mould the pieces into the shapes you want. Place them on a lightly floured baking sheet and cover with a cloth.
11 Leave in a warm place to double in size.
12 Brush gently with eggwash.
13 Bake in a hot oven at 220°C for approximately 10 minutes.
14 Remove from the oven and place the rolls on a cooling rack.

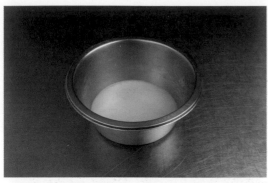
Combining the yeast and liquid

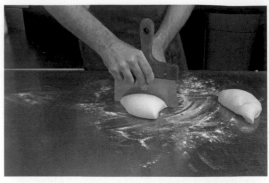
Dividing the dough

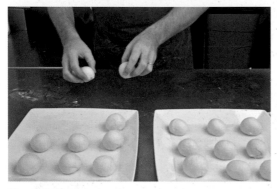
Shaping the dough

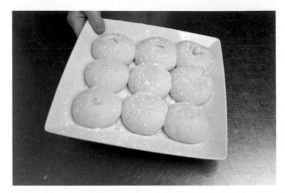
After proving, the dough is twice as big as before

Try something different

Carefully add 50 g of sultanas and 50 g of chopped walnuts at stage 8.

RECIPE

12 Scones

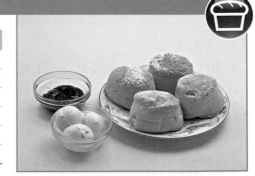
For the scones in the picture, the dough was rolled out 2 cm thick and cut with a 4–5 cm cutter

INGREDIENTS	8 scones	20 scones
Self-raising flour	200 g	500 g
Baking powder	5 g	12 g
Salt	Small pinch	Large pinch
Butter or margarine	50 g	125 g
Caster sugar	50 g	125 g
Milk or water	65 ml	175 ml

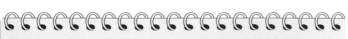

Because of the small amount of fat in the dough, it is essential that you mix gently and handle the dough lightly to produce a light scone.

Cooking

1 Sieve the flour, baking powder and salt into a basin.
2 Gently rub in the fat until the mixture has a sandy texture.
3 Dissolve the sugar in the liquid.
4 Gently and lightly mix in the flour.
5 Divide the dough into two.
6 Using as little flour as possible, gently roll out the dough or cut it with a cutter into rounds 1½ cm thick.

7 Place the dough on a lightly greased baking sheet.

8 Cut a cross with a sharp knife halfway through the rounds.

9 Brush with milk and bake at 200°C for 15–20 minutes.

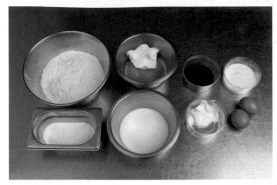
All the ingredients, ready for cooking

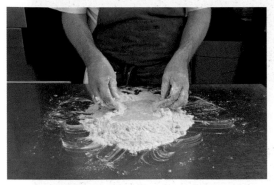
Mixing the ingredients together

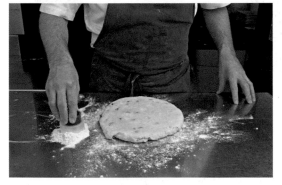
Dipping the cutter in flour before it is used

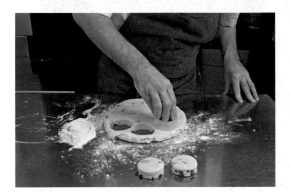
Using a cutter to make rounds from the dough

Try something different

For fruit scones, add 50 g (125 g) washed and well-dried sultanas to the mixture.

For wholemeal scones, use half self-raising flour and half wholemeal flour.

Making other desserts and sweet snacks

RECIPE

(13) Steamed sponge pudding

INGREDIENTS	6 portions	12 portions
Butter or margarine	100 g	200 g
Caster or soft brown sugar	100 g	200 g
Eggs, medium, well beaten	2	4
Flour	150 g	300 g
Baking powder	10 g	20 g
Milk	A few drops	Several drops

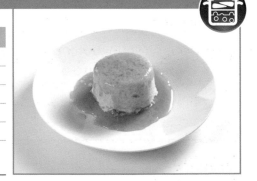

Cooking

1 Cream the fat and sugar in a bowl until almost white.

2 Gradually add the eggs, mixing vigorously.

3 Sieve the flour and baking powder. Lightly fold this into the mixture and a little milk if necessary. It should be dropping consistency (this means that if you lift a spoonful of the mixture and turn the spoon on its side, the mixture will drop off).

4 Place the mixture in a greased pudding basin or individual moulds.
5 Cover securely with greaseproof paper or foil and steam for 1–1½ hours.

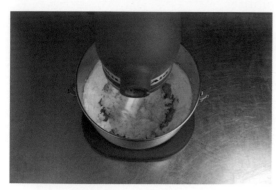

Creaming the butter and sugar together

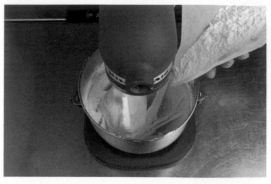

Adding the other ingredients

Serving suggestion

Turn the puddings out of the moulds to serve accompanied with a suitable sauce, e.g. jam, lemon, chocolate, golden syrup.

Try something different

For vanilla sponge pudding, add a few drops of vanilla essence and serve with custard.

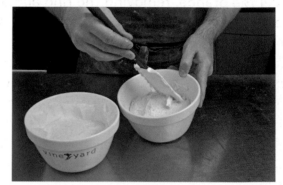

Placing the mixture into pudding basins

For jam sponge pudding, add a good measure of jam to the moulds before putting in the mixture. When cooked and turned out there should be an appetising cap of jam on top. Serve with custard.

For fruit sponge pudding, add dried fruit to the mixture – raisins, sultanas, currants or a mixture of all three. Name the pudding accordingly, e.g. raisin sponge pudding.

RECIPE

14 Fresh fruit salad

Get ready to cook

Make the syrup by boiling the sugar and water. Cool it and pour it into a bowl. Add the lemon juice.

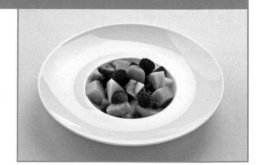

INGREDIENTS	4 portions	10 portions
Orange	1	2–3
Dessert apple	1	2–3
Dessert pear, ripe	1	2–3
Grapes	50 g	125 g
Cherries, in season	50 g	125 g
Banana	1	2–3
Stock syrup		
Caster sugar	50 g	125 g
Water	125 ml	375 ml
Lemon, juice of	½	1

Preparation

1 Peel the orange, removing the rind and all white pith. Cut into segments and remove any pips. Do this over a bowl to catch the juice. Put the orange segments into the bowl with the juice.

2 Cut the apple and pear into quarters. Remove the core, peel and cut each piece into 2–3 slices. Place in the bowl with the oranges and cover with juice.

3 Cut the grapes in half and remove any pips. Peel them if the skin is tough.

4 Remove the stones from the cherries and leave the cherries whole.

5 Mix all the fruit together carefully and chill in the refrigerator.

6 Just before serving, peel the banana, cut it into slices and mix it with the rest of the fruit.

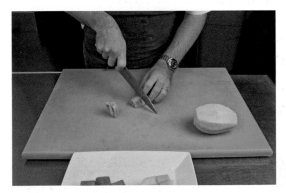

Carefully slicing a kiwi

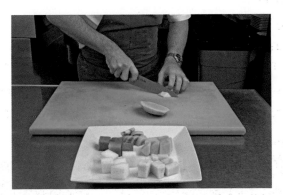

Carefully cutting a mango

Try something different

Other fruits that can be used include pineapple, melon, mango, strawberries, apricots, etc. All fruits *must* be fully ripe.

15 Winter smoothie

Get ready to cook
Prepare, wash and dry the fruit.

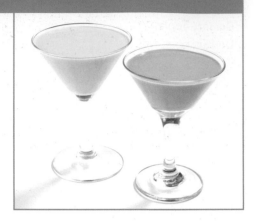

Smoothies are a popular, healthy drink that is quick and easy to make. Simply prepare some ripe fruit and liquidise in a food processor for around 30 seconds.

There are many ready-prepared products available, but the majority of these contain sugar and are made from fruit concentrates. Home-made smoothies are the best.

To make a smoothie the fruit should be:

- fully ripe and sound — not over-ripe or damaged
- picked, peeled where necessary (e.g. pineapples, apples, pears) and washed.

When fruit is fully ripe it is naturally sweet, so usually no extra sweetener is required. If a little extra sweetness is required, add a little honey.

INGREDIENTS	4 portions	10 portions
Frozen berries	400 g	1 kg
Cranberries, blueberries, blackcurrants		60 g
Semi-skimmed milk	600 ml	1½ litres
Natural yoghurt	1250 ml	2500 ml

Preparation

Blend the milk, berries and yoghurt in a liquidiser or use a hand blender.

If the mixture is too thick, use fruit juice to thin it.

Serving suggestion

Serve in suitable glasses.

Try something different

Other fruits you could use include strawberries, raspberries, blackcurrants, grapes, bananas, oranges, mangoes, apples, peaches and passion fruit.

For a richer, milkshake-type drink, add single cream.

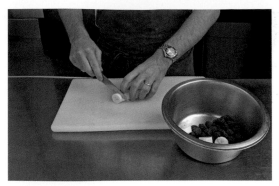

Preparing fruit for a smoothie

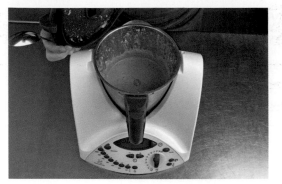

The smoothie has a 'smooth' texture after blending

Activity

Try the following combinations and discuss:

- 100 g strawberries or any soft fruit, 1 banana
- 100 g peeled, chopped pineapple, 2 tbsp honey
- 1 banana, 200 g raspberries, 125 ml single cream.

RECIPE

16 Apple crumble

INGREDIENTS	4 portions	10 portions
Crumble filling		
Bramley apples	600 g	2 kg
Sugar, granulated or brown	100 g	250 g
Cloves	1	2
Topping		
Butter or margarine	50 g	125 g
Plain flour	150 g	400 g
Soft brown sugar	100 g	250 g

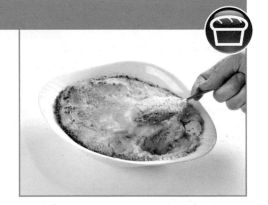

Cooking

1 Peel, core and slice the apples.
2 Cook them gently with a few drops of water, sugar and clove in a covered saucepan.
3 Place the cooked apple in a pie dish or in individual moulds. Remove the cloves.
4 Make the topping by lightly rubbing the fat into the flour. Combine this with the sugar.
5 When the fruit is cool, sprinkle on the topping and bake at 190°C for about 30 minutes, until lightly browned.

Serving suggestion

Serve with custard, cream or vanilla ice cream.

Try something different

Try some fruit combinations, such as:

- apple and blackberry
- apple and gooseberry
- apple and rhubarb.

Try some topping variations:

- add a little spice, e.g. cinnamon, nutmeg, mixed spice, ground ginger
- use half flour and half porridge oats.

RECIPE

17 Pancakes with lemon

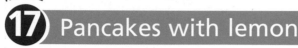

When making a batch of pancakes, keep them flat. Pile them onto a warm plate, sprinkling a little sugar in between each. Fold them when ready for service. Lightly sprinkle them again with sugar and dress nearly overlapping on service plates.

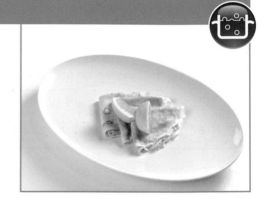

INGREDIENTS	4 portions	10 portions
Flour	100 g	250 g
Salt	Small pinch	Pinch
Egg	1	2–3
Milk	¼ litre	625 ml
Butter, melted or a light oil	10 g	25 g
Light oil for frying		
Sugar, caster	50 g	125 g
Lemon	1	2

Cooking

1 Sieve the flour and salt into a basin.
2 Make a well and add the milk, gradually incorporating the flour from the side of the bowl.
3 Beat vigorously with a wooden spoon or plastic spatula, or whisk to a smooth batter. This should be thick enough to just coat the back of a spoon.
4 Mix in the melted fat.
5 Heat the pancake pan and clean it thoroughly.
6 Add sufficient oil just to thinly coat the pan. Heat this until it begins to smoke.
7 Add just enough mixture to thinly coat the pan.
8 Cook for a few seconds until brown.
9 Turn over and cook the second side for half the time.
10 Turn onto a warm plate, sprinkle with sugar, fold in half then fold again.

Serving suggestion

Serve two pancakes per portion with a quarter of lemon (remove the pips).

Try something different

If a thicker pancake is required, add another 20–60 g flour to the recipe.

Use orange segments in place of lemon.

Spread the pancakes lightly with warmed jam and roll them up.

18 Banana and coconut mini pancake

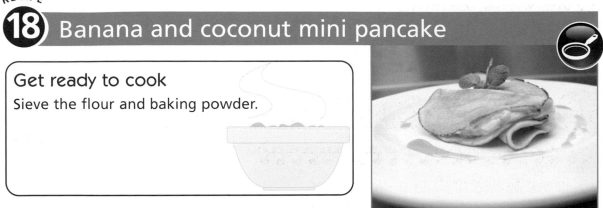

Get ready to cook

Sieve the flour and baking powder.

INGREDIENTS		4 portions	10 portions
Eggs		2	5
Caster sugar		100 g	250 g
Water		65 ml	160 ml
Coconut cream	} combined	100 ml	250 ml
Water		100 ml	250 ml
Plain flour, sieved		150 g	375 g
Baking powder		½ tsp	1 tsp
Margarine for greasing			
Yellow colouring		2 drops	3 drops
Ripe banana flesh, mashed		100 g	250 g
Coconut, grated		80 g	200 g

Cooking

1 Whisk the eggs and sugar together until well mixed. Add the water and mix well.
2 Add the coconut milk, flour and baking powder. Mix well and pass through a strainer.
3 Heat up a griddle and grease it with some margarine to prevent sticking. Pour a small ladleful of batter onto the griddle and let it cook until it stops bubbling.
4 Spoon some banana flesh and grated coconut on top.

Serving suggestion

Fold the pancake in half and serve hot.

19 Rice pudding with dried fruit and nuts

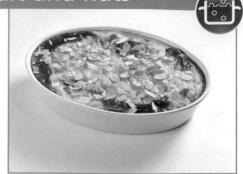

INGREDIENTS	4 portions	10 portions
Milk, whole or skimmed	½ litre	1½ litres
Rice, short grain	50 g	125 g
Caster sugar	50 g	125 g
Vanilla essence	2–3 drops	6–8 drops
Butter	12 g	30 g
Dried fruit	50 g	125 g
Nuts	50 g	125 g
Nutmeg, grated		

Cooking

1 Boil the milk in a thick-bottomed pan, stirring occasionally to stop the milk from burning.

2 Add the washed rice and stir to the boil.

3 Simmer gently, stirring frequently until the rice is cooked.

4 Remove from the heat and mix in the sugar, vanilla, butter and dried fruit and nuts.

5 Pour the mixture into a pie dish, lightly grate with nutmeg and brown under a grill (salamander).

Try something different

Use any mixture of dried or candied fruits, cut into small dice, and lightly toasted sliced almonds.

20 Semolina pudding (Asian style)

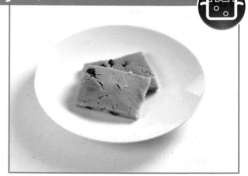

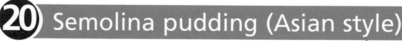

This is called Rava Kesart in India

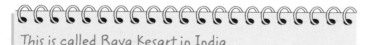

INGREDIENTS	12 portions
Caster sugar	100 g
Water	180 ml
Milk	60 ml
Cinnamon, ground	½ tsp
Ghee or vegetable oil	2 tbsp
Semolina	80 g
Sultanas	1 tbsp
Almonds, flaked	1 tbsp
Almonds, blanched and toasted	12

Cooking

1 Grease a 19 cm × 29 cm rectangular tray.

2 Mix the sugar, water, milk and cardamom in a suitable pan.

3 Stir over heat without boiling until the sugar dissolves. Remove from the heat.

4 Heat the ghee or vegetable oil in another pan and add the semolina. Stir for 1 minute, coating the semolina with the ghee or vegetable oil.

5 Add the milk mixture to the semolina and cook, stirring until the mixture thickens and leaves the sides of the pan. Stir in the sultanas and flaked almonds.

6 Pour the mixture onto the greased tray. Mark it into 12 sections. On each section place a toasted, blanched almond. Cover and refrigerate until firm.

7 When cold and firm, cut into 12 portions.

Serving suggestion

Alternatively the semolina pudding may be served warm straight from the cooking pan.

RECIPE

21 Banana loaf

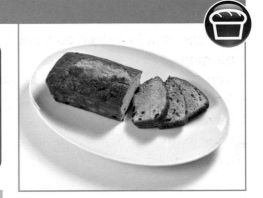

Get ready to cook

1 Beat the egg.

2 Peel and mash the banana.

INGREDIENTS	10 portions
Soft brown sugar	125 g
Margarine, butter or vegetable oil	140 g
Eggs, beaten	2
Baking powder	12 g
Wholemeal flour	200 g
Cinnamon	⅛ tsp
Ripe bananas, mashed	2
Sultanas	50 g

Cooking

1 Cream together the sugar and margarine, butter or vegetable oil.

2 Slowly add the beaten egg and beat well after each addition.

3 Sift the baking powder with the wholemeal flour.

4 Gradually add the flour with the baking powder to the sugar, margarine and egg mixture.

5 Carefully incorporate the mashed bananas and the sultanas. Gently mix well.

6 Place the mixture into a bread tin approximately 20 cm × 12 cm lined with silicone paper.

7 Bake in an oven at 180°C for approximately 30 minutes.

8 Remove and allow to cool. Cut into portions.

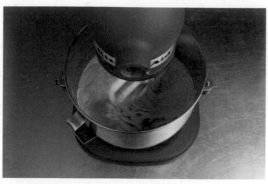

Creaming the butter and sugar

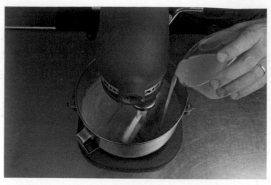

Adding the egg

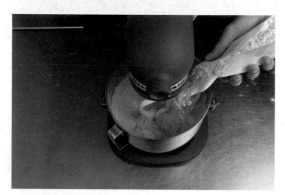

Gradually adding flour

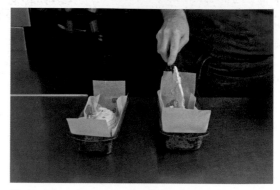

Placing the mixture in a loaf tin

22 Polenta and ricotta cake with dates and walnuts

Get ready to cook

1 Prepare a 20 cm tin lined with baking parchment.

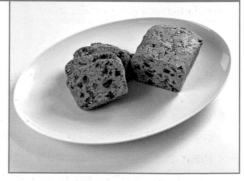

INGREDIENTS	10 portions
Polenta maize flour	200 g
Self-raising flour	200 g
Baking powder	1 tsp
Cinnamon, ground	2 tsp
Caster sugar	225 g
Ricotta cheese	250 g
Melted butter, margarine or vegetable oil	100 g
Water	200 ml
Walnuts, chopped	50 g
Dates, chopped	175 g
Demerara sugar	1 tbsp

Cooking

1 Sift the polenta flour, self-raising flour, baking powder and cinnamon into a bowl.
2 To the flour mixture add the caster sugar, ricotta, butter or vegetable oil and water. Whisk well until it is all blended together.
3 Fold in the walnuts and dates.
4 Mix well and pour into the baking tin. Smooth the top of the mixture.
5 Sprinkle with demerara sugar. Bake in a preheated oven at 170°C for approximately 1½–2 hours.

RECIPE
23) Crème caramel

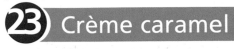

Adding a squeeze of lemon juice at step 1 will stop the caramel from forming crystals.

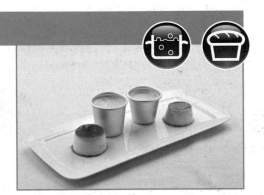

INGREDIENTS	4–6 portions	10–12 portions
Water	125 ml	250 ml
Granulated or cube sugar	100 g	200 g
Milk, whole or skimmed	½ litre	1 litre
Eggs (medium), beaten	4	8
Caster or unrefined sugar	50 g	100 g
Vanilla essence (or a vanilla pod)	3–4 drops	6–8 drops

Cooking

1 Place the granulated sugar and three-quarters of the water in a thick-based pan. Allow it to boil gently. Do not shake or stir the pan.
2 When the sugar has turned a golden-brown caramel colour, add the rest of the water. Bring the mixture (caramel) back to the boil.
3 Pour the caramel mixture into the bottom of individual dessert moulds.
4 Place the beaten eggs, caster sugar and vanilla essence (or pod) in a clean bowl.
5 Warm the milk and whisk it into the egg mixture.
6 Strain the mixture, then pour it into the moulds to fill them.
7 Place the moulds in a roasting tin half full of water. Cook in the oven at approximately 160°C for about 40 minutes.
8 Remove from the oven and allow to cool.
9 When completely cold, loosen the edges of the crème caramel with your fingers. Shake the mould firmly and then turn it out on to a plate.
10 If there is any caramel left in the bottom of the mould, pour it around the dessert.

There are lots of words that you will hear and read in the kitchen that you may not be familiar with. These are specific to cooking and many of them are French in origin. As you work through the book you can refer back to this list to check any cookery words that you do not understand.

Aromats – Fragrant and appetising-smelling herbs and spices, e.g. mint with new potatoes and peas, cloves in apple pies.

Au gratin – The final finish on certain dishes, e.g. macaroni cheese, cauliflower cheese. The dish is sprinkled with grated cheese and/or breadcrumbs, and browned either under a grill or in a hot oven.

Bain-marie – A large container of hot water, usually attached to the kitchen range, in which foods (e.g. soups, sauces, mashed potatoes) can be kept hot without fear of burning.

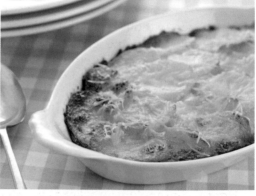

Baste – To spoon the cooking fat or liquid over food (e.g. roast joints of meat and poultry) during cooking to keep it moist and succulent.

Beat – To mix fat and sugar rapidly until the mixture is light and aerated and almost white. A method used when making many pastry products. 'Beat' is also used sometimes for whipping egg whites to incorporate air, e.g. when making meringues. See *Whisk*.

Blanch and refresh – To place food into cold water, bring it to the boil then put it into a sink under cold running water to refresh. Used for e.g. bones for stock, meat or poultry for white stews. Tomatoes can be skinned more easily if they are placed in boiling water for ten seconds and then refreshed.

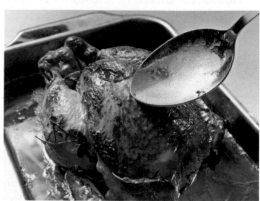

Blend – To take various ingredients and gently mix (blend) them, e.g. rubbing fat into flour when making pastry, selecting and mixing spices for a savoury dish. Also the mixing (blending) of food (e.g. a soup or sauce) to produce a smooth texture.

Bouquet garni – Often abbreviated to BG in recipes, this is a small bunch of herbs (e.g. parsley stalks, thyme and bay leaf) tied with string in between two pieces of leek and/or celery. It is also known as a faggot and is used to give extra flavour to certain dishes, e.g. soups, sauces, stews.

Brine tub – A mixture of water, saltpetre, salt, bay leaf, juniper berries, brown sugar and peppercorns. It is used for pickling or curing meats (e.g. silverside of beef) for periods of up to ten days in a refrigerator.

Brunoise – To cut food into small dice (see page 271).

Buffet – A selection of foods (hot and/or cold) on display, which customers may help themselves to or be served, e.g. cold meats, salads, pastry items, hot food and accompaniments.

Casserole – An earthenware, porcelain or metal ovenproof dish with a lid, in which many different foods (e.g. casserole of chicken) can be cooked and, in some cases, be served from. It is also the method of cooking food slowly in the oven in a casserole dish.

Chinois – A conical strainer used for straining foods in small quantities (as opposed to a colander, which is used for larger quantities). The mesh may be fine or coarse. Coarse chinois are also used for passing soups and sauces.

Chop – To roughly cut meats, poultry and vegetables on a chopping block or chopping board. If hard substances like bones are being chopped, then a chopper should be used on a chopping block. If soft foods such as onions and vegetables are being chopped, then a sharp knife and a chopping board should be used. Chopping is less precise than cutting and more pressure is applied.

To chop an onion:

1 Peel it with the root pointing away from you. Cut it into fine slices without going through the root.

2 Turn the onion so that the root is pointing to one side or the other, depending on whether you are right or left handed. Now slice across the onion three or four times, without going through the root.

3 Finally, slice along the length of the onion again, without going through the root. The onion will fall into small chopped pieces with the root left.

Cocotte – A porcelain or earthenware dish used both for cooking and serving certain foods, e.g. eggs in cocotte.

Combine – To combine all ingredients into one piece after initial mixing, e.g. pastry.

Concassé – This describes something that is coarsely chopped, e.g. peeled and deseeded tomatoes, parsley, coriander.

Consistency (adjust) – The consistency of soups, sauces and stews should be neither too thick nor too thin, so it may need to be adjusted when finishing these foods.

- Hot sauces should have a light consistency, just coating the back of a spoon.
- Thick soups can be slightly thicker.
- Cold sauces, such as mayonnaise, are usually made thick and, according to their use, may be left thick or thinned.

Cook out – To carefully cook the flour in a roux, sauce, soup or stew so that it cooks but does not take on too much colour.

Cordon – To neatly arrange a thread or thin line of sauce onto a finished plate of food, e.g. strawberry sauce around a strawberry meringue.

Correct – To lightly season a dish with salt and possibly pepper and other condiments. When the dish is finished, it should be tasted for flavour and, if necessary, extra seasoning added. It should then be tasted again until the flavour is considered to be correct. See also *Seasoning*.

Court-bouillon – A flavoured liquid of water, salt, onion, carrot, parsley stalks, bay leaf, thyme, peppercorns and vinegar used for the deep poaching of certain oily fish, e.g. whole salmon.

Crème fraiche – A mixture of whipping cream and buttermilk heated to 24–29°C. It is served as an alternative to whipped cream with many dishes, e.g. fruit salad.

Crêpes – These are simply pancakes.

Croquettes – Cooked food (e.g. duchesse potato, chicken) moulded into cylinder shapes, coated in flour, beaten egg and fresh white breadcrumbs (pané) and deep fried.

Croûtons – Small, neat pieces of fried or toasted bread served with certain soups and in some salads.

Crudités – Small, neat pieces of raw vegetables (e.g. carrot, celery) served with a savoury dip as an appetiser before a meal.

Cure – To salt and smoke (dry method) meat. The term is mainly applied to bacon. Curing gives the bacon a keeping quality (allows it to be kept for longer). Another method of curing is to soak the meat in brine. This can be followed by smoking. If the bacon is soaked in brine but not smoked, it has a milder flavour but less keeping quality.

Cut – To cut various foods (vegetables, meat, etc.) into pieces of the required size or shape. A sharp medium-sized

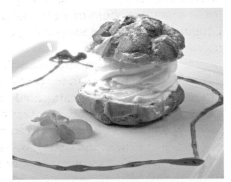

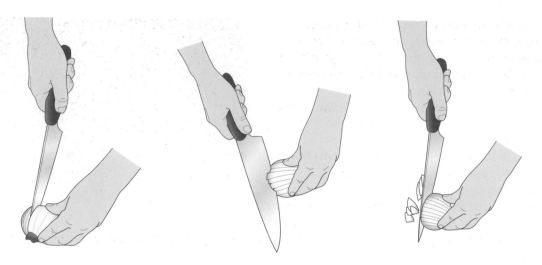

knife is normally used. Cutting is a more precise and delicate process than chopping. As a hygiene precaution, different-coloured chopping boards should be used for the various foods to prevent the risk of cross-contamination.

Deglaze – To swill or rinse out with stock a pan in which food has been roasted or fried. All the flavours from the food are dissolved in the stock and used in the accompanying sauce or gravy.

Dilute – To mix a flour (e.g. cornflour or arrowroot) in water before using it to thicken a sauce or gravy.

Drain – To place food (e.g. cooked vegetables) in a colander to allow the water to drain away.

Eggwash – A mixture of beaten egg with a little milk. It is used to brush on pastry or bakery goods before cooking, in order to give them a shiny and appetising gloss. Also used when coating fried foods. The food (e.g. fish) is coated in flour, then eggwash and then fresh white breadcrumbs before it is fried.

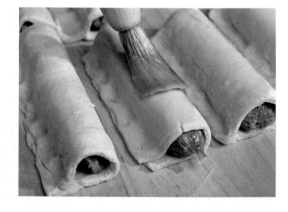

Escalope – A thin slice of meat, e.g. pork, turkey.

Farce – A stuffing of various ingredients made according to the food it is to be used with, e.g. fish, meat. A stuffing should be a complement to the food and contain herbs and/or spices.

Flake – To break into small pieces, e.g. cooked fish.

Flan – An open pastry tart with a filling that can be sweet (e.g. treacle, fruit) or savoury (e.g. quiche).

Garam masala – A combination of hot spices that includes large black cardamoms, cinnamon, black cumin, cloves, nutmeg and black peppercorns. The mixture should be used sparingly and is usually put into foods towards the end of their cooking period. It can also be used as a final light sprinkle over cooked foods, e.g. cooked meats, vegetables, soups.

Garnish – The final trimming or addition to a plate or dish of food, e.g. watercress and fried potatoes with a steak.

Glaze – A stock reduced down slowly by gently simmering until it reaches a slightly thick consistency. The flavour, at this stage, should be very strong. It is then kept in suitable containers in the refrigerator and used in small quantities to strengthen soups, sauces, etc. that lack flavour. Commercial glazes are also available, e.g. Jardox, Marmite.

Grate – To use a food grater to cut foods (e.g. cheese) into fine pieces.

Hors d'oeuvre – An appetising cold or hot first-course dish (starter) or a small selection of dishes, e.g. melon, crab salad.

Jardinière – Vegetables cut into small batons (see page 271).

Julienne – Vegetables cut into fine strips (see page 271).

Jus-lié – A gravy thickened with arrowroot diluted in water, used for many dishes, e.g. chicken casserole.

Knead – Kneading is a technique when making strong doughs (e.g. for bread, buns). When the dough is first mixed it is sticky. It has to be worked and manipulated in a strong way (kneaded) until it is smooth.

Lardons – Small chunky pieces of streaky bacon. These are usually shallow fried to a golden-brown colour and used as a garnish in many dishes and salads, e.g. baby spinach salad, braised beef.

Liquidise – To make various foods (e.g. soups, smoothies) into a thickish, smooth mixture using a food processor.

Marinade – A mixture used to flavour and tenderise food. There are two types of marinade.

1 A wet marinade is a rich, spicy, pickling liquid (made of red wine, oil and vinegar, herbs and spices). Meats (e.g. beef) are soaked in the mixture to give them flavour and to make them tender

2 A dry marinade is a mixture of herbs and spices that can be sprinkled on to the meat (e.g. chicken kebabs) and moistened with lemon juice.

   To marinate means to flavour food with a marinade.

Menu – A list of all the dishes available in the establishment. Menus are written in many different ways according to the place where the food is eaten. They often include a great deal of other information, e.g. price, menu policy. It is a good idea to start collecting menus as a great deal of information can be obtained from them.

Mirepoix – A mixture of roughly cut onions and carrots, a sprig of thyme and a bay leaf used as a base for certain dishes, e.g. stews.

Mise-en-place – The basic preparation that needs to be done before the service begins. There is an old saying that can be used to describe this: 'a place for everything and everything in its place'.

Mixing – Combining ingredients (e.g. for soups, salads, cakes) to produce the correct consistency, texture, blend and finish.

Mousse – A light dish that can be sweet or savoury, e.g. raspberry mousse, chicken mousse.

Napper – (Pronounced *nappay*) to lightly coat food with a sauce or liquid.

Pané – Describes food (e.g. fish) that has been coated with flour, eggwash and fresh white breadcrumbs before frying.

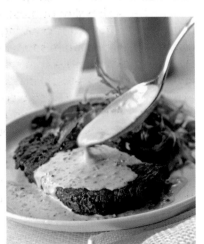

Passing – Forcing a liquid (e.g. sauce) through a suitable meshed conical strainer (a chinois). Passing should not be confused with straining, in which the cooked food is poured into a colander in order to drain off the liquid.

Piquant – Pleasantly sharply flavoured, such as when a sauce is made piquant by adding vinegar (e.g. balsamic) and/or vegetables (e.g. gherkins pickled in vinegar) to add sharpness.

Plat du jour – A menu term that literally means 'dish of the day'. It is a dish that has been freshly prepared for the daily menu and usually changes daily.

Prove – A term applied to making yeast doughs. After the dough has been mixed it is covered and left in a warm place to double in size (to prove).

Pulses – Dried peas and beans, of which there are more than twenty varieties.

Ragoût – A stew; the term is usually applied to a beef stew.

Reduce – To reduce the quantity of a stock by gentle simmering. This concentrates the flavour (makes it stronger).

Refresh – To place hot food under cold running water, e.g. meats and bones should be refreshed after they have been blanched.

Roux – A basic mixture of fat or oil and flour that is cooked and used for thickening a variety of sauces, e.g. béchamel, velouté.

Salamander – A grill that heats from above.

Sauté – To toss in fat or to shallow fry, e.g. sauté potatoes, chicken sauté.

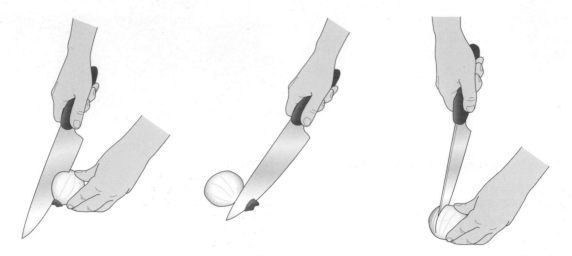

Score – To cut lightly through the fat (e.g. of rack of lamb) or the skin (e.g. of loin of pork) with a small sharp knife before cooking.

Seasoning – Salt and possibly pepper (not all customers like pepper) added to a dish to enhance flavour. White pepper should be added to light-coloured sauces and milled black pepper to dark sauces. Seasoning should be added lightly – customers can add more if they wish to. Take care if you are using convenience stocks – allow for the salt base of MSG (monosodium glutamate), which is frequently used in these, i.e. add less salt.

Separate –

1 To separate the yolk of an egg from the white by using the two halves of the eggshell.
2 If a thickened sauce separates, it breaks down, e.g. the ingredients of mayonnaise may separate if, for some reason, it fails to mix properly (see page 157).

Shred – To slice vegetables into very fine strips. Contrast with 'chopping'. To shred an onion:

1 Peel it and cut it in half.
2 Remove the root.
3 With the root pointing away from you, slice the onion into very fine strips.

Simmer – To boil a liquid and then lower the heat so that it is bubbling gently (just below boiling). Many foods are spoiled by boiling them rather than simmering them.

Skim – To remove any fat or scum (which may contain impurities) from the surface of a simmering liquid (e.g. stock). If you do not skim frequently, some of the fat or scum may boil into the liquid and spoil its flavour.

Straining – See *Passing*.

Sweat – To cook vegetables (e.g. cut vegetables for a soup) with a little fat in a covered pan without colouring. This is an important process that, if carried out correctly, improves the quality and flavour of the dish.

Washing – Washing your hands thoroughly before, during and after handling foods should be an in-built discipline for all food handlers (see page 81). Certain foods need to be washed carefully in cold, fresh water. Vegetables lifted freshly from the soil need to be washed in this way as one speck of dirt can be sufficient to cause food poisoning.

Whisk –

1 To mix thoroughly as in certain sauces, e.g. mayonnaise.
2 To beat thoroughly to incorporate air, e.g. egg whites for meringues.
3 To whisk cream to incorporate air and increase its volume.
   A whisk is also the piece of equipment used to do the whisking.

Index

NOTES page numbers for recipes are in **bold**

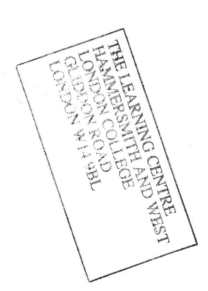